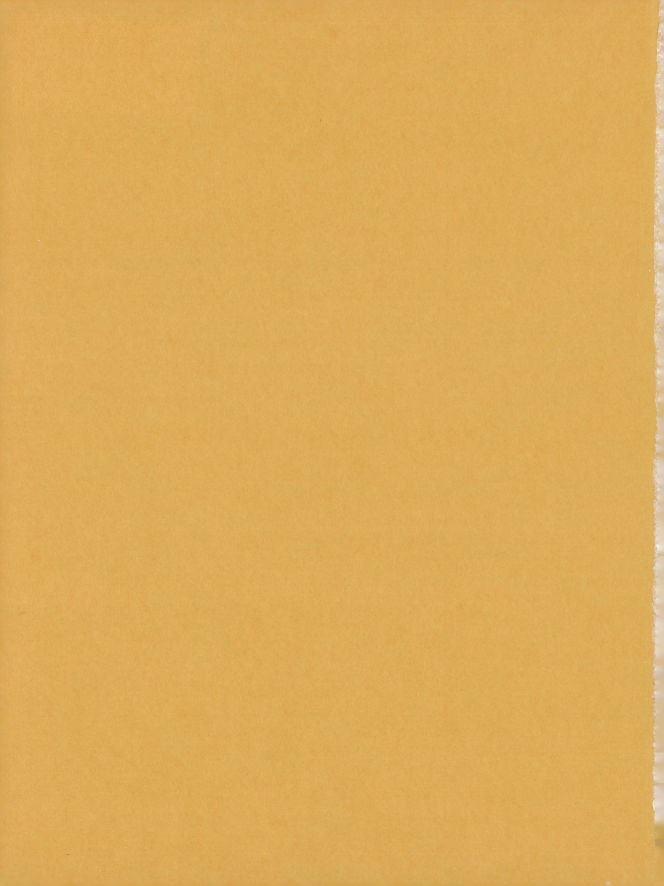

www.wadsworth.com

wadsworth.com is the World Wide Web site for Wadsworth and is your direct source to dozens of online resources.

At *wadsworth.com* you can find out about supplements, demonstration software, and student resources. You can also send e-mail to many of our authors and preview new publications and exciting new technologies.

wadsworth.com
Changing the way the world learns®

Principles and Applications of Assessment in Counseling

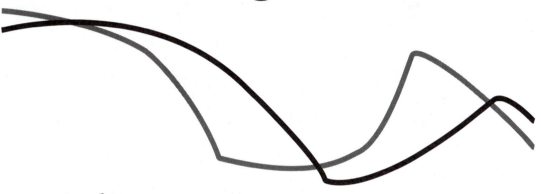

Susan C. Whiston
University of Nevada, Las Vegas

Brooks/Cole
Thomson Learning.

Australia • Canada • Mexico • Singapore • United Kingdom • United States

Counseling Editor: Eileen Murphy
Editorial Assistant: Julie Martinez
Marketing Manager: Jenny Burger
Signing Representative: James Gaughan
Project Editor: Tanya Nigh
Print Buyer: Mary Noel
Permissions Editor: Bob Kauser

Production Service: Pre-Press Company, Inc.
Compositor: Pre-Press Company, Inc.
Cover Designer: Bill Stanton
Cover Image: Source: Eyewire
Cover Printer: R. R. Donnelley/Crawfordsville
Printer/Binder: R. R. Donnelley/Crawfordsville

Printed in the United States of America

3 4 5 6 7 03 02 01

For permission to use material from this text,
contact us:
Web: www.thomsonrights.com
Fax: 1-800-730-2215
Phone: 1-800-730-2214

For more information, contact
Wadsworth/Thomson Learning
10 Davis Drive
Belmont, CA 94002-3098
USA
www.wadsworth.com

International Headquarters
Thomson Learning
290 Harbor Drive, 2nd Floor
Stamford, CT 06902-7477
USA

UK/Europe/Middle East/South Africa
Thomson Learning
Berkshire House
168-173 High Holborn
London WC1V 7AA
United Kingdom

Asia
Thomson Learning
60 Albert Street #15-01
Albert Complex
Singapore 189969

Canada
Nelson/Thomson Learning
1120 Birchmount Road
Scarborough, Ontario M1K 5G4
Canada

Library of Congress Cataloging-in-Publication Data
Whiston, Susan C., 1953–
    Principles and applications of assessment in counseling / Susan C. Whiston.
        p.   cm.
    Includes index.
    ISBN 0-534-34849-1 (alk. paper)
    1. Counseling.   2. Psychodiagnostics.   I. Title.
BF637.C6W467   1999
150'.28'7—dc21

99-16349
CIP

 This book is printed on acid-free recycled paper.

To Tom
whose assessments I don't always agree with,
but whose assessments I always respect

Brief Contents

Contents

Preface

The intent of *Principles and Applications of Assessment in Counseling* is to assist the counselor in being a more effective clinician through the use of sound assessments. I will argue that assessment is an integral part of the counseling process and that practitioners need refined assessment skills. The following are some brief examples of how assessment can be used in counseling.

- A 12-year-old boy is referred to a school counselor or a counselor in an agency because his parents are concerned that he is getting mostly Ds in school. In assessing and conceptualizing the client problem, it might be helpful to have information from intelligence and achievement tests.

- A 34-year-old man has worked in construction all his adult life and can no longer work in this field because he is paraplegic as a result of a car accident. Results from an interest inventory and a current aptitude assessment could assist the counselor in understanding this individual and could facilitate the search for a different career.

- A 17-year-old girl reports that she feels lost and depressed. Furthermore, she feels pressured to make decisions about her future when she doesn't have any idea what career she wants to pursue. A counselor might use a combination of career measures, such as an interest inventory, an aptitude test, and a values instrument. The counselor might also use a personality inventory to explore the level of the girl's depression.

- A 58-year-old woman has been referred to counseling by her physician because she has stomach problems that appear to have no physiological base. The clinic's staff psychiatrist evaluated this client, giving an assessment of symptoms and a personality inventory. The psychiatrist recommended that counseling focus on the woman's problems with anxiety. A counselor who is knowledgeable about the instruments used by the psychiatrist could expedite the sessions by using the information already gathered.

- An 8-year-old girl who has been in only special education classrooms has been "mainstreamed" into a third-grade class for instruction in mathematics. The girl is having some difficulties with social skills and was referred for counseling on this issue. A counselor might acquire some helpful information on how best to intervene with this girl by examining the existing testing information (e.g., intelligence testing and adaptive skills assessment).

- A couple has been married for 15 years, but now they report that all they do is "bicker" and feel continually annoyed with each other. A counselor might use a marital satisfaction inventory to explore the degree of conflict and to identify areas of dissatisfaction. The counselor might also use a personality inventory with the couple to investigate similarities and differences in their personalities.

- A family seeks family counseling because the two adolescent children were recently arrested for possession of cocaine. The counselor might use a structured interview to assess the drug use of the adolescents. In addition, the counselor might use a family assessment to gain some insights into the dynamics of the family.

In order to use assessment techniques appropriately, a counselor needs to have a solid foundation in measurement. Section I of this book focuses on the underlying principles of any type of psychological assessment. This section of the book addresses the basic concepts of measurement and the fundamental methods used in assessment. In order to evaluate and use any assessment, a clinician needs to understand these foundational concepts. For readers who may tend to be a little phobic about statistics, there will be a few formulas. The intent of this book is not to turn its readers into statisticians; in fact, readers are encouraged to focus on concepts rather than on the mathematical calculations. For example, when a standard deviation is provided in the manual, the practitioner will not need to calculate the standard deviation. The clinician, however, will need to understand how the standard deviation was calculated and what it means. In order to use many instruments, counselors need to understand some basic statistics that *describe* individuals' scores. Chapter 2 includes a discussion of the two basic types of assessment instruments and methods used in scoring instruments. Clinicians need to understand the psychometric qualities of assessment instruments. The term *psychometric* typically means the measures of mental processes or psychological constructs. The psychometric qualities generally considered are *reliability* and *validity*. Chapters 3 and 4 cover the topics of reliability and validity and how these concepts are important in both evaluating and using instruments. Chapter 5 focuses on the selecting, administering, scoring, and communicating of assessment results.

Section II of the book builds on the foundations established in the first section by exploring specific methods and areas of client assessment. Clinicians can use numerous methods of client assessment, such as interviews, informal tools, and standardized instruments. No matter what type of assessment strategies a counselor selects, these tools must be both reliable and sound. Chapter 6 discusses initial assessment in counseling, focusing on topics related to the initial interview and assessment methods that can be used in the first session with a client. Chapters 7 and 8 address the assessment of human cognitive abilities—Chapter 7, the measure of intelligence or general ability; and Chapter 8, achievement and aptitude assessment. Counselors are expected to have knowledge of these areas and to be able to interpret the results from instruments that measure them. Because of rapid changes in our society, many individuals are seeking career counseling. Assessment is often a part of career counseling, and that area of assessment is addressed in Chapter 9. Chapter 10 addresses personality assessment and many of the methods used to assess personality. The last chapter in this section, Chapter 11, focuses on assessing couples and families, and describes the dynamics that occur within families.

Section III of this book presnets topics related to application and issues related to assessment interventions in counseling. Generally, this section concerns methods for applying assessment information and emphasizes pertinent issues related to the use of assessment results. Chapter 12 addresses methods in which assessment information can be used in counseling. In this chapter, three central ways are identified: for treatment planning, as a therapeutic intervention, and to evaluate counseling services. In some settings, the clinical decision-making process requires a formal diagnosis. Chapter 13, on diagnosis and assessment, is followed by Chapter 14, which is related to the use of assessment with special populations. Chapter 14 focuses on multicultural issues related to assessment because the research clearly indicates that a counselor needs to consider the client's race, socioeconomic level, disabilities, and culture in interpreting or using any assessment information. Ethical and legal issues also need to be considered when a counselor uses a test or assessment tool. These issues are discussed in Chapter 15. In the field of counseling, technological advancements have led to rapid changes in assessment and appraisal techniques. With these changes, counselors need to remain aware of the strengths and limitations of computerized or technological applications. Chapter 16 addresses these technological applications and then moves on to consider future trends and issues related to assessment and appraisal in counseling. With the advent of the twenty-first century, it is useful to be clear about the ways the field is changing and how those changes will affect the ways that counselors assess clients and how counselors use assessment information in a therapeutic manner.

Acknowledgments

I would like to acknowledge a number of individuals who assisted in different ways with this book. First, I would like to express my appreciation to the personnel at Brooks/Cole-Wadsworth Publishing Company for their support of this book. I am particularly indebted to Eileen Murphy who had a significant influence on this project from the initial stages through the completion of the book. In addition, I am grateful to the anonymous reviewers who provided helpful comments and suggestions.

I also wish to thank my colleagues and the administration at the University of Nevada, Las Vegas, who awarded me a sabbatical leave to write this book. A special thanks goes to Fred Kirschner who reviewed all of the chapters and provided detailed suggestions. I also appreciate the reviews of Josephine Bonomo, Pam Eastburg, and Sue Sinicki, who provided a student's perspective on the content.

I also want to acknowledge my family. My children, Jen, Michael and Matthew, who assisted in many household tasks during the writing of this book. The person, however, that provided the most support during this process was Tom Sexton. I truly appreciate his continual personal and professional support.

Susan C. Whiston

Principles and Applications of Assessment in Counseling

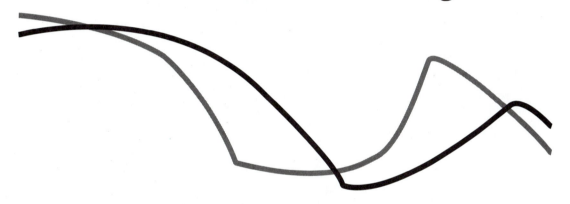

Principles of
Assessment

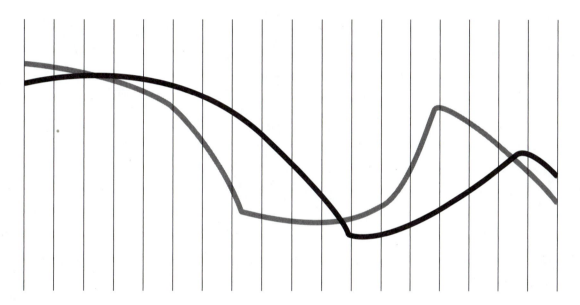

CHAPTER 1

Assessment in Counseling

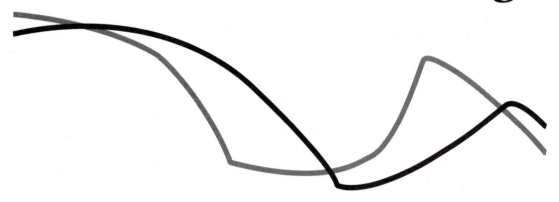

By their very nature, humans are complex; and the more pieces of the human puzzle the clinician can access, the more likely it is that the counselor will have a clear image. As with a jigsaw puzzle, if the counselor only has a few pieces of the puzzle, it is hard to figure out what the whole picture is. Formal and informal assessment techniques can assist counselors in gathering "puzzle pieces," which facilitate a more comprehensive view of clients. Counselors with numerous methods for accessing client information have more material to use in a therapeutic manner than does a clinician with limited assessment skills.

As a counselor you will regularly assess clients. Assessment may address what the client's issues are, how prevalent their problems, whether counseling can be beneficial, what their strengths are, and what skills they already possess. Assessing people is not something entirely new to you; you have probably been doing assessment on an informal basis for many years. When they walk into a class for the first time, many individuals begin to casually assess their fellow classmates. You may have assessed individuals' personalities or interests at a social gathering. Assessment of other individuals is a part of everyday life; it is also a part of the counseling process. In the 1930s and 1940s, counseling and assessment were virtually synonymous (Hood & Johnson, 1997). Although most clinicians do not currently see counseling and assessment as synonymous, client assessment does continue to play a crucial role in the counseling process.

What Is Assessment?

Before pursuing the topic of assessment in counseling, it is important to discuss what the term "assessment" precisely means. The *Standards for Educational and Psychological Testing* (American Educational Research Association, American Psychological Association, & National Council on Measurement in Education, 1985) is one of the primary authoritative sources in this area. These standards define the term **assessment procedure** as "any method used to measure characteristics of people, programs, or objects" (p. 89). A term closely associated with assessment is **psychological test,** which Anastasi and Urbina (1997) define as an objective and standardized measure of a sample of behavior. Cronbach's (1990) definition is similar, with a test being a systematic procedure for observing behavior and describing it with the aid of numerical scales or fixed categories. In reviewing these definitions, there are some commonalities. All the definitions discuss getting a *measure* or using some type of measurement. In assessment, counselors often want an indication of quantity (e.g., How depressed is the client? Are the test scores high enough to get into Harvard?). In simple terms, many assessment questions are related to whether there is a lot of "something" or just a little.

The issue of quantity leads to the next topic: the "something" that is being measured. In counseling, practitioners are often interested in human constructs such as emotions, intelligence, personality factors, self-esteem, and aptitudes. These constructs, however, cannot be directly measured. For example, an individual cannot give a pint of emotions as they can a pint of blood. Humans, for the most part, indicate their emotions by their behavior: their statements, or even answers they give on a questionnaire. It is important to remember that speaking and responding to a questionnaire are behaviors. Even when people take a test, their behavior is sampled in a certain area. Therefore, all that can be gathered are *samples of behavior* for most of the areas about which counselors want to gather information. In very rare instances, a clinician may use a physiological measure, such as pulse rate, as a measure of anxiety. Hence, when we assess other people, we observe a sample of their behavior and *infer* certain meanings from that sample. Two important questions should arise. First, is the sample of behavior indicative of how the person usually behaves? And second, are the inferences we are making correct?

If the counselor's intent is to obtain a sample of behaviors and make some inferences or clinical decisions, then it makes sense that the counselor should be careful about the manner in which he or she obtains the behavior sample. Being careful becomes even more important when the counselor is comparing individuals for selection, placement, or other purposes. This care is related to a third point that is common in the definitions related to assessment: an objective or systematic measure of behavior. As an example, let's say a counselor only wants to work with motivated clients. This counselor would need to gather samples of behaviors that reflect each client's level of motivation. In this case, the counselor could decide that a direct approach is good and she could ask the clients if they are motivated. To the first client, she might ask, "Are you motivated to try some different things in counseling?" To the second client, she might ask, "Are you motivated?" With the third client, she might say, "You do not seem very motivated." This counselor's ways of gathering a sample of behavior would probably affect the behaviors of the clients! Thus, in assessment, the manner of gathering behavior samples needs to be objective, standardized, and systematic.

The focus in this book is assessment and appraisal in counseling, but it adheres to the traditional definition of psychological assessment. In order to be fair to the clients, assessment needs to be systematic and objective. With assessment in counseling, clinicians are in essence gathering samples of client behaviors and making inferences based on those behaviors. Therefore, when evaluating available assessment tools, clinicians should focus on the methods or procedures used for gathering the sample. As an example, a counselor interviewing a client needs to consider what behaviors are being sampled and whether these behaviors are typical of the client. The counselor also needs to consider the inferences he or she is making and the evidence (or validity) of those inferences.

The final aspect of assessment is measurement. If a counselor is assessing a client, he or she is attempting to measure some aspect of the client. Even if the question is whether or not the client has some attribute, the assessment involves measurement. For instance, determining whether or not a client is suicidal involves measuring the degree to which suicide indicators are present.

A distinction is sometimes made among the words **assessment, appraisal,** and **testing.** "Assessment" is the broad term that implies the evaluation of individuals through a process that may involve test results and other sources of information. In this book, the terms "assessment" and "appraisal" are used interchangeably, based on the opinion that both assessment and appraisal include the use of formal and informal techniques, not just standardized tests. Assessment and appraisal are terms applicable not just to formal psychological evaluation; in this book they are defined as procedures used to gather information about clients, which is then used to facilitate clinical decisions and provide information to clients. A distinction needs to be made between **tests** and **instruments.** The term "test" is often reserved for an individual instrument where the focus is on evaluation. Many instruments that counselors use are not evaluative; such as scales, checklists, and inventories designed to provide information. In this book, the term "instrument" will include tests, scales, checklists, and inventories. In this discussion of assessment and appraisal in counseling, there may be terms with which you are unfamiliar. In this case, the Glossary at the end of the book may be helpful.

Assessment Is Integral to Counseling

Some counseling students wonder if they really need training in assessment. Consider, for a moment, the counseling process and the essential steps in counseling. Although the counseling process is quite complex, it includes the following four broad steps:

1. Assessing the client problem,
2. Conceptualizing and defining the client problem,
3. Selecting and implementing effective treatment,
4. Evaluating the counseling.

It is important that counselors skillfully assess the client's problem because if this assessment process is incomplete or inaccurate, the entire counseling process can be negatively affected. Assessment skills, however, are not just needed in this first step; they are important throughout the counseling process. A counselor may be extraordinarily skilled at conceptualizing a problem, but if the clinician is using limited information, the conceptualization process will be hampered. During the conceptualizing stage, counselors need to continually assess a client to be sure they are adequately conceptualizing and defining the client's problem. The third step of implementing treatment is based on the previous assessments. Counselors do not provide one generic treatment; they gear their interventions to each individual client. If the problem is incorrectly defined, the chances of selecting an appropriate treatment are quite low. Finally, once the treatment is provided, counselors need to assess or evaluate whether it was effective. So, once again, the practitioner needs assessment skills. Therefore, just as counselors need effective communication skills, they also need effective assessment and appraisal skills in order to help clients. Assessing clients is an integral part of the counseling process; it is not a distinct area where some counselors administer tests.

Are There Benefits to Using Formal Assessment Instruments?

Occasionally, counseling students have indicated that they never intend to use formal assessment tools. Although informal assessment methods can often be appropriate, automatically rejecting the use of formal assessment instruments may restrict a counselor's effectiveness. Some studies have documented that counseling outcome is enhanced when testing is incorporated into the counseling process (Sexton, Whiston, Walz, & Bleuer, 1997). Duckworth (1990) contends that when "good" tests are used, the counselor can gain insight into the client more rapidly than when relying on counseling alone. If problems are delineated in an efficient manner, treatment can be initiated sooner. Similar to a physician incorporating medical testing to aid in the healing process, Duckworth suggests that tests enrich the counseling process in the following ways.

Testing as an aid to focusing on developmental issues. Counseling is developmental in its focus, and there are instruments that assess a client's developmental level (e.g., measures of career maturity and cognitive development). There are other instruments that, although not designed to measure developmental level, can provide information on issues that may impede developmental growth. Rather than using tests to diagnose unchangeable personality factors, counselors can use instruments to identify factors that can be altered—factors such as family dynamics, changeable personality factors, environmental stresses, coping strategies, and learning styles. Instruments can not only be used to identify limitations; they can also reveal strengths that may facilitate the change process. Furthermore, instruments can be used to chart clients' developmental changes during the counseling process or to measure change at the end of counseling. Sharing with clients the testing results that show progress can have a potent effect, because some clients put more stock in the results of an instrument than they do in verbal feedback.

Testing as an aid to problem solving. According to Duckworth (1990), the objective information provided in formal testing can be useful in problem solving. Clients often come to counseling after they have tried every way they know how to solve their problems. Providing objective assessment information can sometimes help clients identify new methods of solving their problems or clarify ways in which they may be contributing to their problems. For some clients, instruments like the Myers-Briggs Type Indicator, which provides information on how people perceive and process information, can be helpful in understanding the problem-solving methods they use. Many clients have the resources for resolving their problems, but they may have difficulty identifying and utilizing those resources. Assessment results may help them identify their own resources and learn new methods for using them.

Testing as an aid in decision making. Clients often come to counseling for assistance in making decisions, posing questions such as: Should I drop out of school? Should I get a divorce? or Should I change careers? Increasing the amount of information a client can use in decision making generally enhances the decision-making process. Selecting instruments that generate information about occupational choices, career interests, and family dynamics can often assist clients in making major decisions. Using assessment information to aid clients in decision making does not always necessitate administering tests. Often clients have taken assessment instruments during previous educational experiences or in other situations that can be used in counseling. As an example, one client based his decision to pursue a job on his ACT (American College Testing) scores that he had taken two years before.

Testing used in a psychoeducational manner. Duckworth's (1990) final category in which tests can facilitate the counseling is related to tests as psychoeducational tools. Specifically, she contends that tests can engage clients in a psychoeducational experience. Tests can teach people about themselves, thereby encouraging personal growth. A woman client recently reported that taking an interest inventory at age 31 had a major impact on her personal development. This experience began the process of better understanding herself and the importance of different roles in her life. As Duckworth noted, tests can be a psychoeducational tool in counseling when clients receive results that stimulate insight, understanding, and action.

Fredman and Sherman (1987) propose that clients often benefit from formal assessment because these instruments provide a different avenue of reaching the client. They contend that counselors should sometimes get away from providing a totally auditory experience and add visual, kinesthetic, and tactile dimensions to their sessions. They suggest that testing can add a visual experience that often inspires more confidence than do spoken words. They have found that this visual experience often motivates clients to take action about a conflict or problem.

Do Counselors Ever Use Formal Assessment Strategies?

There are numerous indications that counselors view formal assessment strategies as a significant aspect of their work. Elmore, Ekstrom, and Diamond (1993) surveyed members of two divisions (the American School Counselor Association and the Association for Assessment in Counseling) of the American Counseling Association (ACA). They found that 73 percent of the respondents indicated that tests were very important or important in helping them carry out their work. In a more recent survey of these groups, only 9 percent of the respondents indicated they never were involved in activities related to interpreting scores from tests/assessments or used the information in counseling (Elmore, Ekstrom, Shafer, & Webster, 1998).

Counselors in different settings use many of the same assessment instruments. Bubenzer, Zimpfer, and Mahrle (1990) found that community mental health counselors were most likely to use the Minnesota Multiphasic Personality Inventory, the Strong–Campbell Interest Inventory, the Wechsler Adult Intelligence Scale—Revised, the Myers–Briggs Type Indicator, and the Wechsler Intelligence Scale for Children—Revised. School counselors indicated that they were most likely to use the Wechsler Intelligence Scale for Children, the

Preliminary Scholastic Aptitude Test, California Achievement Test, Differential Aptitude Tests, and the Strong–Campbell Interest Inventory (Elmore et al., 1993). It appears that counselors working in diverse settings need to be competently trained in the use of these commonly used instruments.

What Do Counselors Need to Know About Assessment?

Because assessment is an integral part of counseling, it is crucial that practitioners become competent in this area. Table 1.1 contains a list compiled by researchers of the minimum competencies for proper test use (Moreland, Eyde, Robertson, Primoff, & Most, 1995). These competencies can be coalesced into two major themes, the first being related to knowledge of the test and its limitations. Some of the specific elements of this theme concern acknowledging the need for multiple sources of convergent data, keeping up with the area, and consulting on interpretations. Gathering multiple sources of information is important to appropriate client assessment. It is unwise to base decisions on the results from one assessment because no instrument can perfectly measure complex psychological factors, and sometimes circumstances influence results. As an example, a client enters counseling reporting she has been feeling fatigued, guilty, and depressed, with some suicidal thoughts. The counselor administers a depression inventory and the results indicate a very low level of depression. If the counselor had made therapeutic decisions based solely on the results of the depression inventory, the client would have been ill served. In this illustration, the client was confused by the instructions and reversed the Likert scale that indicated the severity of the symptoms of depression. The client believed she was indicating great difficulty on many of the items, while in fact her answers reflected that those symptoms were not present. The counselor in this case gathered multiple sources of information that were not consistent with the depression inventory. This inconsistency led the counselor to question the client about the inventory, which revealed the reversal of the scoring scale. Using multiple assessment strategies also provides more comprehensive and clinically rich information, which can be beneficial. It is clear counselors should always use multiple assessment techniques and/or instruments.

The second major theme related to test usage identified by Moreland et al. (1995) concerns accepting responsibility for the competent use of the test. Counselors need to learn the skills related to competent assessment and know the limits of their own competency. No counselor should ever administer any assessment instrument to a client without the necessary knowledge and training, because clients may be harmed. Anastasi (1992) suggests that the major reason for the misuse of tests is inadequate or outdated knowledge about the statistical aspects of testing and about the psychological findings regarding the behavior that is the target of the assessment. Therefore, counselors need knowledge about

TABLE 1.1

Minimum competencies needed for proper test use

1. Avoiding errors in scoring and recording

2. Refraining from labeling people with personally derogatory terms like *dishonest* on the basis of test scores that lack perfect validity

3. Keeping scoring keys and test materials secure

4. Seeing that every examinee follows directions so that test scores are accurate

5. Using settings for testing that allow for optimum performance by test takers (e.g., adequate room)

6. Refraining from coaching or training individuals or groups on test items, which results in misrepresentation of the person's abilities and competencies

7. Willingness to give interpretation and guidance to test takers in counseling situations

8. Not making photocopies of copyrighted materials

9. Refraining from using homemade answer sheets that do not align properly with scoring keys

10. Establishing rapport with examinees to obtain accurate scores

11. Refraining from answering questions from test takers in greater detail than the test manual permits

12. Not assuming that a norm for one job applies to a different job (and not assuming that norms for one group automatically apply to other groups)

Source: Moreland, Eyde, Robertson, Primoff, & Most, *American Psychologist*. 1995, 50, 14–23. © 1995 by the American Psychological Assn. Reprinted by permission.

measurement concepts, an understanding of the psychological area being assessed, and understanding about the specific instrument being used.

If counselors want to continue to provide mental health services to clients, they must be educated in the area of assessment and properly trained and supervised in the use of specific instruments. As Clawson (1997) documented, numerous states have attempted to restrict the use of psychological tests to licensed psychologists. For example, the Louisiana State Board of Examiners in Psychology has sued a licensed professional counselor to keep him from using psychological tests. These efforts are likely to increase unless counselors can prove that they are competent and trained in the use of assessment procedures. If counselors lose the right to perform assessment, they will also lose the right to be able to diagnose, because assessment is crucial to diagnosis (Clawson, 1997). Most managed health care organizations require that a diagnosis be made before they will reimburse practitioners. Therefore, if counselors lose the right to assess in a state, they will be eliminated from the private practice market in that state.

The key to counselors retaining assessment and diagnosis privileges is training and competency. If counselors are not well trained in assessment, clients can be harmed. This book is an introduction to assessment that is geared toward counselors-in-training and is designed to encourage counseling students to become well-educated assessment providers. Counselors must be able to evaluate assessment tools and determine which instruments are appropriate for specific clients. The evaluation process continues even after appropriate instruments have been identified because counselors must determine the best instruments for specific situations. In addition to evaluation skills, counselors need to know how to use instruments appropriately. Competent use of assessment tools involves determining what inferences can be made and understanding how to interpret results appropriately. The intent of this book is not only to provide selection and evaluation skills, but also to provide information on the appropriate use of assessment tools and interventions in counseling. Thus, the focus is two-pronged: one related to evaluating and selecting assessment tools skillfully and the other concerned with using assessment instruments and interventions appropriately.

History

In order to understand current assessment techniques and instruments, counselors need information about the history of assessment. This brief excursion into the development of assessment is designed to provide a context for understanding the current state of this field. Through knowledge about relevant issues and about why and how some instruments were developed, we can become good consumers of current assessment techniques and tools.

Early Testing

Assessment is not a new phenomenon; testing has been around for many centuries (Anastasi, 1993; Bowman, 1989). There is some evidence that the Greeks might have used testing around 2,500 years ago. The Chinese used a civil services examination 2,000 years ago. Even with this early Chinese examination, there were discussions of the effects of social class, cheating, and examiner bias (Bowman, 1989). In general, however, English biologist Francis Galton is credited with launching the testing movement. Galton did not set out to initiate testing, but in his study of human heredity he wanted a way to measure human characteristics of biologically related and unrelated individuals. Galton believed that sensory discrimination tests could be used as a measure of individual intelligence. He based this opinion on the premise that all information is conveyed through the senses and, thus, the more perceptive a person is, the greater the information that is accessible for intelligent judgments and actions. Galton also made a significant contribution in the area of statistics. The commonly used statistical technique of correlation came from his work in heredity and "co-relations."

Another prominent figure in the early testing movement was American psychologist James McKeen Cattell. Cattell was a student of Wilhelm Wundt, who is credited with founding the science of psychology but was also interested in measuring psychological constructs. Wundt's purpose was somewhat different from Galton's in that he and his colleagues were interested in identifying factors common to human beings. Drawing from the work of Galton and Wundt, Cattell expanded testing to include memory and other simple mental processes. Cattell was the first to use the term "mental test," but his mental tests were quite simple—not strongly related to estimates of school achievement or to other criteria now considered indicative of intelligence (Anastasi, 1993).

1900 to 1920

In 1895, Binet and Henri published an article criticizing most available intelligence tests as being too sensory oriented. Binet was given the opportunity to develop his ideas when the French Minister of Public Instruction appointed him to a commission studying educationally retarded children. The result was the first version of the Binet–Simon scale, published in 1905. The instrument was administered individually to examinees. It was, however, a simple instrument with only 30 items and a norming group of 50. The Binet–Simon scale was different from previous measures of intelligence as it focused on assessing judgment, comprehension, and reasoning. The instrument was revised in 1908 to incorporate a ratio of mental age level to chronological age level, which was labeled the intelligence quotient (IQ). For many years this method of calculating intelligence quotient was utilized, although, as we will see in later chapters, there are some problems associated with this method for determining IQ. Binet's instrument was translated and adapted in several countries. One of these adaptations was by L. M. Terman at Stanford. It became known as the Stanford–Binet scale, which was first published in 1916. The Stanford–Binet included many new items and revised many items from Binet's work. It also was restandardized on an American sample of around 1,000 children and 400 adults.

While individually administered intelligence tests were being developed, there was also some interest in group testing. Group testing became particularly interesting to military experts in the United States during World War I. Army psychologists worked quickly to develop a group-administered intelligence assessment for use in selection and classification of personnel. The army used a multiple-choice format, which had only recently been introduced by Otis. These first group-administered intelligence tests were known as Army Alpha and Army Beta. Army Alpha was used for routine testing, while Army Beta was a nonlanguage instrument designed for use with recruits who were illiterate or did not speak English. Shortly after the end of World War I, the army released these two instruments for public use.

1920s and 1930s

During this same early period of instrument development, theoretical discussions were also occurring concerning the characteristics of intelligence. Spearman (1927) proposed that intelligence consisted of two types of factors (i.e., one that pertained to general tasks and another that pertained to specific tasks). Thurstone (1938), on the other hand, proposed that there was no general factor of intelligence but rather seven primary mental abilities. With the increased interest in measuring intelligence, there was also continuing debate considering the definition and makeup of intelligence.

In this time period, interest in testing was not restricted to intelligence testing alone. At the end of World War I, there was an interest in identifying those men who were not emotionally capable of serving in the armed forces. The army once again developed the prototype, but this time the group test focused on personality assessment and was called the Woodworth's Personal Data Sheet. This self-report inventory was also released for civilian use, and it spurred the development of other self-report personality inventories. In 1921, Rorschach described the technique of using inkblots as a tool for diagnostic investigation of the personality. His methods did not have an immediate impact, but years later these early writings had a major influence on clinical assessment.

During this period, private industries began to see that tests could be used for selecting and classifying industrial personnel. Special aptitude tests were developed, primarily for use in clerical and mechanical areas. This time period also saw the development of vocational counseling instruments. E. K. Strong published the first version of the Strong Interest Blank in 1927. Another individual active in the development of interest inventories for vocational counseling was G. Frederic Kuder, who first published the Kuder Preference Record-Vocational in 1932.

The 1920s also marked the publication of the first standardized achievement battery, the Stanford Achievement Test, in 1923. This instrument was designed to provide measures of performance in different school subjects as compared to a single subject. In addition, students' performance could be compared to a broad achievement standard of students from schools in various parts of the country. In the mid-1800s there was a move from oral achievement examination to written essay testing. By the 1930s, there was considerable evidence concerning the difficulties with written essay examination, particularly due to the lack of agreement among teachers in grading essay items. The desire for more objectivity in testing promoted the use of more objective items and the development of state, regional, and national achievement testing programs.

In other words, the period of the 1920s and 1930s saw rapid advancement in many areas of testing. As testing quickly grew, people began to need a resource for identifying and evaluating testing instruments. The first edition of the *Mental Measurement Yearbook* was published in 1939 to fill that need. Oscar Buros established these yearbooks as a resource for test users, as they provide information about instruments and also critique the properties of the instruments.

1940s and 1950s

Although there were efforts to produce quality personality assessment tools, there was dissatisfaction with many of these instruments because they were somewhat transparent and could easily be faked by an examinee. Projective techniques, such as the Rorschach, became more popular during this time. With projective techniques, the client responds to a relatively unstructured task, and his or her response is then evaluated. The increased use of projective techniques did not, however, hamper the development of self-report instruments. In the early 1940s, a prominent personality instrument, the Minnesota Multiphasic Personality Inventory (MMPI), was developed by Hathaway and McKinley. The MMPI incorporated validity scales, which assessed the degree to which individuals portrayed themselves in an overly positive or negative way. Also, the MMPI contained items that were empirically selected and keyed to criterion, rather than items that appeared to measure different aspects of personality.

During this period, standardized achievement tests became well established in the public schools. Although there were single aptitude tests before this time, most of the multiple aptitude batteries appeared after 1940. Multiple aptitude batteries could indicate where an individual's strengths and limitations were (e.g., did an individual have higher verbal aptitude or higher numerical aptitude?). The development of multiple aptitude batteries came late compared to other assessment areas, and this was directly related to the refinement of the statistical technique of factor analysis.

With the increased use of assessment instruments in the 1930s and 1940s, problems associated with these instruments began to emerge. As criticisms of assessment rose, it became clear that there was a need for standards with respect to the development and use of instruments. The American Psychological Association published the first edition that defined standards. In later years, three organizations—the American Educational Research Association, the American Psychological Association, and the National Council on Measurement in Education—collaborated on *Standards for Educational and Psychological Testing*. These standards have been revised and they continue to serve as a significant resource in the evaluation and appropriate use of appraisal instruments. These standards are in the process of being revised again, and a new edition is expected to be published shortly.

As assessment became more established, individuals began to see that centralized publication of tests would be convenient for consumers, as well as quite possibly profitable. For example, the testing functions of the College Entrance Examination Board (CEEB), the Carnegie Corporation, and the American Council on Education merged to form the Educational Testing Service. With the centralization of some publishing, electronic scoring became more cost effective. Electronic scoring fostered scoring procedures that were more complicated, and scoring became less prone to errors. Assessment became increasingly sophisticated during this period in assessment history.

1960s and 1970s

This period is marked by an examination and evaluation of testing and assessment. The proliferation of large-scale testing in the schools, along with the increased use of testing in employment and the military, led to widespread public concern. Numerous magazine articles and books questioned the use of psychological instruments and uncovered misuses of these instruments. Assessment instruments were particularly scrutinized for ethnic bias, fairness, and accuracy. This scrutiny uncovered many limitations of existing instruments, particularly concerning the use of some instruments with minority clients.

An interesting paradox occurred during the 1970s. While there was substantial concern about the use of tests, there was also a grass roots movement that encouraged more testing: "minimum competency" testing. This movement grew out of concern that high school students were graduating without sufficient skills, and the public wanted to ensure that children reached a minimal level of competency before they graduated. Many states enacted legislation that required students to pass a minimum competency examination before they could be awarded a high school diploma (Lerner, 1981). There was also legislation at the national level that had a significant impact on testing. In 1974, the Family Educational Rights and Privacy Act was passed, which mandated that parents and children older than 18 had the right to review their school records. This legislation also specified topics that could not be assessed without parental permission.

As the country was beginning to take advantage of advances in technology, the field of assessment was also changing. Computers began to be utilized, particularly for scoring. Near the end of the 1970s, the field began to explore the interactive nature of computers and methods for using computers to administer, score, and interpret assessment results.

1980s and 1990s

The use of computers in appraisal really blossomed in the 1980s. With the increased availability of personal computers, clients were able to take an assessment instrument at the computer and receive the results immediately. Computers could be programmed to adapt the order of items depending on the previous answer of the client. For example, if a client got one item correct, then the next item could be more difficult; but if a client got the item wrong, the next item could be easier. There also was an increase in computer-generated reports. Rather than having psychologists write the reports, many agencies and schools used reports written by computers.

Earlier criticisms led to many instruments being revised during this period. For example, the developers of the MMPI–2 attempted to eliminate many of the shortcomings of the MMPI. The most widely used instrument to assess children's intelligence, the Wechsler Intelligence Scale for Children—Revised (WISC–R), was revised (WISC–III). The adult version of the Wechsler scale (WAIS) was revised twice during this period. New instruments were produced that were designed to be sensitive to cultural diversity (e.g., Kaufman Assessment Battery for Children). Issues related to cultural bias and a sensitivity to multicultural influences that began in the 1960s and 1970s continued to be researched and discussed. Many professional organizations began to realize that standards for multicultural counseling and assessment needed to be developed.

A major testing movement in the 1990s has been authentic assessment. The purpose of authentic assessment is to evaluate using a method consistent with the instructional area and to gather multiple indicators of performance. Authentic assessment has had a major influence on teachers' assessments of students' academic progress (Fisher & King, 1995). Teachers often use portfolio assessment, where multiple assignments are gathered and evaluated. Rather than using only one multiple-choice test, teachers would evaluate multiple essays, projects, and/or tests that are designed to represent the material being taught.

As we look to the next century, it is difficult to predict the future issues and trends in assessment. Technology and the Internet will indubitably have an influence on assessment in counseling, and innovative methods of assessment can be developed. It may be that assessment will not take place as much in the counselor's office, but that many clients may participate in some assessments through the Internet. Multicultural issues will certainly be a focus of research in the assessment area. Identifying methods of assessing individuals with different cultural backgrounds is complex, and hopefully the field will make strides in this area. There are many indications that counselors will need to be more accountable and provide effectiveness data. Thus, counselors may need to incorporate outcome measures into their counseling in order to measure their effectiveness.

Types of Assessment Tools

In order to learn about the effective use of assessment tools in counseling, a practitioner needs to understand some of the basic types of assessment instruments. Assessment and testing are topics that often arise when counselors consult with other professionals (e.g., psychologists, social workers, and teachers). The field of mental health is moving more toward a multidisciplinary team approach to treatment; and if counselors want to continue to be a part of this multidisciplinary team, they need to understand the nomenclature of assessment. Although there are many different ways in which appraisal instruments are classified, the following provides an overview of some common categories and terms used.

Standardized vs. nonstandardized. In order for an assessment device to be a standardized instrument, there must be fixed directions for administering and scoring the instrument. In addition, the content needs to remain constant and to have been developed in accordance with professional standards. If the instrument is comparing an individual's performance to that of other individuals, the instrument must be administered to an appropriate and representative sample. A nonstandardized instrument has not met these guidelines and may not provide the systematic measure of behavior that standardized instruments provide.

Individual vs. group. This distinction concerns the administration of the instrument. Some instruments can be given to groups, which is often convenient and takes less time than administering an instrument to one person at a time. With group administration, however, it is difficult to observe all the examinees and to note all of their behaviors while they are taking the instrument. Often a substantial amount of information can be gained by administering an instrument individually and observing the client's nonverbal behaviors. Some well-known psychological instruments are only administered individually in order to gather relevant clinical information.

Objective vs. subjective. This categorization reflects the methods used to **score** the assessment tool. Many instruments are scored objectively; that is, there are predetermined methods for scoring the assessment and no judgments are required by the individual doing the scoring. Subjective instruments require that the individual make professional judgments in scoring the assessment. For example, many multiple-choice tests are objective instruments, with the scoring completed by noting that the individual's response is correct or incorrect. Essay tests are usually subjective instruments because the person grading these exams must make some judgments about the quality of the answers. Objectively scored instruments attempt to control for bias and inconsistencies in scoring. In counseling, however, we are often interested in exploring issues in people's lives, which are not easily assessed using only objective methods.

Speed vs. power. This classification concerns the difficulty level of the items. In power tests, the items in the examination vary in difficulty, and more credit may be given for more difficult items. A speed test simply examines the number of items completed in a specified time. The determination of a test as a speed or a power test depends on the purpose of the assessment. If we want to know how quickly people can do some task, then a speed test is appropriate. If we want to determine the mathematical abilities of an individual, then a power test is needed.

Verbal vs. nonverbal. In recent years, counselors have become increasingly aware of the influences of language and culture on assessment. Instruments that require examinees to use verbal skills can be problematic for individuals whose primary language is not English. Imagine that you are being tested and you read the following instructions: "Da prodes test ti moras zavoriti ovu knjigu i zafpati." Many people would flunk this test because they would not be able to read the Bosnian instructions that say, "In order to pass this test you must close this book and take a nap." (I know that some readers would be more than willing to oblige with these instructions now that they understand the translation!) Even when a test does not involve verbal skills, if the instructions are given orally or must be read, it is still a verbal instrument. Some people prefer the term nonlanguage instead of nonverbal to denote instruments that require no language on the part of either the examiner or examinee. Another term related to this topic is **performance tests.** Performance tests require the manipulation of objects with minimal verbal influences (e.g., putting a puzzle together, arranging blocks in a certain design). Sometimes there is not a clear distinction between a verbal and nonverbal test. It is difficult to design instruments that have no language or verbal components; hence, with some clients, the counselor may need to determine the degree to which language and verbal skills influence the results. In multicultural assessment, the practitioner needs to consider the degree to which both culture and language influence the assessment results.

Cognitive vs. affective. Cognitive instruments are those that assess cognition: perceiving, processing, concrete and abstract thinking, and remembering. Typically there are three types of cognitive tests: intelligence or general ability tests, achievement tests, and aptitude tests. **Intelligence tests** are sometime called **general ability tests** because the term "general ability" does not have the same connotation as "intelligence" tests. Intelligence/general ability instruments typically measure the ability to think abstractly, solve problems, understand complex ideas, and learn new material—abilities involved in a wide spectrum of activities. Intelligence is a complex phenomenon but, as Sternberg (1985) said, it is essentially related to how "smart" the individual is. **Achievement tests** are measures of acquired knowledge or proficiency. These instruments measure the extent to which the individual has "achieved" in acquiring certain information or mastering certain skills. Individuals are often assessed to determine if they have acquired knowledge or a skill after they have received instruction or training. Classroom tests of a single academic subject are the most common form of achievement tests. Whereas achievement tests measure whether an individual has acquired some knowledge or skill, **aptitude tests** predict an individual's performance in the future. Achievement tests and aptitude tests can be similar in content, but their purposes are different. Aptitude tests do not measure past experiences, but rather judge an individual's ability to perform in the future—to learn new material or skills.

Affective instruments, as compared to cognitive assessments, assess interest, attitudes, values, motives, temperaments, and the noncognitive aspects of personality. Both informal and formal techniques have a dominant role in affective assessment. In the area of formal instruments, practitioners most frequently use personality tests. There are two types of personality instruments: structured instruments and projective techniques. **Structured personality instruments** are like the Minnesota Multiphasic Personality Inventory–2 (MMPI–2), where individuals respond to a set of established questions and select answers from the provided alternatives. With **projective techniques**, individuals respond to relatively ambiguous stimuli, such as ink blots, unfinished sentences, or pictures. Because the tasks are nonstructured, they provide the examinee more latitude in responding. It is theorized that these nonstructured responses are "projections" of the individual's latent traits. Projective techniques are often more difficult for the examinee to fake. The examiner, however, needs to be extensively trained in order to use these instruments appropriately.

Identifying Appropriate Assessment Strategies

Determine What Information Is Needed

Counselors want to select only assessment strategies and tools that are suitable and appropriate for the clients they are assessing. The first step in the process is to determine what information would be useful. An assessment tool is only helpful if it provides needed and useful information. So, before we can evaluate whether an instrument will be useful, we need to first determine what information is needed. This can involve identifying the information needed for a specific client or more general information that is typically needed by most counselors in an organization.

Analyze Strategies for Obtaining Information

Once a counselor has identified the needed client information, the second step is to determine the best strategies for obtaining that information. Part of selecting the best strategy for obtaining the necessary information is to take stock of existing client information. By appraising existing information, the counselor will avoid wasting time duplicating existing information. For example, in career counseling with a college student, there probably are multiple sources of information on abilities (e.g., entrance exams such as the SAT or ACT, high school grades). Once the counselor has surveyed information he or she already has or can easily access, the next step is to determine the strategies for obtaining any additional information that is needed. A primary decision is whether information can best be gathered through formal or informal techniques. Often both formal and informal assessment tools provide an optimum situation, because the strengths of one method complement the other and they together provide in-depth analysis of clients. The counselor also needs to consider which assessment method would be most suited to the client or clients (e.g., paper and pencil self-report, behavioral checklist, computer assessment). Analyzing the attributes of the clients before selecting an instrument will facilitate appropriate assessment selection. Counselors also need to consider their own professional limitations and the types of instruments that they can ethically administer and interpret.

Search Assessment Resources

Once the counselor identifies the information needed and the most effective strategies for gathering that information, then the counselor can move to perusing existing instruments. Duckworth (1990) suggested that, whenever possible, the client should be involved in the selection of instruments. This does not mean that the counselor should provide a detailed lecture on choices of instruments with psychometric information. Instead, the counselor can engage the client in a brief discussion of possible avenues to pursue.

It is impossible for any practitioner to be familiar with the thousands of published and unpublished assessment tools in the counseling realm. In addition, it is not always simple to identify possible instruments to use. There is no one source that describes every formal and informal assessment tool that has ever been developed or used. Practitioners, therefore, often need to use a variety of sources and technologies to begin to develop a list of possible tools. Counselors should search existing assessment resources on a regular basis, because new instruments may be more appropriate and existing instruments are often revised. A counselor would not want to use an older version of an instrument when a newer and improved version is available.

General Assessment Resources

One of the most important assessment resources is the *Mental Measurements Yearbooks* (MMY). This series of yearbooks contains critiques of many of the commercially available psychological, educational, and career instruments. The first yearbook was published in 1938 by Oscar K. Buros, who continued to spearhead the publication of subsequent yearbooks until his death in 1978. Each yearbook extends information in the previous yearbooks by reviewing instruments published or revised during a specific time period. The latest version is the *Thirteenth Mental Measurements Yearbook* (Conoley & Impara, 1998), which contains reviews for more than 400 newly published or revised instruments. The yearbooks provide information on the purpose of the instrument, for whom the instrument is appropriate, its costs, and the publisher. In addition, the yearbooks contain reviews and critiques by noted authorities in the assessment field. The reviews and critiques provide an overview of the instrument's strengths and limitations.

Another resource published by the Buros Institute is *Tests in Print,* which is useful in attempting to identify possible tests by content area. *Tests in Print* summarizes information on most commercially available tests published in English. The instruments are also cross-referenced with the *Mental Measurements Yearbooks*. The Buros Institute can be accessed through the Internet (Appendix B contains the URL address). Through their Internet site, you can find reference information on the location of information and critiques in the *Mental Measurements Yearbooks* or in *Tests in Print*. If individuals want a specific critique, they can purchase this service and have the information faxed to them. This site also provides the Test Locator, which individuals can use to identify possible instruments.

Another prominent publisher for assessment resources is PRO–ED, which publishes *Tests* and *Test Critiques. Tests* (Sweetland & Keyser, 1991) provides descriptive information on approximately 3,500 instruments in the areas of psychology, education, and business. The information on the instruments in-

TABLE 1.2

Resources for identifying instruments in specific counseling areas

1. Donovan, D. M., & Marlatt, G. A. (1988). *Assessment of addictive behaviors.* New York: Guilford Press.

2. Fisher, J., & Cochran, K. (1994). *Measures of clinical practice: A sourcebook* (2nd ed.). New York: Free Press.

3. Fisher, J., & Cochran, K. (1994). *Measures of clinical practice: A sourcebook Volume 1. Couples, Families and Children.* New York: Free Press.

4. Grotevant, H. D., & Carlson, C. I. (1989). *Family assessment: A guide to methods and measures Volume 2, Adults.* New York: Guilford Press.

5. Impara, J. C., & Murphy, L. L. (1994). *Buros Desk Reference: Psychological assessment in the schools.* Lincoln, NB: Buros Institute.

6. Impara, J. C., & Murphy, L. L. (1996). *Buros Desk Reference: Assessment of substance abuse.* Lincoln, NB: Buros Institute.

7. Kapes, J. T., Mastie, M. M., & Whitfield, E. A. (1994). *A counselor's guide to career assessment instruments.* Alexandria, VA: National Career Development Association.

8. Reynolds, C. R., & Kamphus, R. W. (1990). *Handbook of psychological and educational assessment of children. Vol. 1: Intelligence and achievement.* New York: Guilford Press.

9. Reynolds, C. R., & Kamphus, R. W. (1990). *Handbook of psychological and educational assessment of children. Vol. 2: Personality, behavior, and context.* New York: Guilford Press.

10. Rubin, R. B., Palmgreen, P., & Sypher, H. E. (1994). *Communication research measures: A sourcebook.* New York: Guilford Press.

11. Schutte, N. S., & Malouff, J. M. (1995). *Sourcebook of adult assessment strategies.* New York: Plenum.

12. Toutliato, J., Perlmutter, B. F., & Straus, M. (Eds.) (1990). *Handbook of family measurement techniques.* Newbury Park, CA: Sage.

cludes purpose, costs, available data, and scoring. This same organization has published *Test Critiques,* with the latest volume being *Test Critiques: Volume 10* (Keyser & Sweetland, 1994). This resource provides detailed reviews of instruments, including an overview of practical applications.

Some resources are compendia of instruments within a certain topic area. Table 1.2 lists some of the assessment references related to specific areas of counseling. Table 1.2 is not a complete list, because new resources are continually being published. Therefore, counselors attempting to gather information about instruments in a specific area should also explore other resources.

Counseling journals can be used to identify potential instruments. Some journals are specifically related to assessment and will provide information on appraisal tools. Journals that often include articles or research studies related to assessment in counseling are: *Applied Psychological Measurement, Career Development Quarterly, Journal of Counseling and Development, Journal of Career Assessment, Journal of Counseling Psychology, Journal of Marital and Family Therapy, Journal of Mental Health, Measurement and Evaluation in Counseling and Development,* and *Professional Psychology: Research and Practice.* Many professional organizations publish newsletters that contain information on assessment instruments and issues.

ERIC

Concerning the process of identifying possible testing tools, the *ERIC* Clearinghouse on Assessment and Evaluation (ERIC_AE) can be a very valuable resource. This clearinghouse, which focuses on providing assessment information, is located at Catholic University of America (210 O'Boyle Hall, Washington, DC 20064, tel. (800) 319-5120). Individuals can access a vast array of information through the Internet (URL: http://eric.net.) or the gopher site (gopher.cua.edu then click on Special Resources). One extremely valuable source is the Test Locator, which is a joint project of the ERIC Clearinghouse on Assessment and Evaluation, the Educational Testing Service (ETS), the Buros Institute of Mental Measurement, the Region III Comprehensive Center, and PRO–ED test publishers. Through the ERIC_AE sites, counselors can access the ETS Test Collection, which is a database of over 9,500 instruments. This tool can easily be used to generate lists of possible instruments for use with clients and to gather information about the specific instruments on the list. Furthermore, the sites can be used to find references to materials published in the *Mental Measurements Yearbooks* and volumes of *Test Critiques*. Within the Test Locator, a counselor can access a collection of abstracts and descriptions of almost 200 tests that are commonly used with limited-English-speaking students. This resource can be particularly helpful in identifying possible instruments for multicultural assessment. This section of the Test Locator is a project between the Region III Comprehensive Center at George Washington University Center for Equity and Excellence in Education (CEEE) and the ERIC_AE. Besides the Test Locator, other useful information is provided through the ERIC_AE net site. The clearinghouse also publishes materials on assessment, including brief digests on pertinent assessment topics.

Electronic Sources

The assessment field is being dramatically affected by new technology. (This major influence will be discussed in more detail in Chapter 16.) One of the ways in which technology has influenced assessment is in locating possible instruments. The ERIC Clearinghouse on Assessment and Evaluation and the Buros Institute Web sites, as previously discussed, are a couple of the resources available through the Internet. The amount of information on the Internet, however, is exploding; and it is impossible to identify all the pertinent resources available. Appendix B includes the URLs for a number of helpful resources for assessment in counseling. The Internet does not restrict access, so instruments that are located over the Internet may not be sound instruments. No matter how an instrument is identified, it should be properly evaluated before it is used with a client.

Summary

Often the terms *assessment* and *appraisal* have different meanings in the helping profession, depending on the situation and context. This book defines these terms as procedures designed to gather information about clients, including formal and informal techniques. Assessment can involve formal tests, psychological inventories, checklists, scales, interviews, and observations. The degree to which counselors accurately assesses clients will influence the effectiveness of their counseling. Assessment is an integral part of the counseling process, and counselors need to develop proficient assessment skills.

In these times when counselors' competencies in assessment are being challenged, counselors need to demonstrate that they are competent in this area. The development of assessment and appraisal skills involves knowledge of basic measurement techniques and methods for evaluating instruments. Those skills also involve knowledge of the constructs (e.g., intelligence, personality) that are being measured and how to use the results in counseling. Assessment results can sometimes have a dramatic effect on a client; therefore, counselors should strive to assure that appraisal results are used in a professional and ethical manner.

CHAPTER 2

Basic Assessment Principles

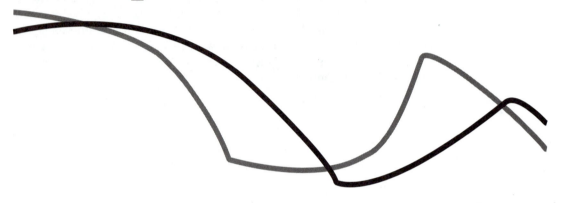

L et's assume that you have just taken a test called the Counseling Aptitude Scale and you received a score of 60 on this fictitious instrument. It is difficult to draw any conclusions based solely on this score of 60. For example, we don't know if the scores ranged from 0 to 60 or if the range was from 60 to 600. Even if the scores on the instrument were between 0 and 60, a score of 60 would mean something different if everyone else taking the instrument had a score of 58. Any score on any instrument is difficult to interpret without additional information. The basic principles discussed in this chapter will help counselors understand assessment scores and results and help counselors begin to know how to interpret those scores to clients.

Measurement Scales

When a counselor uses assessment, he or she is attempting to *measure* some aspect of the client. Measurement typically involves the application of specific procedures for assigning numbers to objects. When some entity is measured, there are rules for how the measurement is performed. As an example, there is a rule on the length of an inch. In measuring any matter, whether we are measuring a person's weight, the temperature outside, the number of lawyers in New York City, or the emotional stability of graduate students, the rules for measuring depend on the precision of the measurement scale. There are four basic types of measurement scales: nominal, ordinal, interval, and ratio scales. Any measurement of a client (whether it is his level of self-esteem or her height) will involve one of these four types of measurement scales. Numbers at different levels or scales of measurement convey different types of information to practitioners (Cohen, Swerdlik, & Smith, 1992). Counselors need to determine the type of measurement scale that is being used in an assessment in order to evaluate the instrument properly. Often statistical tests are used to analyze the psychometric qualities of an instrument. The type of measurement scale will influence the selection of appropriate statistical techniques. Therefore, one of the early steps in evaluating an instrument is to identify the measurement scale used and then determine if the statistical analyses are appropriate for the measurement scale.

The **nominal scale** is the most elementary of the measurement scales and involves classifying by naming based on characteristics. The intent of the nominal scale is to name an object. If this scale is used, there is no indication of amount of magnitude. An example of a nominal scale is when 1 = Democrats, 2 = Republicans, 3 = Libertarians, 4 = No party affiliation. When numbers are assigned to groups, it is not possible to perform many of the common statistical analyses. For example, the average for the above numbers for party affiliation is 2.5, which does not convey any real meaning. With a nominal scale, we can only get a count or a percentage of individuals who may fall into a specific category.

Because an **ordinal scale** provides a measure of magnitude, it often provides more information than the nominal scale. It is possible to tell which scores are smaller or larger than other scores with an instrument that has an ordinal scale. An example of an ordinal scale is a counselor observing a group of children and ranking them from best to worst behavior in the classroom. The ordinal scale allows one to rank or order individuals or objects, but that is the extent of the precision. On the fictitious Counseling Aptitude Scale mentioned earlier, you received a score of 60, while Mason's score was 50 and Rebecca's was 90. Unless we know that there are equal intervals in points throughout the scale, all we can say is that Rebecca did the best, you were in the middle, and Mason performed the worst. With any kind of measurement, unless there are equal units (e.g., inches has equal units), the degree to which there is a difference cannot be precisely determined. It is often difficult to design instruments that measure psychological and educational aspects in equal intervals. Consider the difficulty in developing items for a depression scale where throughout the scoring of the instrument the intervals would always be equal.

In an **interval scale,** the units are in equal intervals; thus, a difference of five points between 45 and 50 represents the same amount of change as five points between 85 and 90. An example of equal intervals is weight; if you gain five pounds it is always the same even if you are going from 115 to 120 or from 225 to 230. In assessment in counseling, many instruments are treated as if there is interval data, such as intelligence tests where the difference between 85 and 100 is the same as between 100 and 115. Many of the statistical techniques that are used to evaluate assessment instruments assume that there is an interval scale. (There are instruments, however, that do not have an interval scale and should not use those statistical techniques.) In evaluating instruments, counselors need to consider whether the scoring results can be classified as an interval scale and whether it is appropriate to use the typical statistical methods that will be addressed later.

A **ratio scale** has all the properties of an interval scale and requires the existence of a meaningful zero. For example, with intelligence, there is no definition of what a score of zero would mean. The results from an intelligence test might be considered as an interval scale but not a ratio scale. In measuring other entities, such as pulse or using the Celsius scale, there are meaningful zeros. Height is an example of a ratio scale because inches are equal units and there is a meaningful zero. With this type of scale, it is possible to do ratios and make conclusions that something is twice as big as something else. For example, a person who is seven feet tall is twice as tall as a person who is three and a half feet tall. With interval scales, such as IQ, those conclusions cannot be made. Thus, we cannot say that someone whose IQ is 200 is twice as smart as someone whose IQ is 100. The level of measurement influences the methods that can be used to evaluate the instrument and, therefore, counselors need to consider the scale of measurement when beginning to examine an instrument.

Norm-Referenced Versus Criterion-Referenced Instruments

In order to interpret a score on any instrument, the practitioner first needs to consider whether it is a norm-referenced or a criterion-referenced instrument. In a **norm-referenced instrument,** an individual's score is compared to other individuals who have taken the instrument. The term *norm* refers to the group of individuals who took the instrument to which any score is compared. A norming group can be quite large, such as a national sample of 2,000 adults who have taken a personality inventory. On the other hand, a norm could be your fellow classmates, such as when an instructor "grades on the curve." Simply speaking, a norm-referenced instrument is when an individual's performance is compared to others' performance.

In a **criterion-referenced instrument,** the individual's score is compared to an established standard or criterion. Criterion-referenced instruments are sometimes called domain- or objective-referenced. With a criterion-referenced instrument, the interest is *not* how the individual's performance compares to others, but rather how the individual performs with respect to some standard or criterion. In criterion-referenced instruments, the results are reported in terms of some specific domain. Therefore, in order to interpret a client's criterion-referenced results, a counselor needs to understand the domain being measured, such as multiplication of two-digit numbers, third grade spelling words, or knowledge of counseling theories. In criterion-referenced testing, the testing often pertains to whether the person has reached a certain *standard* of performance within that domain. For example, do they get 70% of a sample of second grade arithmetic problems correct, do they spell 90% of fifth grade spelling words correctly? Many of the tests you have taken in your academic career have been criterion-referenced tests, where, for example, you need to score 90% or better correct for an A, 80% or better for a B, 70% or better for a C, and so forth.

Sometimes with a criterion-referenced test there is a *mastery* component. In these cases, a predetermined cut-off score indicates whether the person has attained an established level of mastery. For example, a State Department of Education may designate a certain score on a test that all high school students must achieve before they can graduate from high school. Professional licensing examinations for counselors and psychologists are examples of criterion-referenced tests that include a mastery component. In many states, there is a preestablished score on the examination that reflects a necessary level of mastery in order to be licensed as a counselor. Those individuals who do not attain that score are considered not to have mastered the body of knowledge necessary to perform as a professional counselor. Some classroom tests can involve the concept of mastery, such as a teacher wanting to know if a student has mastered the multiplication table for the number 3 before the student can advance to learning the multiplication table for the number 4.

There are several difficulties in developing sound criterion-referenced instruments. First, criterion-referenced tests are designed to measure a person's level of performance in a certain domain. Therefore, we want an instrument that can adequately measure that domain. Let's use an example of a theories and techniques class in a counseling program. A criterion-referenced test for this class would need to adequately measure all the information in the domain of counseling theories and techniques. However, there is no universal agreement within the field about which theories are most important, nor is there complete agreement on which techniques are most effective. Therefore, it is difficult to determine what content should be included in a theories and techniques test. Often with higher-order knowledge areas, it is difficult to determine what is the precise content domain and what content within that domain is particularly meaningful. Anastasi and Urbina (1997) contend that criterion-referenced testing is best for assessing basic skills, such as reading and mathematics at the elementary level.

Another problem with criterion-referenced instruments is determining the criterion for mastery level. This issue centers on what exact score truly indicates that someone has mastered the content. For example, if the mastery level is preset at 90%, does it in effect mean that a person who receives 89% has not mastered the content? What about the person who just made a mistake in marking that resulted in his being below the mastery level? It is often difficult to determine the exact score that indicates someone has indeed mastered that content. The consequences of making mistakes in misidentification often influence the setting of the mastery level. If we are discussing a professional licensing examination (e.g., in counseling), the consequences of misidentification might be quite serious if individuals are considered, by their performance on the instrument, to be competent when in fact they are not adequately prepared to practice. In this case, the cut-off score might be set quite high in order to minimize the number of false positives. Criterion-referenced instruments can be very useful, for they can provide an indication of an individual's level of performance in a certain content domain; yet, there are numerous difficulties in developing sound criterion-referenced instruments.

Norm-Referenced Instruments Interpretation

Let's return once again to our example of the Counseling Aptitude Scale (CAS) and your score of 60. In this example, this fictitious instrument is being used to determine who has more aptitude compared to other individuals in terms of counseling. Because we are comparing the scores of individuals, this is a norm-referenced interpretation. Often with norm-referenced instruments, we use statistics to help us interpret the scores. If we examine the scores in Table 2.1, it would be difficult to actually interpret your score of 60 on the Counseling Aptitude Scale compared to 25 other people's scores by simply looking at the scores. Organizing the scores in a logical manner can facilitate the process of understanding the scores.

By converting the scores into a **frequency distribution** as is reflected in Table 2.2, we can better understand how your score of 60 compares to the others who have taken the fictitious CAS. A frequency distribution is simply where the scores (X) are indicated on the first line and the frequency (f), or number, of people achieving that score is indicated beneath. A frequency distribution provides a visual display that helps organize the data so that we easily see how the scores are distributed. In the frequency distribution in Table 2.2, we can see that the number or frequency of people receiving scores of 10, 20, 80, and 90 is smaller than the number of people receiving scores of 40, 50, and 60.

Sometimes, however, graphing the frequency of scores can provide a better visual display of how a group of people scored on an instrument. Often in assessment, a **frequency polygon** is used because this graphic representation makes the data easier to understand. A frequency polygon is a graph, where on the x, or horizontal, axis the scores are charted and on the y, or vertical, axis

TABLE 2.1

Raw scores on the Counseling Aptitude Scale

Name	CAS Score
Mason	50
Stacy	60
Scott	40
Angelina	70
John	40
Lynne	60
Yi-Tung	70
Marilyn	40
Judge	90
Rebecca	80
Robert	20
Maria	50
Matthew	60
Liz	40
Ophra	50
Jenny	30
David Lee	30
Satish	10
Lisa	60
Juan	50
Louise	50
Steve	20
Terry	40
Pat	50

TABLE 2.2

Frequency distribution for the scores on the Counseling Aptitude Scale

X	10	20	30	40	50	60	70	80	90
f	1	2	2	5	6	4	3	1	1

Note: X is for CAS scores and f is for the frequency of individuals the frequencies of the scores are charted. A point is placed by plotting the number of persons receiving each score across from the appropriate frequency. The successive points are then connected with a straight line. Figure 2.1 is a frequency polygon for the scores on the Counseling Aptitude Scale and reflects a graphic display of the information contained in the frequency distribution in Table 2.2. The frequency polygon makes it easier to see that many more people had a score lower than your 60, but there were some individuals who had scores higher than yours. This frequency polygon also reflects that most of the people had scores between 40 and 60, with the largest number of people receiving a score of 50.

Sometimes with scores from an instrument, we don't want to plot each individual score because there is a large range of scores. For example, we could have an instrument where the range of scores was from 1 to 400, which would make a very large frequency polygon if we plotted each possible score (1, 2, 3, . . . , 398, 399, 400). In this case, we want to make the information more manageable by determining the frequency of people who fall within a certain interval of scores. Figure 2.2 contains a frequency polygon where the scores are grouped into convenient interval classes. As indicated earlier, in a frequency polygon the frequency of persons scoring in that interval is indicated by a point being placed in the center of the class interval. In a **histogram** a column is used, where the height of the column over each class interval corresponds to the number of individuals who scored in that interval. As Figure 2.2 indicates, either a frequency polygon or a histogram can be used to visually display the same frequency of scores, with the choice being related to which one provides the best graphic display.

FIGURE 2.1

Frequency polygon for Counseling Aptitude Scale scores

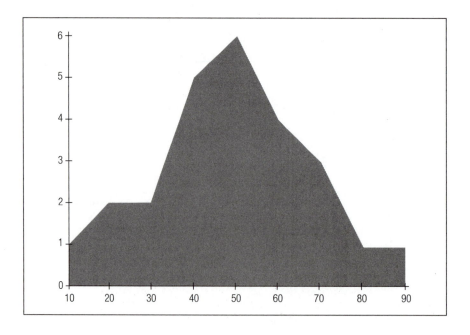

FIGURE 2.2

Frequency polygon and histogram with interval scores

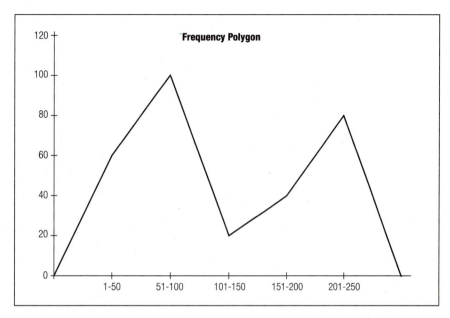

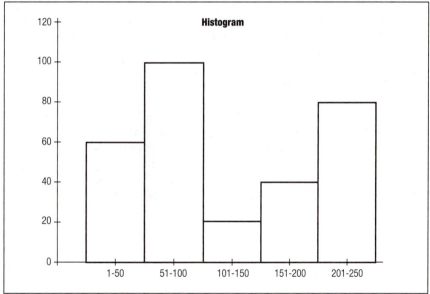

Measures of Central Tendency

Graphing the scores using either a frequency polygon or a histogram can be helpful in understanding how your score of 60 on the Counseling Aptitude Scale compares to others' scores. It also may be useful to have some indication of how *most* of the other people performed on the Counseling Aptitude

Scale. The mode, median, and mean are measures of central tendency that can be useful in interpreting individuals' results on an instrument. The **mode** is the *most frequent* score in a distribution. On the scores on the CAS, the mode or the most frequent score is 50, since both Tables 2.1 and 2.2 reflect that six people received this score, which is the highest frequency of any of the scores. To find the mode, one merely counts the number of people who received each score and the score that has the highest number of people is the mode.

In interpreting your score of 60, you now know that your score is ten points higher than the mode. It might also be helpful to know if your score is above the median or below the median. The **median** is the score where 50 percent of the people had a score below it and 50 percent of the people had a score above it. The median is the score that evenly divides the scores into two halves. The median is determined by arranging the scores in order from lowest to highest and finding the middle number. When we examine the Counseling Aptitude Scale scores, we see that the median is 50. There are 25 scores in the distribution for the CAS that we would need to arrange in order from smallest to largest. We then count to the thirteenth score, since that is the middle point where 12 people (50%) would have a score lower and 12 people (50%) would have a score higher. If you have an even number of scores in a distribution, then there will be no one middle number. In this case, you take the average between the two middle scores. As an example, let's say we have the following scores: 1, 1, 1, 3, 14, and 16. The median would be 2 since that is the average between the 1 and 3, which are the two middle scores in this distribution.

If we examined these same scores of 1, 1, 1, 3, 14, 16, the mode would be 1 and the median would be 2. In this instance, the mode and the median do not really describe the variation in scores very well, because the higher scores of 14 and 16 are not really reflected in either the mode or the median. This is an example of why the mean is a useful measure of central tendency. The mean in the example of 1, 1, 1, 3, 14, 16 is 6, which provides a measure that represents the distribution of scores. The **mean** is the arithmetic average of the scores:

$$M = \frac{\Sigma X}{N}$$

In this book, which will include a few statistical formulas, the mean will always be notated by the letter M and an individual's score or some other data point by X. The Greek symbol Σ stands for sigma and means to sum. N represents the number of individuals in the group. In this formula, we sum (Σ) the scores (X) and then divide by the number of individuals in the group (N) to get the mean or average. In the above example, we would sum the scores ($1 + 1 + 1 + 3 + 14 + 16 = 36$) and then divide 36 by the number of scores ($N = 6$), which is equal to 6. The mean for the scores on the Counseling Aptitude Scale listed in Table 2.1 is 49.2, while the median and the mode are both 50.

Measures of Variability

Knowing the measures of central tendency assists you in understanding what your score of 60 on the Counseling Aptitude Scale means, since you now know that your score is larger than the mean, median, and mode. At this point though, you cannot tell how much above the mean your score is in comparison to other people's scores. For example, it would suggest something very different if the 25 other people who took the Counseling Aptitude Scale all had scores of 60 as compared to the distribution of scores that was presented earlier (see Figure 2.1). It is important that we examine how the scores vary so that we can determine if the person is high or low compared to others and how much higher or lower his or her score may be. For example, the scores of 1, 3, 6, 9, and 11 have a mean of 6 and the scores of 5, 6, 6, 6, and 7 also have a mean of 6. Even though the means are the same, the variations in scores affect how we would interpret a score of 7. Measures of variability provide useful benchmarks because they give us an indication of how the scores vary.

Range

Range provides a measure of the spread of scores and indicates the variability between the highest and the lowest scores. Range is calculated by simply subtracting the lowest from the highest score. On the Counseling Aptitude Scale, the highest score anyone received was 90 and the lowest was 10; therefore, the range is 80 (90 − 10 = 80). Range does provide an indication of how compact or wide the variation is, but it does not assist us in interpreting your CAS score of 60 very well. Range is a simple and somewhat crude measure that can be significantly influenced by one extremely high or low score. More precise measures that provide information about how individuals vary from the mean are often used when counselors interpret scores to clients.

Variance and Standard Deviation

Variance and standard deviation fill this need by providing more precise measures that serve as indicators of how scores vary from the mean. In examining Table 2.3, we might be interested to know how these five scores (1, 2, 3, 4, 5) on the average vary from the mean. In the second column, there is an indication of how each score varies from the mean of 3. If we wanted an average deviation from the mean, we could simply add these numbers together and divide by the number of scores. If we do that, however, what we get is 0. In fact, with any set of scores, by the way we calculate mean, we will always get zero. Therefore, to avoid this problem, we square the deviations and add these together and divide by the number of scores. This number is **variance**, or mean square deviation. In the case of Table 2.3, by adding the squared deviation in the third column and dividing the number of scores, the variance is equal to 2. The problem with variance is that when we square the deviations, they are not in the same measurement unit as the original scores. Therefore, if we take the square root of the variance, then it will take

TABLE 2.3

Illustrations of variance and standard deviation

Score (X)	Deviation (X − M)	Deviation² (X − M)²
1	1 − 3 = −2	−2 = 4
2	2 − 3 = −1	−1 = 1
3	3 − 3 = 0	0 = 0
4	4 − 3 = 1	1 = 1
5	5 − 3 = 2	2 = 4
$\Sigma X = 15$	$\Sigma(X - M) = 0$	$\Sigma(X - M)^2 = 10$
$M = \dfrac{\Sigma X}{N}$	$S^2 = \dfrac{\Sigma(X - M)^2}{N}$	$S = \sqrt{\dfrac{\Sigma(X - M)^2}{N}}$
$M = \dfrac{15}{5} = 3$	$S^2 = \dfrac{10}{5} = 2$	$S = \sqrt{2} = 1.41$

the deviation back to the original unit of measurement. The square root of variance is the **standard deviation,** and it provides an indication of the average deviation in the original unit of measurement. In Table 2.3, the square root of 2 (variance) is 1.41, which is the standard deviation of those scores.

In the area of assessment, we use standard deviation in primarily two ways. First, standard deviation provides some indication of the variability of scores. The larger the standard deviation, the more the scores varied or deviated from the mean. Smaller standard deviations indicate that the scores are more closely grouped together around the mean. Based on the scores presented earlier, the standard deviation for the Counseling Aptitude Scale is 18.74. A counselor cannot ascertain how much variation there is in scores based solely on the standard deviation; however, it is probably safe to say that this standard deviation of 18.74 suggests that there is some variation in scores on the CAS. The second way to use standard deviation involves interpreting individual scores. A standard deviation can provide an indication of whether the score is below the mean, close to the mean, or significantly higher than the mean. We can interpret your score of 60 on the Counseling Aptitude Scale by saying your score is just a little more than one-half of a standard deviation above the mean (60 − 49.2 = 10.8, with one-half a standard deviation = 18.74/2 = 9.37).

Normal Distributions

If the scores on an instrument fall into a **normal distribution** or the **normal curve,** then standard deviation provides even more interpretive information. The distributions of a number of human traits (e.g., weight, height, intelligence, and some personality characteristics) approximate the normal curve. The normal curve has mathematical properties that make it very useful in the interpretation of norm-referenced instruments. The normal curve is bell-

FIGURE 2.3
*A normal
distribution*
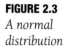

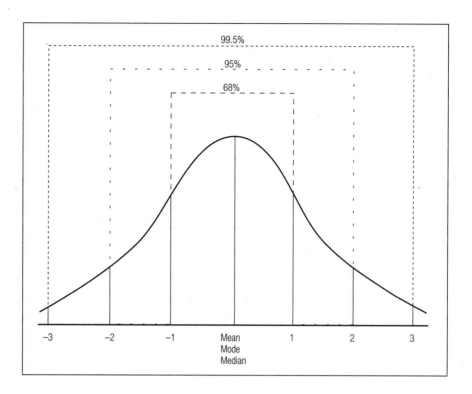

shaped and symmetrical (see Figure 2.3). If the distribution of scores is normalized, there is a single peak in the center and the mean, mode, and median are the same score. The normal curve reflects that the largest number of cases falls in the center range and that the number of cases decreases gradually in both directions. Specifically, 68% of the cases fall between one standard deviation below the mean and one standard deviation above the mean. Ninety-five percent of the cases fall between two standard deviations below the mean and two standard deviations above the mean, while 99.5% of the cases fall between three standard deviations below the mean and three standard deviations above the mean. The percentages of people falling within the different ranges of standard deviations are constant with a normal distribution. In general, the larger the group, the greater the likelihood that the scores on that instrument will resemble a normal curve. If we do have a normal distribution, then counselors can use these percentages to interpret individuals' scores. For example, if an individual score is over three standard deviations above the mean, we know that only a very small percentage of people score there because 99.5% of the individuals score between three standard deviations below the mean and three standard deviations above the mean.

There are times, however, when the scores do not fall into a normal distribution and using the normal curve to interpret scores would be inappropriate. Distributions of scores on an instrument can fall many different ways. They can be multi-modal, which means the distribution has more than one peak.

FIGURE 2.4
*Skewed
distributions*

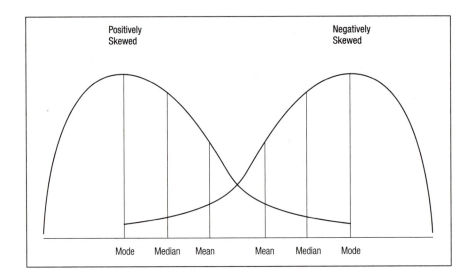

Distributions can also be **skewed** (see Figure 2.4), meaning that the distribution is not symmetrical and the majority of people either scored in the low range or the high range, as compared to a normal distribution where the majority scored in the middle. A **positively skewed distribution** is one in which the majority of scores are at the lower end of the range of scores. A **negatively skewed distribution** is the opposite, where the majority of scores are on the high end of the distribution. The distribution of a criterion-referenced test, where most of the students had scores above 90%, would be an example of a negatively skewed distribution. Some students in an assessment course memorize the difference between a positively and negatively skewed distribution by just thinking that it is the opposite of what makes sense! You may use this technique for learning the difference, but there is a better explanation. If you look at Figure 2.4, you will notice that the mean is more positive as compared to the mode and median in the positively skewed distribution. The opposite occurs with the negatively skewed distribution, where the mean is more negative than either the mode or median. This is why a distribution is labeled either positive or negative, because the mean is skewed positively when the scores are mostly lower, and the mean is skewed negatively when the scores are mostly higher. Determining if the scores on an instrument are skewed is important, because sometimes professionals will interpret scores assuming there is a normal distribution when the distribution is skewed.

Types of Scores

As counselors, we often need to provide clients with interpretations of assessment results. This could be a school counselor interpreting achievement test scores to students or parents; a mental health counselor interpreting a personality inven-

TABLE 2.4

Calculating percentiles for the Counseling Aptitude Scale

X	10	20	30	40	50	60	70	80	90
f	1	2	2	5	6	4	3	1	1
%	4	8	8	20	24	16	12	4	4
Percentile	4	12	20	40	64	80	92	96	99

tory to a client; or a marriage and family counselor interpreting a family functioning inventory to a family. Sometimes the manner in which test results are communicated to the individuals can be quite confusing because clients have little exposure to terms such as normal distribution, percentile, or stanine. Therefore, counselors need to understand the different methods of scoring and become adept at communicating those results in ways that clients can understand them.

The simplest of the scoring methods is the **raw score**, which without any other interpretative data is meaningless. We get raw scores by simply following the rules for scoring. Raw scores are those scores that have not been converted to another type of scoring (e.g., percentile, *T* score). As indicated earlier in this chapter, your raw score of 60 on the Counseling Aptitude Scale actually meant nothing until we began to examine the distribution of scores, measures of central tendency, and measures of variability. When we examine these indicators, we typically have more information with which to interpret a score. Sometimes, however, we want additional information concerning how an individual performed in comparison to the norming group; this is often done by converting a raw score to a **percentile rank** or percentile score. Percentile scores or percentile ranks are the percent of people in the norming group who had a score at or below a given raw score. Percentile should not be confused with common scoring of percentage of items correct.

Percentiles can be determined for any distribution of scores, not just normalized distributions. Table 2.4 reflects how percentiles can be calculated for the scores on the Counseling Aptitude Scale. As you probably noticed, the first two lines of Table 2.4 are the same as the frequency distribution in Table 2.2. We first have to determine how many people out of the group had each score, and then we calculate the percentage of people out of the total group who received that score. For example, for the score of 60, we can see that four people received that score, and 4 divided by the total group (25) is equal to 16 percent. As stated earlier, percentiles are the *percent* of people who received a score at or below a given raw score. Therefore, to get percentiles, we add the percent of people who had a score at or below each of the raw scores. By way of illustration, if we examine Table 2.4 we can see that the percentile for a score of 10 is the fourth percentile. This is because 4 percent of the people received this score ($1 \div 25 = .04$) and there are no people who had a score smaller than this. We would interpret this score to a client by saying, "If 100 people had taken this instrument, 4 people would have a score at or below yours." Let's look at your score (60) and what your percentile would be. The percentage of people who received each of the scores is listed underneath the frequencies.

Thus, in order to determine the percentile, we merely add the percent of people at each score that are at and lower than 60 (4 + 8 + 8 + 20 + 24 + 16 = 80). In interpreting your score of 60, a counselor might say, "Eighty percent of the norming group had a score at or below yours." Another way of communicating this result is to say, "If 100 people took the CAS, 80 of them would have a score at or below yours and 20 would have a higher score." In many ways, using percentiles may help you understand your score of 60 better than some of the other methods we have discussed so far.

Percentiles are used in numerous commonly used counseling instruments that have a normal distribution. Sometimes on instruments like the Differential Aptitude Test (DAT), the results are presented using a percentile band. These bands are based on standard error of measurement, which we will learn about in the next chapter. The percentile bands can be helpful to clients since they can see a range of where they could expect their scores to fall if they took the instrument multiple times.

Although percentiles are easy to understand and provide some useful information, there are drawbacks. Percentiles are not in equal units, particularly at the extremes of the distribution if the raw scores approximate a normal curve. Looking at the bottom of Figure 2.5, you will notice that there is a large difference between the 1st and 5th percentiles, while there would be a very small difference between the 45th and 50th percentiles. With a normal distribution, scores will cluster near the median and mean and there will be very few scores near the ends of the distribution. An example of the lack of equality in units can be seen from the distribution of scores on the Counseling Aptitude Scale. As you will notice in Table 2.4, the difference in percentile scores between the raw scores of 10 and 20 is 8 (12 − 4 = 8). On the other hand, the difference in percentile scores between the raw scores of 40 and 50 is 24 (64 − 40 = 24). Consequently, what was the same 10-point difference in raw scores resulted in remarkable differences in percentile scores. Thus, percentile scores are helpful in providing information about each individual relative position in the normative sample, but are not particularly useful in indicating the amount of difference between scores. In addition, it should be stressed that percentiles are an ordinal scale and cannot be analyzed using statistics that require interval data.

Standard Scores

Standard scores address the limitation of unequal units of percentiles, plus they provide us with a "shorthand" method for understanding test results. Standard scores are different methods of converting raw scores so that there is always a set standard deviation and mean. Standard scores can be used with all types of instruments, such as intelligence, personality, and career assessments. As a result, when we hear that a client has a z score of −1.00 or a T score of 60, we, as professional counselors, will automatically know where that score falls within the distribution without needing more detailed information on that

FIGURE 2.5

The normal distribution and different types of standard scores.

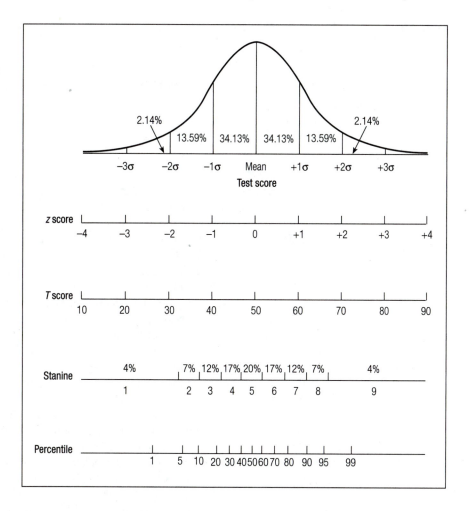

specific instrument (i.e., mean and standard deviation). Standard scores, therefore, provide a quick and easy way to know a client's relative position on an instrument because they describe how many standard deviations a client's score is from the mean.

z Scores

There are various standard scores (e.g., *T* scores, deviation IQs, stanines), but all of them are based on *z* scores. We convert an individual raw score into a *z* score by subtracting the mean of the instrument from the client's raw score and dividing by the standard deviation of the instrument. The formula for computing a *z* score is:

$$z = \frac{X - M}{s}$$

TABLE 2.5

Calculations of z scores

$$M = 75$$
$$s = 5$$

Abby's Score	Keith's Score
$X_1 = 85$	$X_2 = 72$
$z = \dfrac{85 - 75}{5} = 2.00$	$z = \dfrac{72 - 75}{5} = -.60$

In the previous formula, z = standard score, X = an individual's raw score, M = the mean of the instrument or test, and s = the standard deviation of that instrument. Since z scores are standard scores, there is always a set mean and a set standard deviation. With z scores, the mean is always 0 and the standard deviation is always 1. Table 2.5 illustrates the calculation of z scores for two individuals on the same instrument that has a mean of 75 and a standard deviation of 5. Abby's z score of 2.00 indicates that she is two standard deviations above the mean, and Keith's z score of $-.60$ reflects that he is a little more than one-half of a standard deviation *below* the mean. With z scores, it is important to focus on whether the z score is positive or negative, since you would not want to communicate to a client that his or her score was above the mean when in actuality it was below the mean.

If the instrument we are using has a normal distribution, then z scores are called normalized and can provide additional information. We can then visualize on the normal curve where a z score would fall. For example, we can see that Abby's z score of 2.00 is two standard deviations above the mean and we can see that a large percentage of people, 98% to be exact, would have a score at or below Abby's. Keith's z score of $-.60$ is below the mean of 0, and a smaller number of people (27%) have a score at or below his. We can find that exact percentile score for each z score by using the conversion table in Appendix A. This table lists the percentage of people who would fall at or below each z score.

T Scores

T scores are another standard score, with a fixed mean of 50 and a standard deviation of 10. A z score can be converted to T scores by multiplying the z score by 10 and adding or subtracting it from 50. The z score is considered the base of the standard score, since it is used for conversion to another type of standard score. Some test developers prefer T scores because they eliminate the decimals and positive and negative signs of z scores.

Normalized T scores have the same advantages as normalized z scores (see Figure 2.5). T scores are often normalized standard scores, but it is important for counselors to check the manual of an instrument to ensure that this assumption is correct. Some instrument developers will transform the data in order to normalize the distribution. This leads to an interesting dilemma, which concerns the topic of when it is legitimate to transform a nonnormal distribution into a normal distribution and when it is unacceptable to normalize a distribution. Anastasi and Urbina (1997) suggest that transforming a nonnormal distribution should only be done with very large samples and when the lack of normality is related to modest limitations of the instrument. Questions have been raised about some instruments and the transforming of the distribution when the construct is not normalized. As an example, some have questioned whether marital satisfaction in the population really distributes normally; that is, are most couples' levels of satisfaction around the mean with very few people being very unhappy and very happy? Some instruments, such as the Marital Satisfaction Inventory, have been criticized for utilizing transformed *T* scores on constructs that may not be normalized in the population.

Stanines

Another normalized standard score is the stanine scale; *stanine* is a contraction of *stan*dard and *nine*. Stanines range from 1 to 9, with a mean of 5 and a standard deviation of 2 except for the stanines of 1 and 9. Stanines are different from other standard scores because they represent a *range* of percentile scores. Table 2.6 indicates the percentile scores and percentage of people who fall within each of the stanine scores. Raw scores are converted to stanines by having the lowest 4 percent of the individuals receive a stanine score of 1, the next 7 percent receive a stanine of 2, the next 12 percent receive a stanine of 3, and then just keep progressing through the group. Stanines have the advantage of being a single-digit number that many people find easy to use. The disadvantage is that the stanines represent a range of scores, and sometimes people do not understand that one number

TABLE 2.6

Stanine conversions

Stanines	Percentile range	Percentage of individuals
1	1–4	4%
2	5–11	7%
3	12–23	12%
4	24–40	17%
5	41–59	20%
6	60–76	17%
7	77–88	12%
8	89–95	7%
9	96–99	4%

represents various raw scores. Therefore, when information is needed for very important decisions about a client's life, practitioners usually should use more precise measures than stanines.

Other Standard Scores

There are other standard scores, such as deviation IQs and CEEB scores, that are used by mental health practitioners. Deviation IQs are an extension of the ratio IQ (Intelligent Quotient) used in early intelligence tests. The earlier quotients were a ratio of mental age to chronological age times 100 (IQ = MA/CA $\times$ 100). If an individual's mental age were the same as the chronological age, his or her IQ score would be 100. One hundred was considered the benchmark for normal performance. One of the difficulties with the ratio method of calculating IQ is that the method of calculating scores did not produce interval data. Furthermore, different age groups had different standard deviations, so it was difficult to remember all the different standard deviations. Therefore, ratio IQs are no longer used in intelligence tests and deviation IQs are now used instead. Deviation IQs are standard scores where the deviations from the mean are converted into standard scores, which typically have a mean of 100 and a standard deviation of 15. Counselors need to be cautious because some intelligence tests use a standard deviation of 16 and, thus, practitioners must be knowledgeable about the instrument being used.

Another commonly used standard score is the CEEB (College Entrance Examination Board) score. In this standard score, the raw scores are converted into standard scores with a mean of 500 and a standard deviation of 100. Many people are familiar with this standard score, although they may not be familiar with the title "CEEB score," because instruments like the Scholastic Assessment Test (SAT) and the Graduate Record Examination (GRE) use this standard score.

Age or grade equivalent scales. Two developmental scales, age norms and grade norms, are widely used, particularly in educational settings. These types of scales compare a test taker's raw score to the average raw score of individuals at that same developmental level. Students, parents, teachers, and even counselors often misunderstand age or grade equivalent scales. Cronbach (1990) condemned the use of either age norms or grade norms.

Typically with an **age norm,** or an age equivalent scale, the average score of the norming group at that particular age is converted to an age equivalent score. There are two common methods to calculate age equivalent scores. One of these methods is through a procedure called item response theory, which will be discussed in Chapter 4. In item response theory, the items are specifically developed to measure performance at certain developmental levels. The second method of calculating age norms or age equivalent norms is with a norm-referenced approach. With a norm-referenced approach the focus is on comparing individuals to other individuals. Often, rather than comparing the individual with other age level performances, the process simply involves comparing the individuals to other individuals at that same age. The average performance score of 9-year-old children becomes the equivalent of a score of 9. Different age level equivalents are extrapolated depending on whether the individual is above or below the mean. Therefore, when this process is used to determine an age equivalent score, we should not interpret that a score of 12 reported for a 9-year-old student means that the child is functioning as an average 12-year-old. The 9-year-old student is being compared to other 9-year-old children and is performing at a considerably higher level than the average 9-year-old. Because there are different methods for determining age equivalent scores, it is important for a counselor to determine how the score is calculated and whether those age equivalent scores are appropriate to use.

Grade equivalent norms, or grade equivalent scores, are based on the same reasoning as age norms. With grade norms, however, the average score for students in a particular grade is converted into the grade equivalent for that specific grade. Grade equivalent scores are widely used in the area of achievement testing, primarily because they are easy to communicate. It is often easier to say a child is performing at the sixth grade, second month (6.2) level than at the 79th percentile. Parents and others like grade equivalent scores because they have more of a context to interpret those scores. For example, at a party a parent can simply brag that little Jimmy is already reading at the fourth grade level and he is only in first grade. The problem with this is Jimmy is probably not reading at the fourth grade level; rather his score indicates that he performed substantially higher than the average first grader. Moreover, a reading test for first graders may not even include any items that are truly fourth grade reading items. Grade equivalent scores are typically extrapolated scores based on average performance of students at that grade level. Therefore, Jimmy's grade equivalent score does not indicate that Jimmy should be placed in a fourth grade class for reading.

Helping professionals need to be aware of other problems with age norms and grade norms. One of the most pressing problems is that age and grade equivalent scores are often used because professionals believe that these scores communicate results effectively when, in actuality, they typically only confuse people. The information age and grade equivalent scores communicate is often ambiguous because there is no universal agreement on what constitutes age or grade achievement. For example, does eleventh grade mathematics include trigonometry or a combination of algebra and geometry? Thus, one person's interpretation of a grade equivalent could be very different from another's interpretation. A second problem is that learning does not always occur in nice equal developmental levels. Let's take the example of reading. Consider whether the difference in reading that typically occurs between first and second grades is equal to the change that takes place between seventh and eighth grades. Many people would contend that the change that takes place between first and second grades is far greater than the change between seventh and eighth grades and, therefore, we do not have equal units of measurement in age or grade norms. Another problem with age and grade equivalent scores is that instruments will vary in the scoring. One publisher's test could give a child a sixth grade, eighth month score (6.8), while another publisher's instrument could result in a score of 7.1. The two scores may be related to small differences between the instruments, but consumers of the scores may have very different interpretations of scores that are really not all that discrepant. Another problem with age or grade equivalent scores is that teachers or administrators may expect all students to perform at or above the age or grade level. Teachers have been reprimanded because students have had scores below grade level. These misconceptions fail to take into account that the instruments are norm-referenced and the expectations are that fifty percent of the students will fall above the appropriate age or grade score and fifty percent will fall below this score. Therefore, expecting all students to fall above the mean is unrealistic in most classrooms, and inappropriate given norm-referenced testing.

Age and grade equivalent scores are often misunderstood, and counselors can be particularly helpful to parents or guardians by assisting them in understanding these scores. A case in point is Justin, who was a ten-year-old who had both academic and behavioral problems in school. Justin's parents entered counseling because they were having a major disagreement over whether to have Justin repeat the fourth grade. The father anticipated that the counselor would automatically agree with him concerning the need for Justin to repeat the grade when the counselor saw his test scores taken at the beginning of fourth grade, where Justin had a reading grade equivalent of 3.4 (third grade, fourth month) and a language arts grade equivalent of 3.8. The counselor explained to the parents that Justin was only slightly behind the average performance of fourth graders in language arts and a little more behind in reading. After working with the family for a few sessions and talking to Justin's teacher, the counselor realized that there were a number of complex issues that were influencing Justin's academic and behavioral problems. Through the counseling, the parents began to look at their parenting styles and different methods they could use to assist Justin with his schoolwork. Although this case is an example of a situation in which the score is below grade level, parents also react to scores above grade level and want their child to be placed in a higher grade based on their grade equivalent scores.

Evaluating the Norming Group

In using a norm-referenced instrument it is not only important to consider what type of scoring is most appropriate (e.g., percentiles vs. *T* scores), but it is also important to determine whether the norming group is suitable for the client(s). You may wonder what is the best type of norming group, with the answer to that question being "it depends." The adequacy of a norming group depends on the clients being assessed, the purpose for the assessment, and the way in which that information is going to be used. Hence, there are *no* universal standards for what constitutes a good norming group, but rather the determination of an adequate norming group rests with the practitioner who is using the instrument.

One way to evaluate a norming group is to examine the methods used for selecting the group. In general, more credence is given to a sample that is drawn in a systematic method. In statistics, we often use the word *sample* to refer to the group that is actually being tested. This sample is drawn from the larger group of interest, the *population*. Returning to the Counseling Aptitude Scale example, the population would be the large group of all counseling students in the United States. It would be very difficult to have a norming group that included all of these counseling students and, therefore, we might draw a sample of these students that would represent this larger population. One method of selecting this sample would be to draw a *simple random sample*. In a simple random sample, every individual in the population has an equal chance of being selected. Hence, if we wanted to use simple random sampling procedures with the Counseling Aptitude Scale, we would have to give every counseling student in the United States an equal chance of being selected. Ensuring that every counseling student is entered into the pool from which the sample is drawn would be an extraordinarily difficult task.

In the area of appraisal, a *stratified sample* is often used. In a stratified sample, individuals are selected for the norming group based on certain demographic characteristics. Instrument developers may want their norming group to match the percentage of African Americans, Hispanics, Native Americans, and Asian Americans in the nation. They would need to actively recruit a sufficient number of people for their norming group so that the proportions of individuals from these ethnic groups match the proportions found in the latest reports from the United States Census Bureau. Other demographic variables that commonly influence the gathering of stratified samples are gender, socioeconomic level, geographic location, amount of education, marital status, and religion. Sometimes an instrument will incorporate a stratified sampling technique for a specific purpose, such as selecting children with certain learning disabilities or including a specified proportion of both depressed adults and nondepressed adults. If a stratified sample is used, the counselor should evaluate not only the adequacy of the sample, but also the methods used for recruiting the sample. For instance, there are some instruments for adults where the developers have recruited primarily college students rather than a wider sample of adults.

Another sampling strategy commonly used in the assessment field is *cluster sampling*. This process involves not selecting individuals, but rather using existing units. By way of illustration, let's assume we are developing a measure of self-esteem for elementary age children. It would be unusually arduous to attempt a random sample and list all the elementary children even in one state. Therefore, the instrument developers might use a cluster sampling technique and list all the elementary schools in a state and randomly select elementary schools. The specific elementary students would not be randomly sampled;

instead, larger units (i.e., elementary schools) would be randomly selected using cluster sampling.

When a counselor uses a norm-referenced instrument, the interpretation is restricted based on the particular normative population from which the norm was derived. Counselors, therefore, need to have knowledge about the characteristic of the norming group in order to use the instrument appropriately. The size of the norming group should be sufficiently large to provide a solid comparison. Furthermore, the norming group should be appropriate for the counselor's clients. This is particularly important with multicultural assessment. If there are discrepancies between the norming group and the client, the counselor needs to closely examine whether the results are valid.

Summary

This chapter summarizes some of the basic methods in which instruments are categorized, scored, and interpreted. In examining an instrument, it is important to determine if it is a norm-referenced versus a criterion-referenced instrument. Norm-referenced instruments compare an individual's performance to other people's performance on the instrument. On the other hand, criterion-referenced instruments compare an individual's performance to an established standard or criterion. In regard to norm-referenced instruments, statistics assists us in organizing and interpreting the results. Frequency distributions are charts that summarize the frequencies of scores on an instrument. Frequency polygons and histograms graphically display the distribution of scores so that practitioners can easily identify trends. Measures of central tendency (i.e., mode, median, and mean) provide benchmarks of the middle or central scores. The mean or average score is often used in interpreting appraisal results. The measures of variability (i.e., range, variance, and standard deviation) indicate how scores vary and where an individual's score may fall in relation to others' scores. Standard deviation is the most widely used measure of variability. Standard deviation has some important qualities if the distribution approximates the normal curve. With a normal distribution, 68 percent of the norming group will fall between one standard deviation above the mean and one standard deviation below the mean. In addition, with a normal distribution, the mean, mode, and median all fall at the same point.

There are numerous methods of transforming raw scores in norm-referenced instruments. Percentiles provide an indication of what percentage of the norming group had a score at or below a client's. Standard scores convert raw scores so that there is always a set mean and standard deviation. These scores express the individual's distance from the mean in terms of the standard deviation of the distribution. The most basic standard score is the z score that has a mean of 0 and a standard deviation of 1. Counselors need to be careful when they are using instruments that incorporate age equivalent or grade equivalent norms and to know precisely how the results should be interpreted. Furthermore, counselors need to fully examine the norming group of any instrument and understand the strengths and limitations of that group.

CHAPTER 3

Reliability

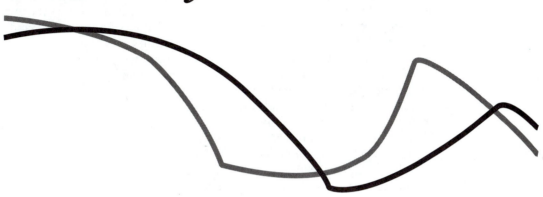

In Chapter 1 there was a discussion of the importance of examining an instrument's psychometric qualities in order to determine if it is appropriate to use. One psychometric indicator of the quality of an instrument is its **reliability.** Reliability concerns the degree to which an instrument's scores are free from errors of measurement. In appraisal, we typically assume that the traits or constructs being measured are stable and that fluctuations are due to error in the instrument. Of critical concern in assessment is the amount of error in any instrument. Reliability coefficients can be calculated to provide an indication of the amount of measurement error in the instrument. Counselors can then use these reliability coefficients in two ways. First, reliability coefficients can be useful in selecting instruments, as practitioners want to use instruments with the most amount of reliability and the least amount of error. Second, reliability coefficients can also be used in the interpretation of results to the client. In this chapter, we examine the theory behind reliability, how reliability coefficients are calculated, and how counselors can use these coefficients in their work with clients.

Classical Test Theory

Some people may have taken an assessment device, for example a test for a class, and believe that the test didn't adequately measure their knowledge in the area. For instance, a person may have felt physically ill or had a disagreement with his or her spouse just before the test. It might also be that the test questions were vague or not particularly well written. On the other hand, some people have also had the experience where they have done better on a test than they really thought they would. They may have guessed right on a couple of questions or the instructor may not have asked many questions on the content that was covered on the day they didn't come to class. In either case, the scores on the test didn't reflect their actual knowledge, or, to state it in another way, there was some *error* involved in the test scores. In terms of reliability, classical test theory is built on this premise: that any result from an appraisal device is a combination of an individual's true ability plus error (Crocker & Algina, 1986).

Reliability is often thought to be an indicator of consistency, but theoretically it is based on the degree to which there is error within the instrument. Classical test theory suggests that every score has two hypothetical components: a true score and an error component. In Figure 3.1 this relationship is presented, where *Obs.* represents the observed score, *T* signifies the true score, and *E* represents the error. In the field of assessment, no one has been able to develop a perfect instrument, so all instruments are a combination of a true measure and some degree of error. The pertinent question is how much of any score is true and how much is error? Figure 3.1 shows how in theory we progress from the simple concept of the observed score being equal to our true score plus error to reliability being a ratio of true variance to observed variance. Therefore, when we are reading an instrument's manual and the authors of the instrument include a reliability coefficient, we use classical test theory to interpret that coefficient. A reliability coefficient of .75 would indicate that 75 percent of the variance is true to observed variance. As Figure 3.1 also indicates, 1 minus the ratio of error variance to observed variance is equal to reliability ($1 - x = .75$) and, therefore, we can determine that the ratio of error variance to observed variance is .25 ($1 - .25 = .75$). Thus, we use a reliability coefficient to give us an *estimate* of how much of the variance is true variance and how much is error variance. It must be remembered that this is only an estimate; our methods of calculating reliability are not sophisticated enough to tell us how much in actuality is true variance and how much is error variance. Thus, as we will see later in this chapter, there are different methods for calculating reliability; however, with all these different methods for calculating reliability coefficients, we use classical test theory to interpret the reliability coefficients.

FIGURE 3.1

Classical test theory and reliability

- According to classical test theory, reliability is based on the concept that every observation (e.g., test score, instrument result, behavioral observation) is a combination of an individual's true score plus error.

$$Obs. = T + E$$

- Based on the above, theorists then proposed that the variance of the observation or score would be equal to the variance of the true score plus the variance of error.

$$S_O^2 = S_T^2 + S_E^2$$

- In order to make the above equation into something that can be used to determine reliability, we can divide the variance of the true on both sides of the equation

$$\frac{S_O^2}{S_O^2} = \frac{S_T^2}{S_O^2} + \frac{S_E^2}{S_O^2}$$

- Since anything divided by itself is equal to 1, the equation then becomes:

$$1 = \frac{S_T^2}{S_O^2} + \frac{S_E^2}{S_O^2}$$

- Theoretically, we can now take the variance of error to the variance of observed off both sides of the equation.

$$1 - \frac{S_E^2}{S_O^2} = \frac{S_T^2}{S_O^2} + \frac{S_E^2}{S_O^2} - \frac{S_E^2}{S_O^2}$$

- Since anything minus itself is zero, we are then left with the equation of:

$$1 - \frac{S_E^2}{S_O^2} + \frac{S_T^2}{S_O^2} = \text{Reliability}$$

- Based on theory, a measure of reliability provides an estimate of the amount of true variance to observed variance. Therefore, if we are reading in a test manual that an instrument has a reliability coefficient of .80, using classical test theory we interpret it as 80 percent of the variance is true to observed variance. In using the other side of the above equation, we can also see that 1 minus the error variance to observed variance is equal to reliability. Therefore, we can conclude that 20 percent of the variance is error variance ($1 - .20 = .80$).

Reliability and Unsystematic Error

In technical terms, reliability is an estimate of the proportion of total variance that is true variance and error variance. This error variance is only *unsystematic error* and does not include systematic error. Reliability is calculated using the consistency of scores obtained by the same individuals, whereby variations in scores provide an estimate of error. Examining the difference between systematic and unsystematic error should clarify this distinction. *Systematic* means there is a system, where methods are planned, orderly, and methodical. *Unsystematic* means the lack of a system, where occurrences are presumed to be random. An example of systematic error is when a test question contains a typographical error and everyone reads that same error. Reliability would not measure that error because it is systematic. Systematic errors are constant errors that don't fluctuate. Unsystematic errors are those errors that are not consistent, such as a typographical error on just one person's test.

Unsystematic errors can arise from a variety of sources. Sometimes there are situations where an error arises in the administration. As an example, a school counselor may be responsible for the administration of the Scholastic Assessment Test (SAT) at one school and may not read the instructions correctly to those students, while students at other schools receive the correct instructions. There may be problems with the facilities during the administration of an instrument, where the room is too hot, cold, or noisy. The examiner's demeanor can vary due to illness or a lack of sleep and this may result in unsystematic error. Illness, fatigue, and emotional factors can all affect an individual's performance on an assessment instrument. The construction of the items on the instrument may be vague and people may vary in how they interpret the items. With any instrument, we want to know the degree to which unsystematic error is a problem, and reliability provides us an estimate of the proportion of unsystematic error.

Correlation Coefficients

Reliability is *calculated* based on the amount of consistency between two sets of scores (e.g., give a group an instrument once, then wait a period of time and test them again to see if the scores change). Often when individuals want to examine consistency, they use the statistical technique of **correlation.** Correlation provides an indication of consistency by examining the relationship between scores. Figure 3.2 shows an example of a small class who took a test once and then a week later took it again. In this example, there is a perfect positive correlation (+1.00) since everyone in the class got the same score and the same rank the second time as they did in the first administration. The second scatter diagram in Figure 3.2 reveals a negative correlation; whereas the scores on the *x* axis increase, the scores on the *y* axis decrease. In some cases we do not want a negative correlation. For example, with reliability, we wouldn't want those who had the highest scores the first time they took the tests to have the lowest scores the second time they took the test. Nor would we want the reverse, where those who had the lowest scores at first have the highest scores the second time. There are times, however, when a negative correlation is expected. For example, if client hostility were to increase during the counseling process, we would expect that the effectiveness of the counseling would decrease.

The statistical technique of correlation produces a **correlation coefficient** that provides a numerical indicator of the *relationship* between the two sets of data. Remember that correlation is a statistic that is *not* just used to determine reliability but that has multiple uses that involve examining the relationship between two sets of variables. Correlation coefficients can range from -1.00 to $+1.00$. The closer the coefficient is to 1.00 (either positive or negative), the stronger the relationship. On the other hand, the closer the coefficient is to

FIGURE 3.2

Scatterplot for positive and negative correlations

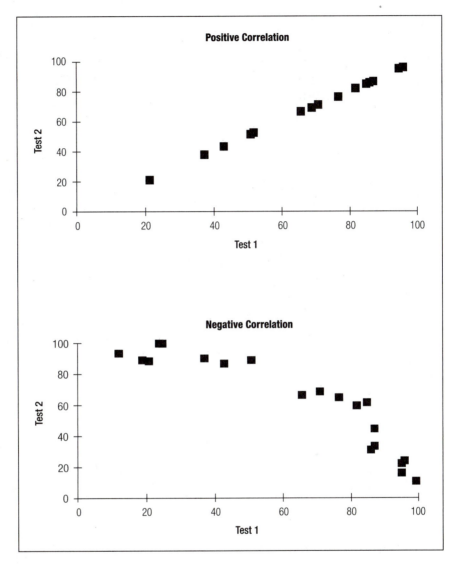

.00, the smaller the relationship. A correlation coefficient of zero indicates the lack of evidence of a relationship. Correlation coefficients can be computed in various ways; the nature of the data determines the appropriate method.

The most common method for calculating correlations is the *Pearson-Product Moment Correlation Coefficient,* which is essentially based on the simple concepts of "a positive times a positive is a positive, a negative times a negative is a positive, and a positive times a negative is a negative; a big times a big is a big, and a small times a small is a small." Figure 3.3 shows how these concepts

FIGURE 3.3

Calculating a Pearson-Product Moment Correlation

	First Administration		Second Administration	
	Raw Score	z Score	Raw Score	z Score
Tom	62	−1.90	80	−.78
Meg	78	−.38	78	−1.10
Dick	75	−.67	91	.94
Joe	84	.19	85	.00
Harry	88	.57	87	.31
Beth	92	.95	78	−.78
Amy	95	1.24	96	1.73

$M = 82$

$$SD = \sqrt{\frac{774}{7}} = \sqrt{110.57} = 10.52$$

$M = 85$

$$SD = \sqrt{\frac{284}{7}} = \sqrt{40.57} = 6.37$$

Product of z scores

−1.90 × −.78 =	1.48
−.38 × −1.10 =	.42
−.67 × .94 =	−.63
.19 × .00 =	.00
.57 × .31 =	.18
.95 × −.78 =	−.74
1.24 × 1.73 =	2.15
	2.86

$$r = \frac{\Sigma z_1 z_2}{N} = \frac{2.86}{7} = .41$$

are used to calculate a correlation coefficient. The formula for the Pearson-Product Moment Correlation is:

$$r = \frac{\Sigma z_1 z_2}{N}$$

In this equation, r represents the Pearson-Product Moment Correlation and $\Sigma z_1 z_2$ characterizes the sum of the product of the z scores (take each person's z score on the first administration and multiply it times the z score on the second test and then add these products together). N in this equation represents the number of individuals. Converting each individual's scores into z scores provides an indication of whether they are above or below the mean. Remember that z scores above the mean are positive numbers and z scores below the mean are negative numbers. We would expect people to be consistent, in that they would either be above the mean or below the mean on both administrations (a positive times a positive and a negative times a negative). Thus, if they are consistent in their performance, that increases the product of the z scores and, thus, increases the correlation coefficient. On the other hand, if they are above the mean one time (a positive z score) and below the mean the second time (a negative z score), then a positive times a negative is a negative and this will decrease the correlation coefficient. The same applies to size of the z scores, because a higher z score (a big) times a higher z score (a big) will produce a larger number than a big z score times a smaller z score. What is important to understand is that scores that are consistent contribute to a larger correlation coefficient (toward either a $+1.00$ or a -1.00) and scores that are inconsistent reduce the size of the correlation coefficient (more toward .00).

There are easier methods for calculating a *Pearson-Product Moment Correlation* that do not require converting every raw score into a z score. The following formula is easier to calculate and will be less time consuming.

$$r = \frac{N(\Sigma XY) - (\Sigma X)(\Sigma Y)}{\sqrt{[N(\Sigma X^2) - (\Sigma X)^2][N(\Sigma Y^2) - (\Sigma Y)^2]}}$$

Even though this formula does not appear to take into consideration the consistency of raw scores, it actually does, because all the methods of calculating correlations take into account whether the two sets of data vary in the same manner. Sometimes with correlations, individuals want more than just an indicator of the relationship and would like to know the percent of common variances between the two sets of data. In this case, they simply square the correlation coefficient to find out the percentage of shared variance between the two variables. This statistic is called the **coefficient of determination** and is represented by r^2. Therefore, if a correlation coefficient is equal to .50, the amount of shared variance is equal to .25 ($r^2 = .50^2$). The amount of shared variance is often represented in a Venn diagram (see Figure 3.4) that visually

FIGURE 3.4

Venn diagram representing percent of shared variance

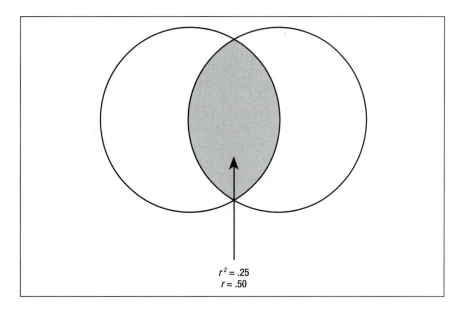

$r^2 = .25$
$r = .50$

represents the amount of overlap between the two variables. Therefore, if there is a large degree of shared variance, there would be a large section where the two circles overlap; however, if r^2 is quite small, then the circles would hardly intersect.

Types of Reliability

The previous discussion of correlation is necessary in order to understand how an estimate of reliability is actually calculated. As you will remember, reliability in theory provides us with an indication of the amount of true variance to observed variance. In everyday counseling, however, it is impossible to get a measure of true variance. Therefore, we often use the statistical technique of correlation to provide us with an estimate of reliability that is based on the concept of consistency (i.e., we would trust that a score is a "true" estimate if a person gets that same score consistently). The following sections provide an overview of the typical methods for estimating the reliability of an instrument.

Test-Retest

A common method for estimating the reliability of an instrument is to give the identical instrument twice to the same group of individuals. With the **test-retest reliability** method, a reliability coefficient is calculated by simply correlating the performance on the first administration with the performance on the second administration. It is expected that the variation in scores between the first and second administrations would be related to unsystematic error since everything else should be the same. The correlation coefficient between the test and retest scores provides us with an estimate of reliability. We then use classical test theory to interpret the coefficient. Therefore, if the reliability coefficient using test-retest is .80, we would interpret it by saying that 80% of the variance is true to observed variance and 20% is error to observed variance. In reliability, we don't square the correlation coefficient or use the coefficient of determination. The reliability coefficient itself is used to evaluate whether to use the instrument or not.

There are some difficulties in using test-retest as a method for determining reliability. One of the major problems is that something could intervene between the first administration and the second administration. For example, a counselor might be interested in developing an instrument to assess clients' potential for having an eating disorder. If this counselor gave the test once, and before he or she could give it again there was a popular television miniseries dealing with eating disorders that many of the group members watched, then that would probably affect their scores on the retest. Instrument manuals should specify the time period between the first and second administrations in a test-retest situation. In general, reliability coefficients tend to decrease as the amount of time between the testing increases. Anastasi (1988) recommended that the time period between the test and retest should rarely exceed six months. Sometimes a test-retest reliability coefficient will be called a *coefficient of stability* when there is a long period between the administrations of the instruments. In this case, the test-retest reliability is providing an indication of the stability of the scores.

The test-retest method of estimating the reliability of an instrument is only appropriate if the following assumptions are met. First, the characteristic or trait that is being measured must be stable over time. If an instrument measured situational anxiety (not trait anxiety), we would anticipate much more fluctuation in scores and the test-retest method would not be appropriate. Trait anxiety is supposedly stable over time and, in this case, test-retest would be an appropriate method for estimating reliability. The second assumption is that there should be no differential in practice effect. With many skills, people become more proficient as they practice, and the first administration of the test could serve as that practice. For example, in a psychomotor test where individuals are required to screw nuts and bolts together, individuals may improve with practice and score significantly higher on the retest. The third, and last, assumption is that there should be no differential in learning between the test and the retest. Exposure to education or psychological interventions between the testings can influence the performance on the second test. Sometimes learning can occur as a result of the first test. For example, sometimes people will simply remember the correct response to an item if the time between the testing is fairly short. In addition, it is not uncommon for people to be bothered by a question and after the test is over to seek the correct answer to the question. Some people may then learn as a result of taking the first test. Therefore, there are instruments where test-retest is appropriate to use and other times when test-retest is not appropriate. As consumers of assessment instruments, counselors need to decipher when the test-retest method is an appropriate technique for determining reliability of an instrument.

Alternate or Parallel Forms

Estimating reliability using **alternate** or **parallel forms** requires that there be *two* forms of the instrument. In this method, individuals are given one form of the instrument initially and then are assessed with a second alternate or parallel form of the instrument. The scores on the two instruments are then correlated, which results in an estimate of reliability. This method avoids the many difficulties of the test-retest method because different forms of the instrument are used. Having two forms eliminates problems associated with individuals just remembering responses; therefore, the forms can be given in immediate succession.

Care should be taken with alternate forms to ensure that that the two forms are truly parallel. Ideally, the two forms of the instrument should be independently constructed to meet the same test specifications. In order for the instruments to be equivalent, there must be the same number of items and the items must be in the same format. Content sampling becomes critical because both forms must adequately sample the content domain equally. Most content domains will vary in terms of difficulty, so instrument developers need to guard against one form being more difficult than the other. In the personality area, we want to ensure that similar questions are addressing the same issue; even subtle wording changes can alter the context in which individuals answer questions. For example, some people would read the questions of "do you fight with your spouse" and "do you argue with your spouse" as being equivalent. Others, however, may interpret "fight" as being physical and "argue" as being verbal. The instrument's manual needs to include evidence that the two forms are truly equivalent.

Although there are many advantages to the alternate-form method of estimating reliability, there are also some difficulties in using this method. Often in the area of counseling, it is difficult to develop even one sound instrument; the efforts required to develop two different but equivalent forms can be monumental. Therefore, alternate, or parallel, forms is a less prevalent method of estimating reliability. Also with alternate forms, the first instrument may have some influence on the administration of the second instrument (e.g., practice effect or learning) that will affect the reliability coefficient.

Internal Consistency Measures of Reliability

All of the following types of estimating reliability use one administration and a single form of the instrument. These methods then divide the instrument in different manners and correlate the scores from the different portions of the instrument. Thus, these forms of reliability examine the instrument "internally" in order to determine its consistency or lack of error.

Split-half reliability. In the **split-half reliability** method, the instrument is given once and then split in half to determine the reliability. The first step involves dividing the instrument into equivalent halves. Splitting the instrument into the first half and the second half is often not appropriate because some tests become progressively more difficult. In addition, warming up and practice effect may influence performance on the first half, while fatigue and boredom may influence performance on the second half. Often an instrument is divided in half by using the scores from the even items and the scores from the odd items. This odd-even splitting will often minimize some of the problems with equivalency, particularly if the items are arranged by order of difficulty. Other methods for dividing the instrument involve selecting items randomly or organizing the items on the instrument by content.

After the instrument has been divided into two halves for each person, the second step involves correlating the two halves. This is problematic, however, since a correlation coefficient is influenced by the number of observations involved in the calculation (i.e., a larger number of observations will generally produce larger correlation coefficients and a smaller number of observations will produce smaller correlation). Therefore, when we split an instrument into two halves and correlate the halves, we are using half the original number of items in the calculation. For example, if an instrument involves 50 items, the split-half method provides an estimate of reliability based on 25 items. Because longer instruments will generally have higher reliability coefficients than shorter instruments, split-half reliability coefficients will be smaller than other methods that use the original number of items. Research has shown that the **Spearman–Brown formula** provides a good estimate of what the reliability coefficient would be if the two halves were increased to the original length of the instrument. Instrument developers often use the Spearman–Brown to correct split-half reliability estimates. The Spearman–Brown formula is:

$$r_{ii} = \frac{2r_{hh}}{1 + r_{hh}}$$

In this formula, the r_{ii} represents the Spearman–Brown corrections of the split-half reliability coefficient. The r_{hh} is the original split-half correlation coefficient. When comparing the reliabilities of different instruments, one should never directly compare a split-half reliability coefficient to a Spearman–Brown reliability coefficient since it would be expected that the Spearman–Brown would be higher. As an example, would you select the ABC Self-Esteem Inventory with a split-half reliability coefficient of .88 or the XYZ Self-Esteem In-ventory with a Spearman–Brown reliability coefficient of .88? You should not assume that these two instruments are equally reliable since the Spearman–Brown is a correction of the split-half. Therefore, you would be correct in selecting the ABC Self-Esteem Inventory because the split-half reliability coefficient of .88 would be increased if the Spearman–Brown formula were used.

Kuder–Richardson formulas (KR 20 and KR 21). The **Kuder–Richardson formulas** are other methods for calculating reliability by examining the internal consistency of one administration of the instrument. The decision to use either the KR 20 or the KR 21 is based on the characteristics of the instrument, specifically if the items are measuring a homogeneous or heterogeneous behavior domain. Let's use the examples of instruments that measure family function to look at the difference between homogeneous and heterogeneous instruments. An example of a homogeneous instrument would be an instrument that measures family function and only assesses the *single* domain of family communication. On the other hand, a heterogeneous instrument would be an instrument where multiple domains are examined, such as an instrument that measures family communication, family cohesion, family adaptability, and family conflict. The KR 20 or the "Kuder–Richardson formula 20" is appropriate for instruments that are heterogeneous. It is purported to be an estimate of the average of all split-half reliabilities computed from all the possible ways of splitting the instruments into halves. The formula for computing a KR 20 is:

$$r_{20} = \left(\frac{n}{n-1}\right)\frac{S_t^2 - \Sigma pq}{S_t^2}$$

In the above formula, r_{20} is the reliability coefficient of the instrument using the Kuder–Richardson 20 formula, n is the number of items on the instrument, and S is the standard deviation of the instrument. The terms p and q are probably new to you. We sum (Σ) the proportion of individuals getting *each* item correct (p) multiplied by the proportion of individuals getting each item incorrect (q). With the KR 20, an individual must calculate for each item the number who got it right and the number who got it wrong. Computers can be of assistance in calculating KR 20s because this method can be quite time consuming.

The formula for the KR 21 is much simpler to compute, but it is only appropriate for an instrument that is homogeneous. The formula for the KR 21 is:

$$r_{21} = \frac{n}{n-1}\left[1 - \frac{M(n-M)}{nS^2}\right]$$

In the KR 21 formula, the r_{21} is the reliability coefficient using the KR 21 formula, n is the number of items, M is the mean, and S is the standard deviation. Sometimes you may see an instrument manual where they have inappropriately used a KR 21 because it is easy to calculate. The KR 21 cannot be used if the items are not from the same domain or if the items differ in terms of difficulty level. In general, the Kuder–Richardson formulas tend to have lower reliability coefficients than the split-half method.

Coefficient alpha. In terms of internal consistency methods of estimating reliability, so far the discussion has only concerned examples where the scoring is dichotomous (e.g., right or wrong, true or false, like me and not like me). Some instruments, however, use scales that have a range such as: strongly agree, agree, neutral, disagree, and strongly disagree. On some personality tests, the answers to questions have different weightings. When the scoring is not dichotomous, then the appropriate method is **coefficient alpha** or **Cronbach's Alpha**. Coefficient alpha (α) takes into consideration the variance of each item. If you would like to calculate a Cronbach's Alpha, see Cronbach (1951). Coefficient alphas are usually low and conservative estimates of reliability.

Nontypical Situations

There are some types of assessment tools for which typical methods of estimating reliability are not appropriate. As consumers of appraisal instruments, it is important for counselors to have an understanding of the assessment areas where special consideration should be taken in determining the reliability of an instrument. One area where typical methods of determining reliability are not appropriate is with speed tests, such as a psychomotor test where the examinees are timed on how many nuts and bolts they screw together. A test-retest would not be appropriate because many individuals (not me, however) will become better at this task with practice. Also, splitting the test in half or using other measures of internal consistency would probably result in nearly perfect reliability. For example, if an examinee got 22 nuts and bolts together in the allotted time, he or she would get 11 even "items" correct and 11 odd "items" correct. Sometimes instruments are split in half and people are given a certain time period to complete each half; then, consistency in performance is examined.

Another area where typical methods for determining reliability may be problematic is with criterion-referenced instruments. As you will remember, criterion-referenced instruments are those in which an individual's performance is compared to a standard or criterion. Criterion-referenced instruments are often used in achievement testing to determine whether the student has achieved a necessary level of performance. For example, a teacher may want to determine whether students have mastered multiplying one-digit numbers before allowing them to proceed toward learning how to multiply two-digit numbers. With criterion-referenced instruments, we would expect that most of the scores would be close to the previously determined criterion or standard. In fact, in some situations all of the examinees continue to receive instruction until the mastery score is achieved. Therefore, in criterion-referenced instruments there is often little variability. Remember the discussion of correlation, when the idiotic phrase "a big times a big is a big, a small times a small is a small" was presented. This phrase applies here to criterion-referenced instruments, as there will be small variations from the criterion score and, therefore, the correlation coefficients will be small because of the lack of variability. Typical methods of determining reliability use correlation, but these methods will frequently result in low reliability coefficients for criterion-referenced instruments. If you are interested in examining the different methods of determining reliability for criterion-referenced instruments, then the following resources may be helpful to you: Berk (1984) and Subkoviak (1984).

Instruments vary in the degree to which the scoring is more objective or subjective. As we will see in the later chapters, there are instruments in which the scoring involves clinical judgment, and some subjectivity is necessary in the scoring of these instruments. With subjectively scored instruments, we are not only interested in whether examinees score consistently, but we're also interested in any scoring differences among the examiners who score the same instrument. If the scoring of an instrument requires some professional judgments, then the instrument developers need to provide information on *interrater reliability*. There are different methods for determining interrater reliability, but the range is the same as other reliability indices (.00 to 1.00).

Evaluating Reliability Coefficients

The evaluation of an instrument's reliability should not be done in isolation. Often, in instrument manuals you will see a range of reliability coefficients rather than just one coefficient. A counselor cannot just look at reliability coefficient(s) and determine whether there is adequate reliability or not. For instance, if you were to examine the reliability coefficient of .91, you might think that it was certainly acceptable. We could even say that this indicates that 91%

of variance is true variance and only 9% is error variance. In order to determine whether an instrument has adequate reliability, we must first examine the purpose for using the instrument. If the results of an instrument could have a substantial impact on an individual's life, then we want an instrument with very high reliability. In many school districts, for example, intelligence or general ability tests are part of the information that is used to determine whether the child can receive special educational services. It would be unfortunate if children did not receive the services they needed because of an unreliable test. As you will see in Chapter 7, some of the widely used intelligence instruments have overall reliability coefficients that are slightly higher than .91. On the other hand, many personality instruments do not have reliability coefficients in the .91 range. Therefore, in evaluating reliability, counselors must examine how they are going to use the instrument and have knowledge about the reliability coefficients of other instruments in that area.

In selecting an instrument, counselors also need to examine the characteristics of their clients and their reliability coefficients. Sometimes an instrument will have acceptable overall reliability but will not be particularly reliable with certain subgroups (e.g., minority clients). As a general rule, instruments that assess younger children are less reliable than instruments for adults. Hence, a counselor could make a mistake and use an instrument that is not particularly reliable for the age group he or she is working with. The reliability coefficients for different ethnic groups or socioeconomic groups may also vary with instruments. Therefore, it is important for counselors to examine not just overall reliability coefficients but also the specific reliability coefficients for pertinent groups.

Standard Error of Measurement

Helping professionals should evaluate the reliabilities of different appraisal tools when selecting appropriate assessment interventions. Reliability, however, is not only useful to practitioners in selecting instruments; it can also be useful in interpreting clients' scores. Reliability is theoretically based on the concept of true score plus error. If a client took a test many times (e.g., 100 times), we would expect that one of those test scores would be his or her true score. **Standard error of measurement** provides an estimation of the range of scores if someone were to take an instrument over and over again. Therefore, with standard error of measurement, a counselor can provide the client with an expected range of where the client's "true score" would fall.

I once had a client who was struggling in his pre-med studies. This client was a junior and his grade point average was a 2.88. He started counseling because he wanted to learn better study skills because he was concerned about not being admitted to medical school with his grades. An assessment of his study skills revealed some minor problems; however, he had developed many effective techniques for studying. During the counseling process, he learned that I was trained to do intelligence assessment and he consistently requested that I test his abilities. I agreed to perform the assessment because the counseling was then focusing on whether he had the abilities to pursue a medical career and have time for other activities. He was finding that he could achieve exemplary grades, but was left very little time for any other activities. He had a family with small children and he truly enjoyed civic activities. Standard error of measurement proved to be very useful in interpreting the results of the intelligence assessment, because standard error of assessment provides an estimated range of where the client's scores would fall if he or she took the test multiple times. For this client, it was expected that 68% of the time his IQ would fall between 110.8 and 117.20. Thus, he was certainly more intelligent than the average person but not in the range that is often considered superior. Providing the range of scores to this client was very helpful because he wanted an estimate of his highest ability. The results of this assessment were consistent with other information that indicated he would need to invest most of his of energy in studying for his current classes. He further concluded that if he were accepted to medical school, it would be enormously difficult and he would have little time for his other priorities.

As indicated earlier, standard error of measurement can provide a range of where people would expect their scores to fall if they took the instrument repeatedly. Standard error of measurement (SEM) is based on the premise that when individuals take a test multiple times, the scores fall into a normal distribution. Thus, when individuals take an instrument numerous times, they tend to score most of the time in a similar fashion to their original score, while dissimilar scores are far less prevalent. In Figure 3.5, the three bell-shaped curves indicate the expected range of scores for Dick, Jane, and Spot if they took an instrument multiple times. Figure 3.6 is an enlargement of Figure 3.5, where we can examine just Dick's expected range. If Dick were to take an instrument multiple times, we would expect that 68% of the time his true scores would fall between 1 SEM below his original score and 1 SEM above his original score. In addition, we could expect that 95% of the time his true score would fall between 2 SEM below and 2 SEM above his score, while 99.5% of the time his true score would fall between 3 SEM below and 3 SEM above his score.

The formula for calculating the standard error of measurement (SEM) is:

$$\text{SEM} = s\sqrt{1 - r}$$

FIGURE 3.5

Dick, Jane, and Spot's range of scores using standard error of measurement

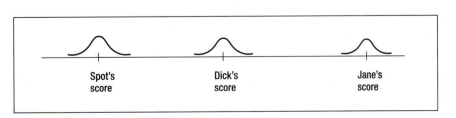

Spot's score   Dick's score   Jane's score

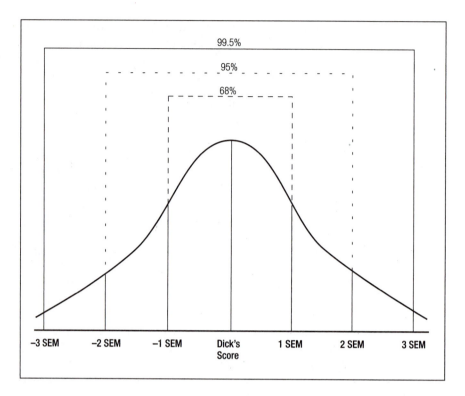

In the previous formula, s represents the standard deviation of the instrument and r is the reliability coefficient. Many readers may be familiar with the Graduate Record Examinations Aptitude Test (GRE), which is an instrument many graduate programs use in selecting and admitting students. There are three sections of the GRE and an individual receives three scores: for the Verbal (GRE-V), the Quantitative (GRE-Q), and the Analytical (GRE-A). The scores range from 200 to 800. In order to understand how standard error of measurement can be used, let's use the example of Anne, who was disappointed in her performance on the GRE Verbal section, with a GRE-V score of 430. Often, the standard error of measurement is provided in the instrument's manual and the counselor does not need to calculate the SEM. In this case, we will calculate the standard error of measurement as an example. Means and standard deviations for GRE scores vary, but for this example we will say the mean is 500 and the standard deviation is 100. The reliability coefficient for the GRE-V is .90 (Educational Testing Service, 1997). Therefore, the standard error of measurement would be: $100 \sqrt{1 - .90} = 100\sqrt{.10} = 100(.32) = 32$. We would then add and subtract the standard error of measurement to Anne's score to get the range. A counselor could then tell Anne that 68% of the time she could expect her GRE-V score to fall between 398 ($430 - 32$) and 462 ($430 + 32$). If we wanted to expand this interpretation, we could use two standard errors of measurement ($2 \times 32 = 64$). In this case, we would say that 95% of the time Anne's score would fall between 366 ($430 - 64$) and 494 ($430 + 64$). If we wanted to further increase the probability of including her true score, we would use three standard errors of measurement and conclude that 99.5% of the time her score would fall between 334 ($430 - 96$) and 526 ($430 + 96$). This information might be very helpful to Anne if she were considering applying to a graduate program that only admitted students with GRE-V scores of 600 or higher. If Anne were to take the GRE again, her chances of obtaining a GRE-V score greater than 600 would be quite small. Therefore, a counselor might assist Anne in examining her GRE scores and considering other options or other graduate programs.

Standard error of measurement incorporates an instrument's reliability in determining the range of scores. To illustrate this point, let's say there are two tests that measure intelligence and these instruments have the same mean (100) and standard deviation (15). Joseph took these two instruments and obtained the same IQ score of 94 on both instruments. Since Joseph obtained the same score, one might expect that the range of where we would estimate Joseph's true score to fall would be similar, but this is not the case, because the reliabilities of the two instruments vary. In the first instrument, the reliability of the overall IQ measure is .92, while the reliability of the second IQ test is .71. Therefore, if we calculate the standard error of measurement for the first instrument, we get 4.24 ($15 \sqrt{1 - .92} = 4.24$). With this first intelligence test, 68% of the time Joseph could expect his IQ score would fall between 89.76 and 98.24. On the second intelligence test, the SEM would be 8.08 ($15 \sqrt{1 - .71} = 8.08$). We would expect that 68% of the time Joseph's IQ score would be between 85.92 and 102.08 based on the second instrument. As we see, the range or score band is notably larger for the second test because the instrument is less reliable. Standard error of measurement will always increase as reliability decreases.

Another matter to consider is that the standard error of measurement and reliability coefficients typically do not remain constant and will vary depending on the ability levels of the participants. For instance, the reliabilities of GRE scores have been found to vary across the span of scores (Educational Testing Service, 1997). The *GRE 1997–1998 Guide to the Use of Scores* includes conditional standard errors of measurement (CSEM) that reflect the variation in reliabilities of the scores. As an example, the CSEM for a score of 250 on the GRE-V is 18, while the CSEM for a score of 550 is 34. In using an instrument, it is important that the counselor determine if the instrument's reliability varies depending on ability level, age, or other factors.

An instrument's reliability can be expressed in terms of both the standard error of measurement and the reliability coefficient. The standard error of measurement is more appropriate for interpreting individual scores, while the reliability coefficient should be used to compare different instruments. Providing clients with a possible range of scores is a more proficient method of disseminating results than reporting just one score. Reporting a single score can be misleading since no instrument has perfect reliability. In the cognitive realm, a range of scores is a better indicator of a client's capabilities. People also vary in their personality and other affective dimensions, and using standard error of measurement can assist clients in understanding that variation. For example, a client may not be depressed on the day the results are interpreted and may dismiss information if the counselor provides only a single score indicating moderate depression. Presenting the results as a range takes into consideration the fluctuations in depression and increases the probability that the client will find the results useful. Many instrument publishers are aware of the importance of reporting results using standard error of measurement and they report results using score bands rather than single scores (see Figure 3.7). Counselors should be encouraged, whenever possible, to interpret assessment results using a range of scores based on standard error of measurement.

Standard Error of Difference

The purpose of certain assessment situations is to compare certain aspects within the client. Often in counseling, for instance, a counselor wants to identify a client's strengths and limitations. Sometimes the focus concerns whether the individual has more aptitude in the verbal area as compared to the numerical area. On an achievement test, a parent may want to know if his or her child's score in reading is significantly lower than in other academic areas. Examining differences in factors within a client also applies to personality assessment.

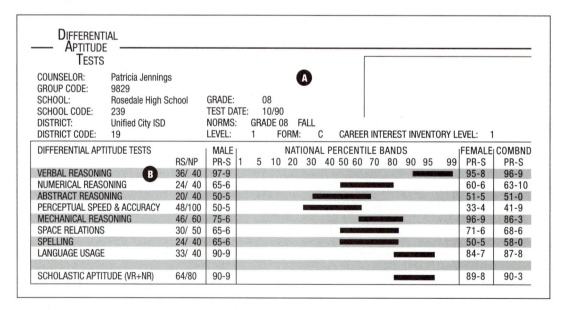

FIGURE 3.7   *Illustration of score bands on the differential aptitude tests*

Many instrument publishers understand the advantages of providing scores using score bands or ranges. Figure 3.7 illustrates percentile bands that are provided in the scoring profile of the Differential Aptitude Tests. In this profile, the band around the percentile score represents 1 SEM below the percentile score to 1 SEM above. With this profile, the counselor can examine strengths and limitations in terms of academic aptitude. In examining Figure 3.7, you will notice that some of the percentile bands overlap, while there is no overlap among other percentile bands. If the bands overlap, the counselor should *not* conclude that these scores are different. Differences can be attributed to areas where there is no overlap between the bands.

With some instruments, the standard errors of measurement are not visually presented and a counselor will need to compute the point difference in order to determine if scores are truly different. In examining differences between two scores, counselors need to take into account the errors of measurement from *both* scores. Examining the standard error of measurement from just one score will not be sufficient to determine the amount of difference actually needed to indicate a meaningful distinction. We can calculate the exact amount of difference needed between scores by using **standard error of difference**. Standard error of difference takes into consideration the standard errors of measurement of both of the scores, as indicated in the following formula:

$$SE_{dif} = \sqrt{SEM_1^2 + SEM_2^2}$$

In the above formula, SE_{dif} is the standard error of differences, SEM_1^2 is the standard error of measurement for the first score squared, and SEM_2^2 is the standard error of measurement for the second score squared. As an example, we may want to examine the differences needed to indicate that there is a difference between a child's Verbal IQ and Performance IQ on the Wechsler Intelligence Scale for Children—Third Edition (WISC–III), which will be discussed in Chapter 7. Sometimes verbal and performance discrepancies are considered in evaluating a child's learning style and the possibility of learning disabilities. The standard error of measurement for the Verbal IQ is 3.53 and the standard error of measurement for Performance IQ scale is 4.54 (Wechsler, 1991). The following is the calculation for the standard error of difference:

$$SE_{dif} = \sqrt{3.53^2 + 4.54^2} = \sqrt{12.46 + 20.61} = \sqrt{33.07} = 5.75$$

Hence, there would need to be a 6-point (rounding of 5.75) difference between a child's Verbal and Performance IQs in order for there to be a meaningful difference. If we wanted to say that there is a *significant* difference, then we would need to incorporate some statistical concepts. Often in statistics, differences are not considered significant unless there is less than a .05 chance that this difference could have occurred by chance. We can achieve this level of significance by doubling the standard error of difference. Thus, on the WISC–III a 12-point difference would be needed in order to determine if the difference between the Verbal and Performance IQs was significant.

Alternative Theoretical Model

Thus far our examination of reliability has only addressed the "true score" model or the "classical" model. The "true score" model is dominant, but a discussion of reliability should also include an alternative model typically called **generalizability theory** or **domain sampling theory.** With a true score approach, the focus is on identifying the portion of the score that is due to true score variance as compared to error variance. In generalizability or domain sampling, the focus is on estimating the extent to which specific sources of variation under defined conditions are contributing to the score on the instrument. According to Cronbach (Cronbach, 1990; Cronbach, Gleser, Rajaratnam, & Nanda, 1972), the instrument given under the exact same conditions should theoretically result in the exact same score. With generalizability theory, the focus is on the degree to which we can generalize scores across alternative forms, test administrators, number of items, and other facets of assessment. Therefore, when reliability information is gathered, there needs to be a description of the "universe." Instead of using the term "true score," the term in generalizability theory is *universe score,* which represents the average of taking the instrument multiple times in the same universe (e.g., same purpose and same conditions). When we use a single score and assume it represents a universe of scores, we are generalizing from it. Cronbach prefers the word "generalize" to "reliability" because the term implies the act of generalizing to a specific purpose rather than an all-inclusive evaluation of the instrument. Thus, with generalizability theory, multiple reliability coefficients or *coefficients of generalizability* are needed. Generalizability theory encourages the study of variations in test scores with the intent of identifying sources of variation. For example, researchers would attempt to identify the portions of the variance that are due to practice effect, examinees' levels of motivation, administrators' styles, and room temperature.

Generalizability theory directs us to consider that reliability is not a stagnant notion, but rather that reliability will vary depending on the purpose, setting, conditions, and use of the instrument. The interest is still in determining the degree to which the instrument is free from error. In fact, using this theoretical approach, a researcher would attempt to identify sources of error and, when it is appropriate, to generalize from the assessment results.

Summary

Reliability concerns the degree to which an instrument's scores are free from errors of measurement. Theoretically, we interpret a reliability coefficient as the ratio of true variance to observed variance. A reliability coefficient of .87 would indicate that 87 percent of the variance is true variance. It is impossible, however, to measure true variance; thus, individuals often calculate reliability using measures of consistency. Some of the common methods for estimating reliability are: test-retest, alternate or parallel forms, and measures of internal consistency (e.g., split-half, coefficient alpha). Reliability coefficients will range between zero and 1.00, with coefficients closer to 1.00 indicating higher reliability. One of the critical steps in selecting psychometrically sound instruments involves the evaluation of instruments' reliability. Evaluating reliability is not a simple task, and counselors need to consider various factors when examining the information on reliability of different instruments.

Reliability is not only useful in evaluating instruments, but it is also helpful in interpreting clients' scores and results. Standard error of measurement is another representation of an instrument's reliability. Standard error of measurement provides a band or a range of where a counselor can expect a client's "true score" to fall. Depending on the confidence level that is needed, a counselor can use standard error of measurement to predict where a score might fall 68%, 95%, or 99.5% of the time. Many professionals in the assessment field encourage counselors to interpret results using a band or range of scores based on standard error of measurement. Professionals should use standard error of difference in order to determine whether the scores on an assessment battery are actually different.

In conclusion, reliability needs to be considered before we can evaluate an instrument's validity. Validity indicates what an instrument measures. If an instrument has a high degree of error then it cannot measure anything well. Therefore, it is important to remember that reliability is the precursor to validity.

CHAPTER 4

Validity and Item Analysis

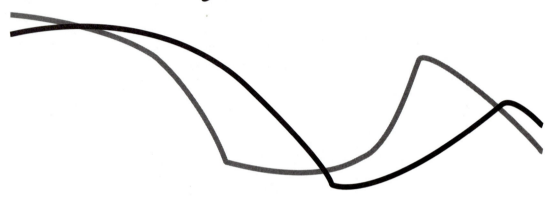

Validity

Validity concerns what the instrument measures and how well it does that task. Validity is not something that an instrument "has" or "doesn't have"; rather, the validation information informs the counselor when it is appropriate to use the instrument and what can be inferred from the results. Validity is an overall evaluation of the evidence and a determination of the degree to which evidence supports specific uses and interpretations. The interpretation of what the scores or results mean is derived from the validity evidence. For example, an instrument's title might indicate that it measures marital satisfaction; however, if we were to examine the validity information we might find that this instrument is only good at predicting the number of arguments between a couple. Some people might contend that the number of arguments a couple has is not a valid indicator of marital satisfaction because some couples, who are deeply dissatisfied, may not even talk to each other, let alone argue. It is important that helping professionals have the skills to evaluate the validity of both formal and informal instruments. In fact, the *Standards for Educational and*

Psychological Standards (AERA, APA, & NCME, 1985) includes the statement "validity is the most important consideration in test evaluation" (p. 9).

The validation of an instrument is a gradual accumulation of evidence that provides an indication of whether the instrument does indeed measure what it is intended to measure. For many instruments, validity information is provided in the instrument's manual. It is not that the instrument is validated, rather it is the *uses* of the instrument that are validated. In later chapters, we will examine instruments that are valid for certain purposes, but the validation information is not supportive of other usages of those instruments. Therefore, before using an instrument, a counselor must evaluate the validation evidence and determine if there is enough evidence to support using that instrument in that specific manner.

Reliability is a prerequisite to validity. If an instrument has too much unsystematic error, then the instrument cannot measure anything consistently. The reverse can be true, however, where an instrument is reliable but not valid. An instrument may measure something consistently but not measure what it is designed to measure. Therefore, reliability is necessary for an instrument to be sound, but high reliability does not guarantee that the instrument is a good measure. In selecting assessment tools, a counselor should first examine the reliability and see if it measures consistently, and then move to *what* it measures and *how well* the instrument measures what it was designed to assess.

Historically, there have been three categories of gathering validation information: content-related, criterion-related, and construct-related evidence. These are general categories that should not be seen as mutually exclusive groups, for there are no rigid distinctions among the three categories. Validity is a unitary concept that involves evaluating all of the accumulated information. The type of instrument and how the instrument is going to be used will influence which type of validation-related information may be more important. In some circumstances content-related evidence may be particularly pertinent, while in other circumstances a counselor would be more interested in criterion-related evidence.

Content-Related Validity

Content-related validation concerns the degree to which the evidence indicates the items, questions, or tasks adequately represent the intended behavior domain. As an example, let's pretend (although it may not be a fantasy for some readers) that you are going to be taking a test over the first part of this book soon. You may study carefully the content in each of the five chapters and feel quite prepared to take the test. You take the test, however, and find that all of the questions address concepts related to reliability! You could then argue that there was a problem with the content-related validity of the test, because, with all the questions coming from one chapter, the behavior domain (basic appraisal concepts) was not adequately sampled or represented. With content-related validity, the instrument developers must provide evidence that the domain was systematically analyzed and ensure that the central concepts are covered in the correct proportion.

With content-related validity, the central focus is typically on how the instrument's content was determined. Content validity evidence is often provided by documenting the procedures used in instrument development. There are common instrument development procedures that are sensitive to content validation issues. Instrument developers should first begin by identifying the behavior domain they wish to assess. At first glance, this seems to be an easy step, while in actuality it is often one of the more difficult steps. In counseling, there are often different theoretical perspectives concerning the areas we wish to assess (e.g., self-esteem, personality, career interests) and no universal agreement on the definitions of these constructs. Let's use an example of developing an instrument to measure client change that may occur as a result of counseling. Consistent with other counseling topics, there are various views on what constitutes client change and how we measure it. Hence, if individuals were attempting to construct a measure of client change, they would need to first define and conceptually clarify this concept. After initially clarifying the concept, these instrument developers would then draw up *test specifications*. Test specifications provide the organizational framework for the development of the instruments. A common first step in test specification is to identify the goals or the content areas to be covered. Considering the example of the client change assessment, we need to bear in mind that client change is a very broad area. The instrument developers would need to consider whether they wanted to measure behavioral change, affective change, or cognitive change. The process of identifying goals and content is helpful because it requires the developers to clearly articulate the intended purpose(s) of the instrument.

The next step in test specification is to precisely state the objectives or processes to be measured. For example, in client change, who will assess the change (e.g., client report, counselor report, or someone else)? Once the objectives have been established, these objectives need to be analyzed and the relative importance of each objective needs to be considered. The developers of the client change instrument would probably want to include more items related to objectives that are of greater importance. Before writing any of the items, the test specification process also involves determining the level of difficulty or abstraction of the items. For example, in the assessment designed to measure client change, the developers would need to determine whether the instrument was going to be for children or adults; the level of complexity of the items; and what would be the appropriate reading level. The manuals of any instrument should describe in detail the procedures used in developing the instrument before any items were written. Developers create a more refined and better quality instrument if significant work is exerted before the items are written.

Another method of providing evidence of content-related validity is by having "experts" review the instrument. Experts usually analyze the degree to which the content of the instrument reflects the domain; whether the weighting of the instrument is appropriate; and the degree to which the content is assessed in a non-biased manner. These experts' critiques of an instrument typically lead to revisions of the instrument. Experts can be scholars in the instrument's area, but they can also be practitioners working in the field. The manual should provide the number of experts, a description of the experts, and an explanation of why these individuals were selected. If experts' judgments were used, then the manual should describe what was done to respond to these judgments.

Content-related validity should not be confused with face validity. *Face validity* is simply that, on the surface, the instrument looks good. Face validity is not truly an indicator of validity and should not be considered as one. An instrument can look valid but may not measure what it is intended to assess. Therefore, a helping professional cannot just examine the questions or items of an instrument and decide to use that assessment tool. Counselors need to evaluate the content validity information provided in the instrument's manual and determine if there is sufficient evidence. The importance of content validity will vary depending on the needs of the counselor. An example of when content validity is important is with achievement tests, where we are interested in how much an individual has learned. We cannot expect someone to learn something unless he or she has had exposure to that information. Therefore, there needs to be a direct correspondence between the information presented and the contents of the assessment. In fact, you may have had the experience in your academic career where you took an achievement test in a class when there was little connection between what was taught and what you were tested on. In this case, the content of the test did not reflect the information taught and you could conclude that there was a problem with content validity.

Criterion-Related Validity

Criterion-related validity is the extent to which the instrument is systematically related to an outcome criterion. With criterion-related validity, we are interested in the degree to which the instrument is a good predictor of a certain criterion. Evidence of criterion-related validity does not apply to every type of instrument because here the focus is on how well the instrument *predicts* to certain behaviors (i.e., the criterion). Instruments where criterion-related validity is important include the Scholastic Assessment Test (SAT), which predicts academic performance in college, or the General Aptitude Test Battery (GATB), which predicts performance in certain occupations. For the SAT, the criterion is academic performance in college, while the criterion for the GATB is performance in certain occupations.

Types of criterion-related validity. There are two types of criterion-related validity: **concurrent validity** and **predictive validity**. The difference between these two types of criterion-related validity is the period of time between taking the instrument and gathering the criterion information. In concurrent validation, there is no time lag between when the instrument is given and when the criterion information is gathered. Prediction is used with concurrent validity in a broad sense, because we are predicting behavior based on the current context. This type of criterion-related validity is used when we want to make an immediate prediction, such as a diagnosis. On the other hand, with predictive validity, there is a time lag between when the instrument is administered and when the criterion information is gathered. If we wanted to develop an instrument that would identify which high school students would graduate from college, we would administer the test while the students were in high school and then we would have to wait until they graduated from college to gather the criterion information. Illustrations of the different types of criterion-related validity are: "Bob is depressed" (concurrent validity) or "Bob is likely to become depressed in the future" (predictive validity).

Criterion characteristics. With instruments that predict, it is important to evaluate not only the psychometric qualities of the instrument, but also the characteristics of the criterion. The criterion is what the instrument is designed to predict (e.g., job performance, personality). An instrument may be highly related to a criterion, but if the criterion is not anything meaningful, then there are not any compelling reasons for using the instrument. We want criteria that are *relevant and useful* for our clients. The criterion should be *reliable* and relatively free from unsystematic error. If there is a large degree of error in the criterion, then there is a very good possibility that the instrument will be unable to predict anything that is useful. Without a reliable criterion, it will be like trying to predict to a target that is always moving. We also want the criterion to be *free from bias.* As an example, if an instrument were developed to predict effectiveness as a fire fighter, the criterion should be an assessment of job performance. It would be a problem if the criterion were supervisors' evaluation of job performance and the supervisors used in this validation study were biased against women fire fighters. Finally, we also want the criterion to be *immune from criterion contamination.* Criterion contamination occurs when knowledge of the instrument influences the gathering of criterion information. For example, criterion contamination may occur if those determining a DSM-IV diagnosis had prior knowledge of a participant's performance on an instrument designed to diagnose. A practitioner could easily be influenced by the information from the instrument and assign a diagnostic label that was consistent with the instrument. In this example, the correlation between the instrument and the diagnostic categories would appear artificially high. Thus, the criterion, in this case, is "contaminated" by the prior knowledge of the individual's performance on the diagnostic instrument.

Methods for establishing criterion-related validity

Correlational Method   The statistical technique of correlation is used to explore the relationship between two variables. Counselors often want to examine the degree to which the instrument and the criterion are related. Because the focus is on the degree to which there is a relationship, it is logical to use correlation to provide an indication of the magnitude of that relationship. The steps in gathering criterion-related validity using correlation are: First, select an appropriate group to use in the validation study. Second, administer the instrument. If this is concurrent validity, the next step would be to collect the criterion data; however, if it is predictive validity, this third step would involve a time lapse where we would wait until it was appropriate to gather the criterion information (e.g., wait until the group finishes college to gather academic performance information). Once the criterion information is collected, the final step is to correlate the performance on the instrument with the criterion information—the result of that calculation being a **validity coefficient**.

Validity coefficients can be helpful to counseling practitioners in two ways. Counselors can compare the validity coefficients from different instruments and select the instrument that has the highest relationship between the instrument and the criterion. Although this sounds quite easy, in practice it can sometimes be complex because different criteria are used. The second way that validity coefficients can be useful in practice is by examining the amount of shared variance between the instrument and the criterion. As you will remember from the discussion of correlation in the previous chapter, a correlation coefficient can be squared, resulting in a *coefficient of determination,* which provides an indication of the amount of shared variance between the two variables. Thus, by squaring the validity coefficient, we get the percent of variance in the criterion that is accounted for by the instrument. In most discussions of validity coefficients, a question arises about the magnitude of the coefficient and how large a validity coefficient should be. Kaplan and Sacuzzo (1997) indicated that validity coefficients are rarely larger than .60 and that we often find them in the .30 to .40 range. Anastasi and Urbina (1997) suggested that they should at least be statistically significant, which means we can conclude that the coefficient had a low probability of occurring by chance.

Regression   The statistical technique of **regression** is another commonly used method for determining the criterion-related validity of an instrument. As we will see, regression is closely related to correlation. It is commonly used to determine the usefulness of a variable or a set of variables in predicting another important or meaningful variable. In appraisal, we are usually specifically interested in whether the instrument predicts some other specific behavior (the criterion variable). For example, does an instrument designed to measure potential suicidal behaviors actually predict suicidal behaviors? Regression is based on the premise that a straight line, called the *regression line,* can describe the relationship between the instrument's scores and the criterion. In Figure 4.1, the scores on an instrument are plotted in relationship to the scores on the criterion. The line that best fits the points is the regression line. Once we have established a regression line, we can then use that line to predict performance on the criterion based on scores on the instrument.

In order to illustrate the concepts of regression, let's pretend that you are interested in an instrument that would predict people's abilities to be "fun" (please note that this is only an illustration). In this example, you are comparing

FIGURE 4.1

Regression line

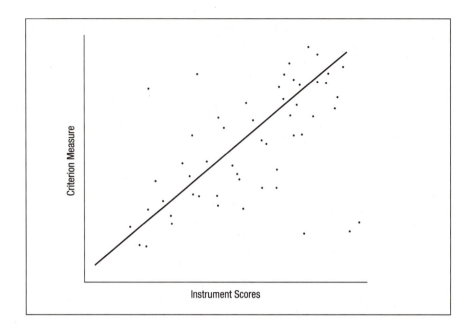

three instruments to use for the screening of friends, neighbors, and co-workers. Figure 4.2 shows three scatter plots that describe the relationship among three instruments and the criterion. In all three of these cases, an individual took one of the three instruments and then friends of that individual evaluated their ability to be fun. Thus, the criterion, which is plotted on the *y* axis, is a rating of "funness." By examining the diagrams in Figure 4.2, we can see that Instrument A is a pretty good predictor because all scores are located near the line. For example, most of the individuals who received a score of 50 were rated as being around 3.00 in terms of funness. On the other hand, Instrument B is not quite as good a predictor because the points are more spread out. With this instrument there is wide variation for those individuals who received a score of 50, with the evaluation of funness ranging from 2.00 to 4.00. There is such a poor relationship between Instrument C and the funness rating (the criterion) that a regression line or a line of best fit could not be determined. In making certain social decisions, you may want more precision in your prediction of "funness" than either Instrument B or Instrument C can provide.

Rarely do we see in assessment a scatter plot as evidence of the predictive ability of an instrument; rather, the evidence is provided in a **regression equation**. This equation describes the linear relationship between the predictor variable and the criterion variable. The regression equation is:

$$Y' = a + bX$$

In this equation, Y' is the predicted score and a is the Y intercept, or the *intercept constant.* The b represents the *slope,* which is the rate of change in Y as a

FIGURE 4.2

Scatter diagrams between scores on three instruments and the criteria for these instruments

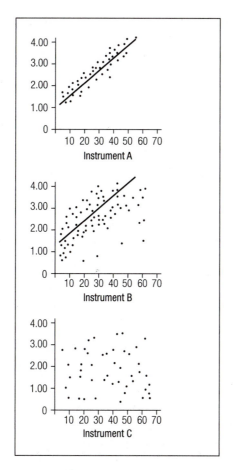

function of changes in *X*. The *X* in the equation is the individual's score on the instrument. The slope is usually called the *regression coefficient* or the *regression weight*. Thus, the instrument developers in the manual will provide information on whether the instrument can significantly predict the criterion (i.e., can the data be fitted into a significant regression equation). While on the subject of regression, note that there is also multiple regression, where there are multiple predictor variables. An example of multiple regression is when the two predictor variables of high school grades and a precollege test (e.g., SAT or ACT) are used to predict academic achievement in college. In multiple regression, the equation is extended to include the additional variables that have different weightings ($Y' = a + bX_1 + bX_2 + bX_3 \ldots$).

Just as no instrument can have perfect reliability, no instrument can have perfect criterion-related validity. As discussed in Chapter 3, we took the lack of perfect reliability into consideration and provided scores in a range using standard error of measurement. The same logic applies with criterion-related validity, where the lack of a perfect relationship between the instrument and the criterion is taken into consideration in the interpretation of the criterion scores by using **standard error of estimate**. Standard error of estimate indicates the margin of expected error in the individual's predicted criterion score as a result of imperfect validity. The formula for standard error of estimate is similar to the formula for standard error of measurement except that the focus of standard error of estimate is on the validity coefficient.

$$Sest = s_y\sqrt{1 - r_{xy}^2}$$

In the above equation for standard error of estimate (Sest), s_y is the standard deviation of the criterion and r_{xy} is the validity coefficient (correlation between the scores on the instrument and the criterion). Standard error of estimate can be used for predicting an individual's performance on the criterion; however, it is more commonly used to look at error around a cutoff point. A developer of an instrument designed to predict suicidal behaviors would want to use standard error of estimate when determining the score in which counselors should be concerned about their clients. Like standard error of measurement, standard error of estimate provides a range of scores, except with standard error of estimate the range is on the criterion.

Decision Theory   Besides the correlational and the regression methods of providing criterion-related validity information, there is a third method that involves the use of **group separation** or expectancy tables. This approach is sometimes referred to as decision theory, because instruments are often used in decision making and this approach evaluates the accuracy of the decision making. Group separation is concerned with whether the scores of the instrument correctly differentiate. For example, do people who score high on the test get the high grades as predicted? Decision theory attempts to assist in the selection and placement process by taking available information and putting it into a mathematical form (see Cronbach & Gleser, 1965). In terms of aiding the decision-making process, we want to know how often the instrument is right (a *hit*) and how often the instrument is wrong (a *miss*). For example, to what extent does the instrument accurately predict those who will succeed in college or in an occupation and accurately predict those who will not succeed. An **expectancy table** is the table that is developed in order to examine whether the instrument differentiates between the groups. An expectancy table can be used in two ways. First, an expectancy table can be used to make decisions, such as admissions or hiring decisions. Second, an expectancy table can be used to provide clients information on the probabilities of succeeding in college or in an occupation given their scores on the instrument.

Let's return once again to the fictitious Counseling Aptitude Scale (CAS) as an example. As you will remember, the Counseling Aptitude Scale is supposed to predict who will be effective counselors and who will not. If we were to develop this instrument, we could use an expectancy table to see: first, if the CAS does predict effective counseling and, second, if we could use the CAS to determine cutoff scores for admission to counseling programs. After we develop the expectancy table, we can then use it to provide potential students an "indication" of how successful they might be as counselors. In order to develop an expectancy table, we have to first find a criterion to use in validating the instrument.

Hypothetically, the Counseling Aptitude Scale will predict counseling effectiveness, which is a difficult concept to measure. Therefore, we might want to use performance in a graduate program in counseling as a criterion (I know some will argue that performance in a graduate program is not a very good measure of people's effectiveness in actual counseling, but let's just go ahead with this as an example). After we have established the criterion of grade point average (GPA) in a counseling program, we next have to gather data. We would take a group of students who had been admitted to a counseling program(s) and before they began classes, we would give them the Counseling Aptitude Scale. We would then sit back and let these students proceed with their counseling program.

As the students graduated, we would gather GPA information to construct our expectancy table. Figure 4.3 shows an imaginary expectancy table for 40 students' Counseling Aptitude Scale scores and their grade point averages. The first table simply charts the students' grade point averages and CAS scores. We would first examine the table to determine if the CAS can differentiate between those students who did well in a graduate counseling program and those who did not perform well.

FIGURE 4.3

Expectancy tables for the Counseling Aptitude Scale

	0–69	70–79	80–89	90–100
A			3	5
B	1	1	5	5
C	4	5	2	
D	3	4		
F	2			

	0–69	70–79	80–89	90–100
A			3	5
B	1	1	5	5
C	4	5	2	
D	3	4		
F	2			

	0–69	70–79	80–89	90–100
A	False Negatives		3	5
B	1	1	5	5
C	4	5	2	
D	3	4	False Positives	
F	2			

In examining this table, we can see that those who did well on the Counseling Aptitude Scale tended to have higher GPAs than those who did poorly on the Counseling Aptitude Scale. We could then examine this table and see how many times the instrument "hit" (was an accurate predictor) and how many times it "missed" (did not accurately predict). Besides evaluating the criterion-related validity of the CAS, examining the hits and misses can also aid us in determining cutoff scores for use in future admissions decisions. Often in graduate school, a student must earn a grade point average of B or above in order to continue in a program. Therefore, in the second table in Figure 4.3, a dark line has been drawn across the B row to indicate which students earned a B or better. As you can see from the second table, 20 students had GPAs above B (1 for 0–69, 1 for 70–79, 8 for 80–89, and 10 for 90–100). If we set the cutoff score at 70 or above (signified by a line), then we would have 30 hits and 10 misses. The 10 misses would be the one person who received a score between 0 and 69 but achieved a GPA of B even though that wasn't predicted, and the 9 people who received a score of 70–79 but their GPAs were below B (5 received a C and 4 received a D average). Now what you need to do is determine the hits and misses if the cutoff score is set at 80 (signified by the dark line) and 90 (signified by the double line). If we set the cutoff score at 80, there are 36 hits and only 4 misses. On the other hand, if we set the cutoff score at 90, there would be 30 hits and 10 misses. Therefore, if the decision was based solely on the most hits and the least misses, then the cutoff score of 80 seems best.

In addition to identifying hits and misses, expectancy tables can provide information about **false positives** and **false negatives**. A false positive occurs when the instrument predicts that the individual has "it" (the criterion) when in fact he doesn't. Thus, if we examine the third table in Figure 4.3, we can see that there are two false positives. The false positives are those two individuals who had scores above the 80-point cutoff but who received a C average in graduate school. A false negative occurs when the instrument predicts that they don't have it when in fact they do. The assessment situation will influence whether individuals should try to minimize the false positives or the false negatives in setting cut-off scores. For example, if an instrument were used to select individuals for a very expensive training program, we might want to minimize the number of false positives. The purpose would be to select only people who would be successful and not spend the money to train people who wouldn't. On the other hand, a false negative can also be quite costly. As an example, take an instrument designed to assess suicide potential. A false negative would mean the instrument would not identify someone as being at risk for committing suicide when in fact he is at risk. A false negative in the case of suicide potential could mean the loss of life. Sometimes expectancy tables are used to identify the individuals who were false positives or false negatives and then identify other characteristics (e.g., personal characteristics, background characteristics) that may contribute to the misclassification. Using the last table in Figure 4.3, we might find it interesting to gather more information about the two individuals who scored between 80 and 89, yet did not achieve a B average in graduate school. There may be characteristics about these individuals that could help in screening those who appear to have counseling potential based on their CAS scores but do not do well in their graduate counseling program.

Expectancy tables are commonly used for selection and placement purposes. They can also be used in counseling to provide probability information to individuals (e.g., What is the probability of achieving a GPA of 4.00 given a Counseling Aptitude Scale score of 49?). The probability information is calculated by determining the percentage of people who fall in certain criterion categories. In looking at Figure 4.3 for example, we see that the probability of achieving an A average with a Counseling Aptitude Scale score of 49 is zero since no one who received a score of 0–69 achieved an A average. There is, however, a 10 percent chance that a person receiving a score of 49 could achieve a B average since 1 of the 10 people who scored between 0 and 69 received a B average. The probability of receiving an A average with a CAS score of 85 is 30 percent since 3 out of 10 people who scored between 80 and 89 achieved an A average.

There are other factors that need to be considered when using expectancy tables to determine cutoff scores for selection or placement purposes. One factor concerns the degree to which the process is selective. A cutoff score in many ways is easier to determine if the process is very *selective*. The opposite is also true, where the selection process is simplified if the intent is to select most individuals and only weed out a few who are extremely low. Another factor that influences the decision-making process is *base rate*. Base rate refers to the extent to which the characteristic or attribute exists in the population. The third factor that influences the decision-making process is the way in which the *scores distribute*. The selection process is considerably more difficult if the scores are grouped closely together as compared to more variability in scoring.

In conclusion, criterion-related validity may be indicated in various ways, such as using both regression and expectancy tables. Instrument developers will often incorporate more than one method to indicate that an instrument is a valid predictor. Furthermore, as we will see, both content and criterion-related validity can be subsumed under construct validity.

Construct Validity

The third major type of validity is **construct validity**, which concerns the extent to which the instrument may measure a theoretical or hypothetical construct or trait. Many of the aspects that counseling addresses are broader, more enduring and abstract kinds of behavior (e.g., anxiety, mechanical aptitude, self-esteem, or intelligence). These constructs are complex phenomena that cannot be simply measured and validated. Furthermore, with many of the constructs in counseling there is no universally defined criterion or agreed-upon content. Therefore, the process of establishing validity for these constructs is more complex and consists of a gradual accumulation of information. An instrument's construct validity cannot be verified through one study, but rather construct validity is demonstrated by multiple pieces of evidence that indicate the instrument is measuring the construct or trait of interest.

The gathering of construct validity information is analogous to the scientific method, where the starting point is the instrument and theories about the trait or construct. On the basis of theory or previous research, predictions are made related to the instrument. These predictions are empirically tested and the results of those empirical tests are either supportive of the validity of the instrument or not. This process is continually repeated and the accumulation of evidence is evaluated in order to determine the construct validity of an instrument. The following are some of the common methods used to provide evidence of construct validity.

There is **convergent evidence** when the instrument is related to other variables that it should theoretically be positively related to. For example, if an instrument is designed to measure depression and correlates highly with another instrument that measures depression, then there is convergent evidence. **Discriminant evidence**, on the other hand, exists when the instrument is not correlated with variables from which it should differ. For example, there is evidence of discriminant validity when an instrument designed to measure depression is not significantly correlated with an instrument that measures trait anxiety. According to Anastasi and Urbina (1997), discriminant validation information is particularly important in terms of evaluating the validity of personality instruments, in which irrelevant variables may influence scores in assorted ways.

Campbell and Fiske (1959) suggested using a **multitrait-multimethod matrix** in order to explore construct-related validity. This procedure involves correlating an instrument with traits that are both theoretically related to the instrument and traits that should be unrelated to the construct being measured. This process also involves correlating the instruments with other instruments that use the same and different assessment methods (e.g., self-reports, projective techniques, and behavioral ratings). The results of these various correlations is a matrix, where we can evaluate the relationship between the instrument and measures of: (a) the same traits using the same testing method; (b) different traits using the same testing method; (c) the same traits using the different testing method; and (d) different traits using different testing methods. Support for the construct validity of an instrument would be indicated when the correlations are higher between the same trait using different assessment methods as compared to different traits using the same methods and different traits using different methods.

Factor analysis is another method used to contribute to the construct validation evidence of an instrument. Factor analysis is a statistical technique used to analyze the interrelationships of a set or sets of data. There are a variety of reasons to use factor analysis, including: (a) exploring patterns of interrelationships among variables; (b) analyzing clusters of variables and identifying variables that may be redundant as indicated by extraordinarily high intercorrelations; and (c) reducing a large number of variables to a smaller number of statistically uncorrelated variables (Agresi & Finlay, 1997). Factor analysis can be used for construct validity by factor analyzing an instrument with other instruments and determining if the instrument intercorrelates with other instruments in the expected manner. For example, a researcher could analyze the factor structure of two achievement instruments. We would find evidence of construct validity if the reading items grouped together, and the mathematics items grouped together, and so on. Factor analysis can also be used to examine how items within an instrument interrelate and group together into one or more factors. Numerous instruments have subscales, and factor analysis can indicate if the items within each of the subscales are related to each other or if there are problems and the items are more related to items in a different subscale.

Meta-analysis is another statistical technique that is being used to demonstrate construct validity. Meta-analysis involves statistically combining the results of many studies to see if there is an overall effect. In assessment, meta-analysis is used to see if the instrument is consistently related to the construct. Using this strategy, researchers combine the results of numerous studies and examine the combined results. The best example of this is Hunter, Schmidt, and Hunter's (1979) meta-analysis, where they used hundreds of studies performed on the General Aptitude Test Battery (GATB) and job performance. They found that the GATB was a very good predictor of job performance using meta-analysis.

Another method used to provide construct validity information is to show evidence of *changes with age.* In many areas related to assessment, it is expected that as individuals mature there will be developmental changes (e.g., reading comprehension, intelligence, and career maturity). Support for the construct validity of an instrument is provided when performance on the instrument changes in accordance with the expected developmental changes. For example, we would expect a fourth grader to have a larger vocabulary than a first grader. Of course, this type of construct-related evidence is only appropriate when there are clear and apparent age changes.

Construct validity information may also be provided when there is evidence of changes due to *experimental interventions.* For example, we may have more confidence in a measure of career maturity if that measure reflects increases after adolescents participate in a career counseling program. In this situation, the researchers need to be careful to show that the interventions are suitable and executed appropriately.

Evidence from *distinct groups* can also contribute to the accumulation of construct validity information. Similar to some of the previously mentioned techniques, the key to this type of validation information is whether the group differences are in the expected direction. For instance, if we were gathering construct validation information on an instrument designed to measure depression, we would expect that the scores for the group of people requesting counseling for depression would be higher than the scores of people who report no depressive symptoms. If the results verify our hypothesis, then this would support the construct validity of the depression inventory.

A comparatively recent contribution to the gathering of construct validity information comes from the field of *cognitive psychology.* The focus on this type of validation information concerns how information is processed and the processes individuals use in approaching tasks. One example in this area is where individuals "think aloud" while taking an instrument. The individuals' verbalizations of their thoughts while taking the instrument are tape-recorded. Researchers then analyze the manner in which they processed the information to see if it is consistent with how the instrument was designed. For example, high school students would verbalize their thoughts as they took a career maturity measure; the researchers would then compare the thoughts to the concepts the instrument was designed to measure (e.g., did the items related to decision making stimulate thoughts concerning the making of decisions). Another example of using concepts from cognitive psychology in gathering construct validity information is the use of computer programs that are designed based on theoretical concepts to simulate an individual's performance. The computer's simulated performance is then compared to the performance of children or adults and similarities and differences in performances are then investigated.

In conclusion, construct validity is indicated by the gradual accumulation of evidence; therefore, it is usually not a clear-cut decision on whether an instrument has construct validity or not. It must be remembered, however, that validation evidence provides the basis for our interpretation of the results. In order to interpret the results of an instrument appropriately, a counselor must evaluate the validity information and determine what can be inferred from the results. Cronbach (1990) suggested that validation should be seen as a persuasive argument, where we are convinced by the preponderance of evidence on the appropriate use of an instrument. An instrument with strong construct validity will attempt to resolve critical uncertainties and explore plausible rival hypotheses. Many times the evaluation of construct validity need not be done by the counselor in isolation, for many instruments have been critiqued by knowledgeable scholars in publications like the *Mental Measurements Yearbook* and *Test Critiques.*

The emphasis in this chapter has been to a degree on formal assessment tools; yet, the concepts associated with validity apply to all types of client assessment. For example, counselors need to consider the concepts of validity when they do an intake interview with a client. In interviewing a client, a counselor needs to consider the content of the interview and the evidence that those questions address the appropriate behavior domain. Furthermore, criterion-related validity also applies to these interviews with clients, because the practitioner often is considering either a formal or informal diagnosis and, also, making predictions about the client's future behavior based on the intake interview. Construct validity is also pertinent because frequently client traits or constructs need to be considered. There is growing evidence to support the contention that practitioners who rely only on intuition and experience are biased in their decisions (Sexton et al., 1997). It may be helpful to practitioners to focus on the concept of construct validity in their informal assessment of clients. Counselors who purposefully analyze an accumulation of evidence will probably make more valid assessments of their clients.

A Comprehensive View of Validity

Some leaders in the assessment field, such as Messick (1995), contend that dividing validity into three types only fragments the concept and that validity should be viewed as a unified consideration. Messick argues that a comprehensive view of validity integrates consideration of content, criteria, and consequences into a construct framework in which the practitioner then evaluates the empirical evidence to determine if it supports the rational hypotheses and the utility of the instrument. Messick suggests that validity is best viewed as a comprehensive view of construct validity. This is not entirely new, as construct validity has traditionally subsumed content and criterion validity. Messick, however, argues that a more comprehensive view of validity should take into account both score *meaning* and the *social values* in test interpretation and test use. Therefore, in evaluating the empirical evidence, the counselor needs to consider both score meaning and the consequences of the measurement. Construct validity is a unifying concept where the counselors examine the evidence considering use, interpretation, and social implications simultaneously. The practitioner should evaluate the evidence to determine if there is a compelling argument that justifies the test use and interpretation. This concept of considering social implications should be particularly relevant to counselors who have the ethical responsibility of working in the client's best interest.

Item Analysis

This chapter includes information on both validity and item analysis. The focus of **item analysis** is on examining and evaluating each item. Consequently, validity evidence concerns the entire instrument, while item analysis examines the qualities of each item. Item analysis is often used when instruments are being developed and, also, when instruments are revised. Item analysis provides information that can be used to revise or edit problematic items or eliminate faulty items. Some of the simpler methods can easily be used to evaluate items in classroom tests, questionnaires, or other informal instruments. There are some extremely complex methods for analyzing items; however, this discussion will include a brief overview of the typical methods used.

Item Difficulty

When examining ability or achievement tests, we are often interested in the difficulty level of the items on the test. The difficulty level of an item should indicate whether an item is too easy or possibly too difficult. **Item difficulty** is an index that reflects the proportion of people getting the item correct. It is calculated by dividing the number of individuals who answered the question correctly by the total number of people.

$$p = \frac{number\ who\ answer\ correctly}{total\ number}$$

An item difficulty index can range from .00 (meaning no one got the item correct) to 1.00 (meaning everyone got the item correct). Item difficulty doesn't really indicate difficulty, but rather how easy the item is, because it provides the proportion of individuals who got the item correct. Let's use an example of an item on a counseling assessment test where 15 of the students in a class of 25 got the first item on the test correct. In this case, we would say the item difficulty (p) is .60.

$$p = \frac{15}{25} = .60$$

There are not clear guidelines on evaluating an item difficulty index. The desired index difficulty level will depend on the context of the assessment. We would need more information to interpret the above index of .60 (interpretation of this item difficulty index might also depend on whether an individual is in the group who got the item correct or the group who got it wrong!). If the intent is to have items that differentiate among individuals, then a difficulty level of around .50 is considered optimum. Some assessment experts have suggested that in multiple-choice items the probability of guessing needs to be considered in determining the optimum difficulty level (Cohen et al., 1992; Kaplan & Saccuzzo, 1997). In other contexts, however, an instructor might be pleased with an item difficulty level of 1.00, which would indicate that everyone in the class was able to comprehend the material and answer the item correctly. Therefore, the determination of the desired item difficulty level depends on the purpose of the assessment, the group taking the instrument, and the format of the item. Calculating item difficulty can frequently provide useful information, because an item that may appear quite easy may confuse students, while a more difficult item may be worded such that the answer can be construed without knowledge of the content.

Item Discrimination

Item discrimination, or item discriminability, provides an indication of the degree to which an item differentiates correctly among the examinees on the behavior domain of interest. For example, have you ever taken a test and felt as if an item didn't discriminate between those individuals that studied hard and knew the material and those individuals who didn't? Item discrimination is not just applicable to achievement or ability tests; we are also interested in whether items discriminate in other assessment areas, such as personality and interest inventories. For instance, we may want to know if individuals who have been diagnosed as being depressed answered an item one way and individuals who do not report depressive symptoms answer the question another way. There are several methods for evaluating an item's ability to discriminate.

One of the most common methods for calculating an item discrimination index is called the *extreme group method*. First, the examinees are divided into two groups based on high and low scores on the instrument (the instrument could be a class test, a depression inventory, or an assertiveness scale). The item discrimination index is then calculated by subtracting the proportion of examinees in the lower group from the proportion of examinees in the upper group who got the item correct or who endorsed the item in the expected manner.

$$d = \text{upper \%} - \text{lower \%}$$

Item discrimination indices that are calculated with this method can range from $+1.00$ (all of the upper group got it right and none of the lower group got it right) to -1.00 (none of the upper group got it right and all of the lower group got it right). An item discrimination index with a negative number is a nightmare for test developers (particularly for instructors with students in the upper group who are vengeful). Like item difficulty, interpretation of an item discrimination index depends on the instrument, the purpose it was used for, and the group taking the instrument. In general, negative item discrimination indices, particularly, and small positive indices are indicators that the item needs to be eliminated or revised.

The determination of the upper group and the lower group with item discrimination will depend on the distribution of scores. If there is a normal distribution, then Kelley (1939) has shown that optimal dispersion is accomplished by using the upper 27% for the upper group and lower 27% for the lower group. Anastasi and Urbina (1997) suggest that with small groups, like the ordinary classroom, the exact percentages to select each group need not be precisely defined but should be generally in the range of upper and lower 25% to 33%.

Another method for determining item discrimination is through the *correlational method*. These correlational approaches report the relationship between the performance on the item and a criterion. Often the criterion is performance on the overall test. Commonly used correlational techniques are the point biserial method and the phi coefficient. A thorough explanation of these techniques would be too lengthy for this discussion, but interested readers are directed to Crocker and Algina (1986). The result of these methods is a correlation coefficient that ranges between -1.00 and $+1.00$, with the positive and larger coefficients reflecting items that are better discriminators.

Item Response Theory

Before moving on to other topics, we need to briefly discuss item response theory (IRT). **Item response theory,** or **latent trait theory,** builds on the concepts of item analysis. The basis for item response theory is different from classical test theory, where the focus is on arriving at one true score and our attempts to control error in the instrument. In classical test theory, the items on the instrument are a sample of the larger set of items that represent the domain, and we get an indication of the individual's performance based on the combined items. In item response theory, the focus is on each *item* and establishing items that actually measure one ability or the respondent's level of a latent trait. Item response theory rests on the assumption that the performance of an examinee on a test item can be predicted by a set of factors called traits, latent traits, or abilities. In application, the latent trait does not actually exist, for the trait or ability could be a measure on a test, the student's age, or the student's grade level. Using an item response theory approach, we get an indication of an individual's performance based not on the total score, but *on the precise items* the person answers correctly. As an example, with a traditional approach we might say a score above 70 indicates that the student is reading at the sixth grade level. With an item response approach, the students would need to answer items 5, 7, 13, 19, 20, 21, and 24 correctly in order to achieve a score indicating they were reading at the sixth grade level. The goal with this approach is to develop items that assess sixth grade reading. Item response theory involves the scaling of items, and these procedures require quite sophisticated mathematical analyses. A thorough discussion of IRT is not appropriate for this book, and interested readers are directed to Hambleton, Swaminathan, and Rogers (1991), Lord (1980), and van der Linden and Hambleton (1997).

IRT suggests that the relationship between examinees' item performance and the underlying trait being measured can be described by a monotonically increasing function called an *item characteristic function* or an *item characteristic curve* (Hambleton et al., 1991). To construct an item characteristic curve, an instrument developer would start by constructing an item that he or she believes will measure the ability of interest. The developer would then give the item to an appropriate group or groups and then plot the results for each item using an item characteristic curve. With an item characteristic curve, the instrument developer plots on the horizontal axis a measure of trait or ability (e.g., age or grade level) and the probabilities of getting the item correct are plotted on the vertical axis. The probabilities are obtained by determining the proportion of persons at different levels who passed an item. Figure 4.4 shows a simplified example of plots of item characteristic curves. In this example, the trait or ability is measured by chronological age and the proportions of 6-year-olds, 7-year-olds, 8-year-olds, and 9-year-olds that answered the questions correctly are the probabilities. With a "good" item, we would expect the probability of getting the answer correct would increase as the underlying trait (e.g., age) increases. The probability of a 7-year-old getting item "a" right is very high (over 90%), while the probability of getting item "b" right is around 50%. The item curves are plotted from mathematical functions derived from the actual data.

There are different models of IRT and the mathematical functions to plot the item characteristic curves vary. The most common model of IRT involves examining item difficulty. Figure 4.4 shows item characteristic curves that are plotted based on item difficulty and percent of individuals who get the item

FIGURE 4.4

Hypothetical item characteristic curves

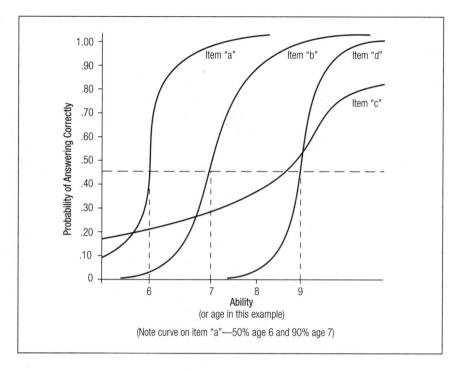

correct. Good items results in a somewhat slanted *S* shape. With this one parameter model, the point on the ability axis where there is a 50% (.50) probability of getting the item correct is typically considered the pivotal point.

Item response theory is based on the concept that each item has nuisances or error variables that escape standardization (van der Linden & Hambleton, 1997). Therefore, we need to control the error for each item, which can be done mathematically (similar in concept to Analysis of Covariance where we statistically control a variable). More complex models of item response theory consider more parameters than just item difficulty. A parameter that is often included is the slope of the curve, which provides an indication of how well the item discriminates. Steeper slopes indicate the item is a good discriminator and flat slopes reflect that it doesn't discriminate very well. In Figure 4.4, item "c" does not discriminate as well as the other items. What is sometimes called the location is the place where the probability of getting a correct response is .50. An item where 50% of the fourth graders get it right would be considered a fourth grade item. In Figure 4.4, item "a" would be a 6-year-old item, item "b" would be 7-year-old item, and item "c" would be a 9-year-old item, and item "d" would be a 9-year-old item. Many models also consider the basal level, which is an estimate of the probability that a person at the low end of the trait or ability scale will answer correctly. Also, many models of item response theory take into consideration the liability of guessing. The combination of parameters produces item characteristic curves that are evaluated to determine the suitability of the item. Consistent with the simpler model, the slanted *S* curve is desired in the item characteristic curves of the more complex models.

Instruments developed with an item response approach are not evaluated the same as those with classical test theory approach. An item response approach to instrument development will theoretically result in an instrument that is not dependent on a norming group. Therefore, the methods for determining standard error of measurement are different. Rather than a classical approach, where standard error of measurement applies to all scores in a particular population, with IRT the standard error of measurement differs across scores (Embretson, 1996).

There are numerous approaches in using item response theory in instrument development and the methods are becoming more sophisticated (van der Linden & Hambleton, 1997). The applications for item response theory are certainly promising. Item response theory is having an influence on large-scale testing programs, particularly in the area of achievement. Another application concerns building item banks, which include items that are scaled to different levels. Publishers have assembled some item banks for fractions, decimals, and long division (Cronbach, 1990). These sophisticated item banks can provide useful information in terms of identifying individuals' academic strengths and limitations. Because of the extensive analysis and calibration of the items, item response theory can be particularly useful in the development of criterion-referenced tests. Item response theory is having an affect on computer administered adaptive testing. In adaptive testing, performance on certain items influences the future items presented to the examinee. For example, if students cannot multiply a one-digit number by a one-digit number, it makes little sense to give them numerous questions asking them to multiply two-digit numbers by two-digit numbers. Thus, the computer sorts the questions based on the previous responses given. Item response theory can be particularly useful in achievement and ability adaptive testing, since the calibrated items can be used to quickly pinpoint an individual's ability level and identify possible gaps in knowledge.

Summary

Validity concerns whether an assessment measures what it is designed to measure. It is not the instrument that is validated, rather it is the uses of the instrument that are validated. The validation of the instrument informs the counselor on what he or she can infer from the results. Content validity concerns whether the instrument adequately measures the behavior domain. Criterion-related validity is related to how well the instrument predicts to a defined criterion. There are two types of criterion-related validity: concurrent and predictive. With concurrent is where there is no time lapse between the taking of the instrument and the prediction, while with predictive there is a time lapse. The third type of validity is construct validity, which applies to instruments that measure theoretical constructs or traits. Construct validity requires the gradual accumulation of evidence and can include both content and criterion-related validity. Many different techniques can be used in the process of gathering construct-related evidence. Counselors evaluating the validity of an instrument should examine what the preponderance of evidence indicates about whether that instrument can be used in a specific manner.

Items in well-constructed instruments are also analyzed. Two of the most common methods of item analysis involve determining the item difficulty and the item discrimination indices. Item response theory is also having a substantial influence on instrument development. Item response theory involves the calibration of items to measure abilities or traits.

CHAPTER 5

Instrument Selection, Administration, Scoring, and Communicating Results

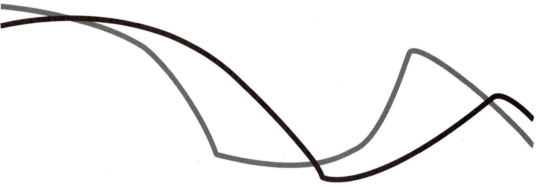

Selection of an Assessment Instrument

A client's life can be adversely affected if a practitioner selects and uses a faulty assessment tool in counseling. Therefore, the selection of an assessment tool or strategy is an important clinical decision. In some counseling situations, the selection of assessment strategies is neglected due to comfort with existing methods and heavy caseloads. Yet, assessment is the foundation of the counseling process, where assessment provides the information to determine future therapeutic goals and interventions. The selection of the assessment methods needs to involve careful consideration and evaluation of existing strategies.

The first step in selecting an appropriate assessment method is to identify possible alternatives. Chapter 1 included procedures for identifying possible assessment strategies. Sometimes counselors select inferior instruments because they have not adequately searched for possible instruments or alternative methods. Once possible instruments and informal strategies have been located, the counselor needs to evaluate them and select the most appropriate assessment method for that counseling situation. Some of the initial information needed to evaluate instruments can be gathered from secondary sources, such as critiques in the *Mental Measurements Yearbooks* and talking to colleagues who use the tool. A thorough evaluation, however, involves carefully examining the instrument's manual. Cicchetti (1994) suggested evaluating the areas of standardization procedures, norming procedures, test reliability, and test validity when selecting a psychological instrument. Some publishers publish specimen sets of instruments that practitioners can purchase in order to review the instruments. Nevertheless, before any instrument is administered to a client, a counselor needs to thoroughly evaluate the instrument with the following in mind.

Evaluating the Instrument

Test purpose. One of the first steps in determining if an instrument is appropriate to use is to ascertain if the purpose of the instrument corresponds to your counseling needs. If an instrument does not measure the behavior or construct of interest, then you don't need to further investigate the psychometric characteristics of that instrument. As said earlier, an instrument is only worthwhile if it provides pertinent information to the counseling process. Sometimes determining an instrument's purpose involves sifting through much of the information in the manual. Occasionally you may find that the purpose stated in the manual is a little different from what the name of the instrument implies. Furthermore, you need to determine if the design of the instrument corresponds to the intended purpose. Some instruments fail to achieve their intended purpose because of problems in construction. In a manual, you should find a description of the purpose and a detailed explanation of how the corresponding behaviors that are related to that purpose will be measured.

Instrument development. Counselors need to closely scrutinize the procedures the instrument developers used in constructing the instrument. Most instruments have a theoretical or empirical base that influences the overall development. If detailed information about the development of the instrument is not provided, then you should be concerned and evaluate the psychometric properties carefully. For many instruments, the development of the actual items plays a central role in the construction of the instrument. Evidence of careful construction of items and evidence of detailed item analysis add credence to the value of the instrument. Counselors should also read the items and consider if they are appropriate for the client(s).

Appropriate selection of norming group or criterion. Depending on the type of instrument, either the norming group in a norm-referenced instrument or the criterion in a criterion-referenced instrument will need to be evaluated. In a norm-referenced instrument, an analysis of the makeup of the norming group is critical. First you need to determine if the norming group is appropriate for your clients. For example, if a counselor is working with adults who did not complete high school, then an instrument that used college students as the norming sample for adults would probably not be appropriate. The practitioner should also evaluate the suitability of the norming sample in terms of age, gender, ethnic makeup, socioeconomic representation, educational level, and geographic location. The ethnic makeup of the norming group is of particular importance and needs to be carefully considered. The size of the norming sample is another consideration in evaluating a norm-referenced instrument. There are no clear rules of thumb in determining the appropriate size of a norming group, but we have more confidence in samples that are large and drawn in a systematic manner.

The evaluation of the criterion in a criterion-referenced instrument involves analyzing the procedures the developers used to determine the criterion. As you will remember, criterion-referenced instruments (not to be confused with criterion-related validity) measure whether the individual has attained a certain level or standard (the criterion). With a criterion-referenced instrument, the evaluation of the criterion is the most important step. In achievement tests, many developers use methods, such as standards from professional organizations, reviews by leading researchers, and studies of curriculum. The manual should supply sufficient documentation to convince the reader that the determination of the criterion was based on suitable information.

Reliability. Students often ask me to tell them how high a reliability coefficient should be to indicate adequate reliability. My answer to their queries is "It depends." There are no clear guidelines in determining what constitutes an acceptable reliability. The type of instrument will affect how we evaluate the reliability coefficients. In Chapters 6 through 11 of this book, the reliability coefficients on some instruments commonly used by counselors are provided in order to furnish a reference. Reliability can be estimated in different ways and some instruments will provide a range of coefficients that were calculated using different methods. In comparing instruments, we need to take into consideration the methods used for determining the coefficients because some methods of determining reliability tend to have lower estimates than other methods. You can also expect to find standard error of measurement in the manual of a well-developed instrument. Another trend to consider when evaluating an instrument's reliability is that reliability coefficients tend to be lower with younger participants. Therefore, you can expect lower coefficients with preschoolers than with adults.

Validity. Evaluating the validity of an instrument involves studying the validation evidence. In examining the validation information, we should not expect to come to a definitive conclusion like the instrument either has validity or does not have any validity. The evaluation of validity involves more the degree to which there is support for particular uses of the instrument. The analysis of validity concerns whether there is a preponderance of evidence to support the use of an instrument in a specific manner or context. The manual should include ample evidence that the instrument is valid for the desired purpose. If there is not ample evidence, then the instrument should be used very cautiously or not at all.

Bias. In the past twenty years, there has been substantial concern about test bias and multicultural assessment. The instrument's authors should provide evidence that the instrument was evaluated for possible bias. Chapter 14 provides an overview of how instruments are typically examined in order to detect possible bias. Some instruments may not be appropriate for certain populations and the manual should address those limitations. If the manual recommends that an instrument not be used with certain clients, then alternate assessments should be explored.

Interpretation and scoring materials. If you determine that an instrument has adequate psychometric qualities, then you want to examine the materials designed to assist in the interpretation of the results. The manual or additional resources should provide the necessary information to interpret the results. With many instruments you can choose from a variety of scoring options and interpretative reports. In examining the interpretative materials, you also need to consider how you are going to use this information in counseling and how it would be most effective to share the information with the client. Some instruments have interpretative booklets that can be given to clients to assist in the counseling process. These booklets should never replace explaining the results, but these types of resources can sometimes be very helpful. Another consideration is how the instrument is scored. Today, many instruments are computer scored, but this can involve having access to an appropriate computer and other equipment (e.g., a scanner). An organization's resources often affect which instruments and scoring services can be considered for use.

User qualifications. In selecting an instrument, practitioners should also consider their own competencies and training. A counselor can only select instruments from the pool that they can use ethically. Counselors must become competent with using a specific instrument before they give it to a client. Instruments vary in the amount of training and experience that is necessary in order to be competent. Some instruments can be used with knowledge gained from studying the manual, while other instruments require supervised instruction on the appropriate use of those devices. One attempt some publishers use to address the variations in needed training is a grading system that classifies instruments based on certain user qualifications. The following are the common levels used:

> *Level A:* These are typically instruments that can be adequately administered, scored, and interpreted by using the manual. The orientation to these instruments is usually left up to the institution or organization in which the individual works. Test publishers will often not send these materials out unless the individual is employed in a legitimate or recognized organization or institution. Examples of instruments at this level are achievement tests and the Self-Directed Search.

> *Level B:* These instruments and aids require technical knowledge in instrument development, psychometric characteristics, and appropriate test use. In order to qualify for Level B, the test user must have a master's level degree in

psychology or education or the equivalent with relevant training in assessment. Examples of instruments at this level are the Myers–Briggs Type Indicator, Suicide Ideation Questionnaire, NEO-PI-R, and the Strong Interest Inventory.

Level C: These instruments and aids require substantial knowledge about the construct being measured and the specific instrument being used. Often the publisher will require a Ph.D. in psychology or education with specific course work related to the instrument. Examples of instruments at this level are, the WISC-III, the Stanford-Binet, the MMPI-2, and Millon Clinical Multiaxial Inventory-III.

The *Code of Ethics and Standards of Practice* (American Counseling Association, 1995) indicates that counselors need to recognize their level of competence and only perform those testing and assessment services for which they have been trained. These standards also indicate that the ultimate appropriate use of an instrument rests with the practitioner. Therefore, if an organization wants a counselor to use instruments in which they are not properly trained, the counselor has an ethical responsibility *not* to perform those assessments. There can be legal ramifications (e.g., losing a professional license or being sued for malpractice) for practitioners who use an instrument that they are not qualified to use.

One of the arguments related to restricting testing and assessment to only psychologists is that unqualified users are using psychological instruments. Qualified and competent use requires more than having the necessary training, for the practitioner must also be knowledgeable about the specific instrument being used. The discussion of instruments in the following chapters of this book will not provide enough information to serve as training for using an instrument. Sufficient knowledge of an instrument is only gained through the thorough examination of the manual and accompanying materials. The counselor must know the limitations of an instrument and for what purposes the instrument is valid.

Practical issues. There are also a number of practical issues that need to be kept in mind when selecting an instrument. In many settings the cost of the instrument plays a role in the decision process. Certainly we should consider whether the instrument provides information that is sufficiently useful to warrant the costs. Some instruments are quite expensive; however, if used appropriately, they can be enormously helpful to clients. Another consideration is time and whether the time investment is worth it. Some clients may be reluctant to spend hours taking numerous assessment tools or some parents may object if instructional time is used for assessment. If, however, they understand the benefits of the assessment, they may be less concerned about the amount of time involved.

In conclusion, the selection of an assessment instrument is an important task. Assessment tools have been used inappropriately in the past, and sometimes this is because professionals have not devoted sufficient time in selecting an appropriate tool for a specific client. A selection decision should not be made without thoroughly examining the instrument and the manual. Figure 5.1 provides some questions to consider when evaluating assessment instruments in counseling.

FIGURE 5.1

Example of a form to evaluate assessment instruments

1. Is the purpose of the instrument clearly stated in the manual?	Yes _____	No _____
2. Does the purpose of the instrument meet my clinical needs?	Yes _____	No _____
3. Do I have the professional skill and background necessary to competently administer and interpret this instrument?	Yes _____	No _____
4. Is there correspondence between the purpose and the behaviors assessed?	Yes _____	No _____
5. Is there evidence that the authors developed specifications for the instrument before the instrument was developed?	Yes _____	No _____
6. Was care taken in constructing and evaluating all of the items?	Yes _____	No _____
7. Do the items seem to be adequate measures?	Yes _____	No _____
8. Did they perform adequate item analysis of all items?	Yes _____	No _____
9. Did they evaluate the items for possible bias?	Yes _____	No _____
10. For norm-referencing instruments, does the norming group seem appropriate for my client(s)?	Yes _____	No _____
11. For norm-referenced instruments, does the size of the norming group appear sufficient?	Yes _____	No _____
12. For norm-referenced instruments, does the norm group appear to represent the pertinent population in terms of the appropriate characteristics?	Yes _____	No _____
13. For criterion-reference instruments, is the criterion clearly stated?	Yes _____	No _____
14. For criterion-reference instruments, was the criterion selected appropriately?	Yes _____	No _____
15. For criterion-reference instruments, is there compelling evidence that the level of expected performance is appropriate?	Yes _____	No _____
16. Has the reliability of the instrument been explored sufficiently?	Yes _____	No _____
17. Does the instrument appear to have adequate reliability?	Yes _____	No _____
18. Does the manual provide the standard error of measurements for all the appropriate scales and subscales?	Yes _____	No _____
19. Does the manual provide validity information?	Yes _____	No _____
20. Is there sufficient evidence for me to feel comfortable in using this instrument for the specific purpose I need?	Yes _____	No _____
21. Does the validity evidence indicate I should be careful in using this instrument with certain clients or in certain situations?	Yes _____	No _____
22. Is there sufficient information and resources for me to feel I can adequately interpret the results of this instrument?	Yes _____	No _____
23. Can the instrument be scored in a manner that fits the situation?	Yes _____	No _____
24. Are there appropriate materials to help the client understand the results?	Yes _____	No _____
25. Is the instrument cost effective?	Yes _____	No _____
26. Can the organization afford to use this instrument?	Yes _____	No _____
27. Are the administration and scoring procedures appropriate for this setting?	Yes _____	No _____
28. Do the benefits of this assessment outweigh the time commitments?	Yes _____	No _____

Administering Assessment Instruments

Many counselors, particularly those in school settings, have the responsibility for administering certain assessment instruments. The administration of instruments is an important task because the results can be invalidated by a careless administration. Furthermore, the behaviors of the administrator of an assessment instrument can have a subtle influence on the examinee's performance. For those of you who appreciate when major points are stressed, the major focus of this section is to *know the administration materials and be prepared!*

It is important for a mental health professional to have read the administration materials before the time of administration. With many instruments, there are pretesting procedures that need to be completed in a required manner. For example, the administration procedures might require that the room be set up in a specific way to minimize the opportunity for examinees to see others' answer sheets. Other procedures might include specific registration procedures, where the examinee must provide two forms of identification in order to sit for the examination. Thus, being prepared for the administration of an instrument should start well before the actual administration.

Due to the importance of test administration, the *Standards for Educational and Psychological Testing* (AERA, APA, & NCME, 1985) devoted an entire section to the topic. In this section, the first standard addresses the importance of the test administrator's carefully following the standardized procedures for administration. Specifically, administrators need to attend to time limits, the methods for administering items and gathering responses, and familiarizing themselves with the testing materials and/or equipment. Many instruments have specific instruction on how the instrument is administered, often including a specific script that is read to the examinee(s). Familiarity with the instructions can save a counselor from a potentially embarrassing situation. Adherence to a time schedule is often part of the administration responsibilities. For example, a careless mistake in timing on the Scholastic Assessment Test (SAT-I) could significantly affect students' scholarship awards and admission into certain colleges. The *Standards for Educational and Psychological Testing* indicate that any modifications to the standardized test administration procedures need to be described in the testing report, with appropriate cautions concerning the possible effects of these modifications. Some standardized instruments will require the test administrator to report any problems or unusual circumstances that occurred during the administration.

An individual administering an assessment instrument also needs to know the boundaries of what is acceptable. For example, instruments vary in terms of what is considered an appropriate relationship and the degree of rapport to have with the examinee(s). Some instruments will encourage a certain degree of reserve, while other instruments will encourage the administrator to be quite warm and encouraging. In terms of knowledge about what is acceptable, the administrator needs to know if there are procedures concerning people leaving to go the rest room, what to do if the administrator suspects cheating is occurring, or what to do if an examinee comes in 30 minutes late. An example of a recent administration problem I witnessed was with a scholastic aptitude test, where some administrators allowed students to use calculators while other test administrators did not allow calculators to be used. The importance of knowing the administrative procedures cannot be emphasized enough. Pre-paring to administer a test or instrument needs to be performed in a methodological manner. A checklist similar to the one illustrated in Figure 5.2 may be helpful.

FIGURE 5.2

Sample checklist for instrument or test administration

Pretesting Procedures

_____ Ensure that all testing materials are kept in a secure place

_____ Read instrument manual to familiarize yourself with all administrative procedures

_____ Check possible testing facilities for size, seating, lighting, & ventilation

_____ Schedule testing facilities

_____ Check to ensure there are no conflicts with arranged testing time(s) and facilities

_____ Send out any pretesting materials that need to be sent

_____ Review testing materials to ensure that all needed materials are available

_____ Arrange for any posting of signs to direct examinees to testing location

_____ Thoroughly study exact procedures for administering the instrument

_____ Read and practice the directions for administering the test

_____ Check stopwatch or other device if time limits are involved

_____ Prepare for questions that might be asked

Immediately Preceding Testing

_____ Make sure that facilities and seating arrangement are appropriate

_____ Organize any registration process

_____ Organize testing materials

Administration of Instrument

_____ Perform any registration duties in the specified manner

_____ Distribute appropriate materials in the specified manner

_____ Administer instrument using the subscribed methods

_____ Adhere to specified time limits

_____ Note any behavioral observation of the client if individually administered

_____ Note any irregularities

After Completion of Testing

_____ Gather testing materials in specified manner

_____ Follow directions specifically for either scoring the instrument or sending the materials to be scored

Effect of the Administrator

Many of you may be required to administer an assessment as a part of your counseling duties. For many years, researchers have attempted to ferret out the influence of the administrator on the examinee's performance. We know that the interaction between two people has an influence on behavior, but the precise ways that the tester may influence those taking the test have yet to be completely understood. We do, however, have some indications of how certain characteristics of the examiner have an influence on an individual's performance on an assessment instrument.

Expectancy effects. An area where there has been considerable research attention concerns the influence of the examiners' expectations on performance. This is sometimes referred to as the "pygmalion effect" as coined by Rosenthal and Jacobson (1968), where teachers' expectations affect the student's performance. The degree to which the expectations have an influence on the examinee's performance is somewhat debatable but, in general, the consensus is that examiner expectations have a small effect (Kaplan & Saccuzzo, 1997). Furthermore, it seems that the expectancy effect may influence the testing in subtle but insignificant ways. One example of this is the research studies that have shown that students who were purported to be "bright" are more likely to receive credit for an ambiguous answer on an intelligence test than students who were alleged to be "dull" (Sattler, Hillix, & Neher, 1970; Sattler & Wingert, 1970). Research has also examined the effect of the expectancies of test administrators that had no scoring responsibilities. Some studies have found the test administrator had an influence (Hersh, 1971; Schroeder & Kleinsaser, 1972), while other studies found the administrator had no influence (Saunders & Vitro, 1971).

Examiner/examinee test-taker relationship. Many researchers (Gelso & Carter, 1994; Sexton & Whiston, 1994) have documented the importance of the counselor-client relationship. It also seems that the relationship between the examiner and the examinee has some influence on the assessment outcome. DeRosa and Patalona (1991) found children performed better when the proctor of the test was familiar. In a meta-analysis, Fuchs and Fuchs (1986) found that, on the average, test performance was about .28 of a standard deviation (about 4 IQ points) higher when the examiner was familiar to the test taker. The difference was slightly more for children from lower socioeconomic levels, indicating the relationship may be more important for these examiners.

The type of relationship and the responses an examiner can make are often covered in the manual. Many instruments are standardized and specifically address the type of relationship the examiner can have with the examinee. We do know that even subtle responses can have either a positive or negative effect and, therefore, it is important for the examiner to know the standardization material and the type of relationship that is acceptable for that instrument.

Race of examiner. There has been substantial research examining the effects of the examiner's race on examinees' performance. There does not appear, however, to be general consensus about the degree to which the race of the examiner has an impact. Sattler (1993) found evidence that examiners do have stereotypes concerning Hispanic children with highly accented English, and that those stereotypes may affect scoring. In general, however, Sattler contended that the influence of the tester's race has a negligible effect on children's performance. On the other hand, Dana (1993) documents that the current Anglo-American format for assessment services requires modification in order to take into account diverse cultural origins. Although Sattler found little evidence of bias, he further stated that examiners cannot be indifferent to the examinee's ethnicity and should be alert to any nuances in the testing situation.

Often examinees' nonverbal behaviors influence the assessment process and interpretation of results. Therefore, differences in nonverbal behaviors across cultures need to be taken into account when performing assessments (Padilla & Medina, 1996). Chapter 14 will address issues related to assessing clients from different cultures and the competencies needed to administer and interpret assessment instruments. Certainly it is important to have knowledge about the examinee's cultural group and research related to using that specific instrument with that cultural group.

The research in the area of the influence of the examiner on the examinee is equivocal; there does, however, seem to be some effect. Examiners should be cognizant of their possible effect and attempt to minimize it. In order not to have an unintended influence on the administration of the instrument, the examiner must be familiar with the administrative procedures and research related to the administration of that particular instrument.

Scoring

Many instruments are scored either by hand or by computer. Some instruments are self-scored, where the client is able to easily score the instruments, typically by adding columns together or counting responses. An example, of an instrument that can be self-scored is the Self-Directed Search (SDS, Holland, Fritzsche, & Powell, 1994). Clients simply count the number of the number items that correspond to Holland's (1985, 1997) six personality types. The manual (Holland et al., 1994), however, warns that scoring errors do occur and that the counselor should take steps to minimize any error. Some practitioners will double-check clients' scoring or others will have the clients recheck their addition.

Often someone other than the client (e.g., the counselor or a clerical employee) scores the instruments. Even if the scoring is quite easy, there are times when it is therapeutically inappropriate to have the client score the instrument. In addition, with many instruments, the hand scoring is somewhat intricate, typically involving placing a template over the answer sheet and counting the answers that correspond to various scales. Accurate scoring must be ensured in order to guard against erroneous findings. There is also research that indicates that even trained clinicians do make mistakes in scoring (Franklin & Stillman, 1982; Ryan, Prefitera, & Powers, 1983). Hand scoring can be tedious and time consuming and, thus, many counselors prefer computer scoring.

Computer scoring, compared to hand scoring, is more accurate, rapid, and thorough (Wise & Plake, 1990). Computers are not biased and will not unintentionally consider factors such as race or gender in scoring. In addition, computers can be programmed to complete complex scoring procedures that it would take humans weeks to perform. Computers can also be programmed not only to score but also to interpret the results. Computer scoring, however, is not always error free. Humans program the computers to perform the scoring, and errors in programming can result in problems. The *Standard for Educational and Psychological Testing* (AERA, APA, & NCME, 1985) calls for test scoring services to monitor their scorings and correct any errors that might occur. This mandate, however, does not guarantee that all computer scoring programs are sound, because individuals who lack sufficient training could write a program that scores and interprets instruments. Before using a computer scoring service, the practitioners need to investigate the integrity of that service and the steps that were taken to develop the scoring program. Another problem with computer scoring and interpreting is related to the ease in which assessment results can be generated. Some organizations might be tempted to skimp on staff training on an assessment device or allow assessments to be conducted without appropriate professional oversight.

Not all assessments are scored by computers and there are a number of areas where clinician judgment is a part of the scoring process. For example, with some individual intelligence tests, the examiner needs to make some professional judgments. The manuals for these instruments attempt to reduce the ambiguity in these judgments by providing explicit scoring instructions. In the personality area, many of the projective techniques involve professional judgments. For many projective techniques there are systematic methods for scoring the client's responses. Another area where scoring is more unstructured is with performance or authentic assessment.

The terms **performance assessments** and **authentic assessments** are often used interchangeably, but there is a slight distinction between the two (Oosterhof, 1994). Both performance and authentic assessments are typically associated with testing that goes beyond paper and pencil tests to assessment that more closely approximates the skill being measured. All authentic assessments are performance assessments, but the reverse is not always true. Authentic assessments involve the performance of "real" or authentic applications rather than proxies or estimators of actual learning. Authentic and performance assessments are typically associated with achievement testing. Performance assessment, however, has its roots in industrial and organizational psychology (Bray, 1982), where individuals were given activities like the "in-basket technique." With both of these types of assessments, multiple-choice items are avoided and performance on open-ended tasks is evaluated. Many of the strengths and limitations in scoring apply to both performance and authentic assessments, so the term performance assessments will be used.

One of the goals of these types of assessments is to see if knowledge can be applied. For example, instead of giving a multiple-choice test on the rules of grammar, a performance test would involve writing a business letter that is grammatically correct. Another example of performance assessment is observing a student complete a lab experience. Performance assessments seek to assess complex learning and processes, where both the product and the process are assessed. Thus, they involve observation and professional judgments about how the individual performed the tasks (e.g., process of performing a lab experiment) and what was produced by that product (e.g., results of experiment). Performance assessments can sometimes assess those more abstract learning skills that traditional multiple-choice tests cannot adequately measure. There are, however, many difficulties associated with scoring these assessments.

Objectivity in scoring becomes more difficult with the open-ended methods that are typically used in performance assessment. Sometimes the criteria for evaluating these measures is not adequately defined and other factors will influence the judgments that are made. Particularly when process rather than product is being assessed, evaluators may fail to observe some important behaviors or attend to behaviors that are not related to the skills being assessed. Because subjectivity is a part of performance assessment, one needs to attend to multicultural issues in scoring. Evaluators' biases can sometimes seep into their observations and evaluations. The use of checklists and rating scales can increase both the reliability and validity of the scoring of a performance assessment (Oosterhof, 1994). A well-thought-out scoring plan is needed in performance assessment.

Linn, Baker, and Dunbar (1991) argue that just because the measures are derived from actual performance does not guarantee that the results from these assessments are valid. Scoring of these assessments cannot be separated from an analysis of the assessment's validity. One needs to examine whether the stimulus material will invoke the expected response or performance. For example, the instructions to the students may be confusing and their abilities will not be measured because of the quality of that stimulus material. There also needs to be a direct and verified connection between the stimulus material and the skills being assessed. Therefore, the manner in which the assessment is both conducted and scored will need to be evaluated.

Although scoring a performance assessment is more complex than grading a multiple-choice examination, there is research related to methods for ensuring sound measurement (Airasian, 1994; Oosterhof, 1994). The procedures for scoring a performance assessment will be enhanced if:

- The assessment has a specific focus
- The scoring plan is based on qualities that can be directly observed

- The scoring is designed to reflect the intended target
- The setting for the assessment is appropriate
- Checklist or rating scales are used by observers
- The scoring procedures have been field tested before they are used

The previous discussion focused on the scoring of performance assessment, but many of the issues pertain to the scoring of instruments that are not multiple-choice. When subjectivity is involved in scoring, the practitioners need to find methods for ensuring objective assessment. These guidelines also apply to nonacademic assessment, where objectivity is also needed. Hence, practitioners should consider the previously mentioned guidelines with many of the assessment strategies they use with clients.

Communicating Results

Once an instrument is scored, counselors often have the responsibility of disseminating and communicating the assessment results to clients, parents, or other individuals. Communicating the results to clients is often one of the most important aspects of the assessment process. Although counselors are trained in communication skills, the interpretation of assessment results requires specialized knowledge and skills. The communication of results is an important process because if the information is not communicated effectively, clients or others may misperceive the assessment results. For example, a common problem is confusing the percentile with the percentage correct. I once had a client who was initially upset with her performance at the 50th percentile. When she saw her score on the mathematical section of an aptitude test, she began to weep and explain that she was never good in math. As I began explaining that her performance was in the average range, she looked puzzled and questioned my interpretation. As the discussion progressed, I began to see that she believed the score indicated 50% correct even though I was using terms like the 50th percentile. Once the misunderstanding was corrected, the client was pleased with her performance and felt more efficacious about her mathematical skills.

The communication of testing or assessment results should not be perceived as a discrete activity but should be interwoven into the counseling. The reason for using any informal or formal assessment is to answer questions that either the counselor or the client has. Thus, the reporting of the results should be directly connected to the focus of the counseling. Counselors need to be knowledgeable about the instrument and the specific results so that the focus during the interpretation of results can be on the client's questions and reactions.

Research Related to Communication of Results

Surprisingly, there is little research related to how practitioners can best communicate results to clients. Most of the research related to communicating results is related to career counseling, although Whiston, Sexton, and Lasoff

(1998) found a decrease of research interest in this area in recent years. Although the research is limited, general findings indicate that those who receive test interpretations, regardless of the format, do experience greater gains in counseling than those who do not receive an interpretation (Goodyear, 1990). In a meta-analysis of career interventions, Oliver and Spokane (1988) found an effect size of .62 for individual test interpretation and an effect size of .76 for group test interpretation. This means that those who received the test interpretation were around two-thirds of a standard deviation higher on the outcome measures used than those who did not receive the interpretations.

Most of the research that is related to the benefits of clients receiving test information is in the career counseling area. There is, however, a growing body of research that indicates sharing personality assessment information can also be therapeutic. Researchers (Finn & Tonsager, 1992; Newman & Greenway, 1997) have found that providing MMPI-2 feedback increased clients' self-esteem and reduced levels of distress. Some organizations as a part of their intake procedures use instruments for screening and diagnostic purposes. Often this information is not shared with clients, but the research related to test interpretation indicates it would be helpful to provide the results to the clients.

Professionals sometimes want to know whether it is better to interpret results individually or in groups. Interestingly, the research is not conclusive in this area. When given a preference, clients *prefer* to receive results individually. In addition, clients report more satisfaction, clarity, and helpfulness when the interpretation is performed individually as compared to other formats such as groups (Goodyear, 1990). If, however, the cost of interpretation is considered, then the evaluation of whether individual or group is more effective changes somewhat. Krivasty and Magoon (1976) found that individual interpretation was six times more expensive than group interpretation. Some counselors (e.g., school counselors) will use a combination, such as using group interpretation for general interpretive information and then follow up with individual sessions to discuss specific results.

There is limited research related to client characteristics and evaluation of assessment processes and procedures. One result that seems logical is that more intelligent clients tend to remember test results better as compared to less intelligent clients. Also, researchers are beginning to explore the relationship between personality and interpretation of assessment results. Lenz, Reardon, and Sampson (1993) investigated the effect of selected client characteristics (i.e., gender, personality, level of identity, and degree of differentiation) on clients' evaluation of SIGI-Plus. Surprisingly, only personality had a significant influence on their ratings, with the relationship being: as scores on the Social and Enterprising scales increased, individuals' rating of the system's contribution to their self and occupational knowledge decreased. Also, Kivlighan and Shapiro (1987) found that Investigative and Realistic individuals were more likely than other personality types to benefit from a test feedback intervention.

Benziman and Toder (1993) examined whether children in mental health settings would prefer to receive assessment feedback from either the examiner or the therapist as compared to their parents. In this study, the children voiced a strong preference for receiving the assessment results from their parents. Jones and Gelso (1988) found that individuals perceived interpretations that were tentative as being more helpful than interpretations that were more absolute. These individuals also expressed more willingness to see a counselor who used a tentative interpretation approach over one who was more absolute. Worthington et al. (1995) found that married couples gained more from assessment feedback as compared to those who just completed the questionnaire. Goodyear (1990) found mixed results on whether clients who participated more in the interpretative process had better outcomes.

General Guidelines for Communicating Results to Clients

- Before any type of interpretation or communication of results to a client, the counselor needs to be knowledgeable about the information contained in the manual. The validity information is the basis for the interpretation, because this information informs practitioners on appropriate uses and interpretations. Furthermore, most manuals will explain the limitations of the instruments and areas where the clinician should proceed with caution.

- In preparing the client to receive test feedback, Hanson and Claiborn (1998) suggest that the counselor should take time to "optimize" the power of the test (e.g., "This test is useful in particular ways, within particular limits"), rather than allowing the client to "maximize" it (e.g., "The test speaks the truth").

- Interpreting assessment results is part of the counseling process and typical counseling variables (e.g., counseling relationship, interaction between client and counselor) need to be considered. In order to communicate assessment results adequately, counselors need to use effective general counseling skills.

- Counselors need to develop multiple methods of explaining the results. Sometimes the communication of results will involve terms such as standard deviation, normal curve, and stanines that are not familiar to many individuals. Preparing to explain the results in multiple ways is necessary, because some clients will not understand their results using standard psychometric terms. When appropriate, include visual aids, because some people understand better by seeing the results rather than hearing a report.

- Whenever possible the interpretation should involve descriptive terms rather than numerical scores. For example, if a client's score is at the 83rd percentile, explain that if 100 people took this instrument, 83 of them would have a score at or below the client's. It is better to provide a range of scores rather than just one score. The description of the results should be tied to the reason for the assessment. As an example, if a counselor gave a personality inventory to a couple, the counselor would need to explain the rationale for taking the personality inventories and how the results can be useful.

- The assessment results should not be presented as being infallible predictions. When probability information is available, then explain the results in terms of probabilities rather than certainties. There is, however, considerable research that indicates people attribute very different meanings to many of the probabilistic words commonly used in appraisal, such as unlikely, possible, probable and very likely (Lichtenberg & Hummel, 1998). These findings indicate that counselors vary widely in their interpretations of probabilistic statements in interpretative reports. Lichtenberg and Hummel suggest that counselors use numerical descriptors (e.g., there is a 95% chance) rather than verbal ones (e.g., there is a high probability) in order to convey more precise information.

- The results should be discussed in context with other client information. Interpretation should never be done in isolation, but rather, the interpretative process should explore how the assessment information conforms with other pertinent information. A competent interpretation involves analyzing not only the assessment results, but also integrating diverse client information into a comprehensive understanding. Assessment results can be viewed as pieces of a puzzle, but other puzzle pieces have to be used in order to understand the total picture.

- When describing the results, the therapist should involve the client in the interpretation. The client needs to be involved in the process in order to address questions about whether the results make sense or if they fit with other information. The counselor should monitor the client's reaction to the information, which can be best accomplished by having the client provide feedback throughout the process. Asking the client for reactions early in the process will lay the foundation for an interactional interpretation.

- Any limitations of the assessment should be discussed in nontechnical terms. Some clients will only be confused by comments such as "The reliability coefficients are low." The explanation of the limitations needs to be geared toward the level of assessment sophistication of the client. If there are questions related to the instrument's results in terms of the gender, racial background, or other characteristics of the client, then this also needs to be explained to the client.

- The counselor should encourage the client to ask questions during the process. Occasionally clients believe they will appear foolish to their counselors, so they will be reluctant to ask questions. In order to see whether the clients understand the information, counselors can use incomplete sentences, where the client fills in the information or completes the sentence. Counselors need to ensure that clients do not leave confused or ill-informed about the results.

- It is often helpful to summarize the results at the end of the conversation in order to reiterate and stress important points. The summarization process provides a second opportunity for the client to question inconsistent results.

Guidelines for Communicating Results to Parents

The guidelines listed above also apply to communicating assessment results to parents; however, there are some specific issues that arise when interpreting results with parents. Parents frequently receive achievement test information, but they may have little background in testing. In addition, schools sometimes send results home, and these materials may not adequately explain the results. Parents will often seek help in interpreting the results from a school counselor; however, any counselor who works with a family should be prepared to interpret achievement and aptitude testing results. Table 5.1 lists common questions asked by parents that all counselors need to be prepared to answer. Occasionally a parent may ask questions about standardized tests as a method to "break the ice" with a counselor with the goal of discussing other issues. Therefore, when the results are being interpreted, the counselor should provide the parents with opportunities to extend the discussion to other topics.

Increasingly, counselors are members of multidisciplinary teams that collaborate in the delivery of mental health services. As a part of a team, the counselor may have the responsibility of counseling the parents after the child has been diagnosed with a disorder. Examples of the more typical diagnoses a child may receive by a school psychologist or community practitioner are: Mental Retardation, Motor Skills Disorders, Communication Disorders, Pervasive Developmental Disorders, Attention-Deficit/Hyperactivity Disorder (ADHD), Oppositional Defiant Disorder, and Conduct Disorder. In these cases, the parents usually have received an explanation of the testing that was performed, but they are often overwhelmed with all the information presented. As counselors work with the parents on coping and parenting issues, it is important for them to understand the testing and the symptoms of the disorder. If counselors are not part of the multidisciplinary team and do not have access to the testing results, they can gain access to the information by having the parents sign an informed consent form to release the information to them.

Parents often struggle with the news that their child has a disorder and the counselor can be instrumental in helping them adjust to the situation. Many parents have experienced numerous difficulties and frustrations and need to interact with an individual who can empathize with their situation. A family's reaction to the diagnosis of a disability tends to go through five stages: impact,

TABLE 5.1

Questions commonly asked by parents

• Why was my child tested?	• Why are the scores so low?
• What is an achievement test?	• Who was in the comparison group?
• What does criterion-referenced mean?	• What do these results mean for the future?
• What is a general abilities test?	• Who will see these results?
• What are percentile scores?	• Why do you test so much?
• What are stanine scores?	• Could my child have done better?
• Why aren't grade equivalent scores good?	• Where did the questions on the test come from?

denial, grief, focusing outward, and closure (Fortier & Wanlass, 1984). To progress through the stages, the family often needs help in understanding the child's condition. This may involve discussing the assessment report more than once. It is particularly important that the counselor prepare to discuss the results using a variety of techniques. The counselor may also help the parents focus on the child's abilities and not just on the disabilities. The entire family can benefit from understanding that the disability is only one aspect of their child's life. Sattler (1993) also encouraged clinicians to emphasize the active role that they and their child can play in coping with the disability. The counselor should attempt to frame the family's response into an active, coping approach as compared to a succumbing, victim framework.

Focusing on methods for coping does not mean the counselor should ignore the negative emotions the family is feeling. It is often very difficult for parents to hear that their child is, for example, mentally retarded or autistic. Both the parents and the child often are experiencing feelings of guilt and feel that they somehow caused the problems identified in the testing. There are also often feelings of sorrow and loss. Even parents who have been aware of developmental delays and other problems for a period of time tend to experience feelings of loss when confronted with the results of testing. Often these feelings are associated with the loss of the "perfect child" that most parents fantasize about at some point. Counselors, therefore, need to provide a therapeutic environment where issues related to loss, anger, and frustration can be addressed.

In addressing negative reactions to the assessment results, the counselor needs to monitor the parents' reactions so that the child does not internalize their negative reactions. Sometimes, a child will interpret the parents' disappointment in the testing result as disappointment in the child. The child may also be concerned about rejection by his or her peers. Often when psychodiagnostic evaluation is completed, educational interventions are implemented (e.g., the child goes to a resource room or receives other special education services). The child may fear the outgrowth of other children becoming aware of his or her situation. Hence, this may be a time when the child is particularly vulnerable and, at the same time, is unsure of his or her parents' level of affection.

Summary

This chapter examined instrument selection, administration, scoring, and communication of results. Clinicians selecting an inappropriate instrument can have a negative impact on clients. An instrument should not be used with a client until the counselor has thoroughly evaluated the materials. A counselor needs to evaluate the instrument's purpose, the procedures used in constructing the instrument, the appropriateness of the norming group or criterion, the reliability, and the validation evidence. Instruments should also be evaluated for potential bias, particularly in multicultural counseling situations. The qualifications of the practitioner should also be considered in determining whether to use an instrument. It is unethical for a counselor to use an instrument in which he or she has not received the proper training. Some publishers use a three-level qualification system (i.e., Level A, Level B, and Level C). The ultimate responsibility, however, for ethical use of an instrument rests with the test user.

Part of using an instrument appropriately is ensuring that the instrument was properly administered. Counselors often shoulder this responsibility, even in settings such as schools where an achievement test is actually administered by classroom teachers. The key to ethical instrument administration is knowing and following the administrative instructions. Most manuals provide instructions detailing the manner in which an instrument should be administered. Counselors need to follow these guidelines and prepare for potential difficulties. Foresight and planning can often circumvent potential problems in instrument administration.

Accurate scoring must be ensured in order to guard against erroneous findings. Computer scoring is becoming more prevalent than hand scoring for many instruments. Some instruments involve quite intricate scoring and can only be computer scored. With certain types of instruments, the scoring involves professional judgments by the person scoring the results. An assessment area that has been of increasing interest is performance and authentic assessments. Subjectivity can be problematic in these types of assessment, but there are procedures that can be used to enhance the scoring process.

Research findings reflect that those who receive test interpretations, regardless of the format, do experience greater gains in counseling than those who do not receive an interpretation. Communicating the results to clients is often one of the most important aspects of the assessment process. There is surprisingly little research related to the most effective methods for communicating assessment results. In general, it is more effective to integrate the communication of assessment results into the counseling process. Clients prefer to have results interpreted to them individually, but group interpretations appear to be effective and are significantly cheaper.

Assessment results need to be interpreted in context. Part of interpreting in a context involves examining whether the results are consistent or inconsistent with other information about the client. In addition, in order to facilitate understanding, the practitioner should be prepared to explain the results using multiple methods. Clinicians also need to explain results to parents and to assist parents in understanding the results and making informed decisions about their children.

Overview of Assessment Areas

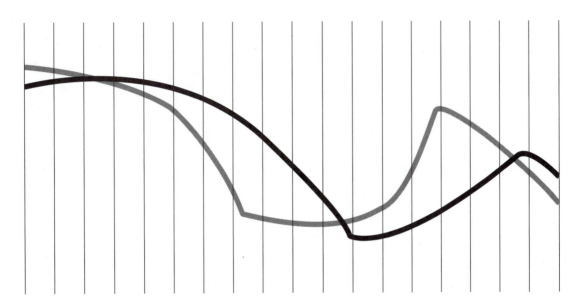

CHAPTER 6

Initial Assessment in Counseling

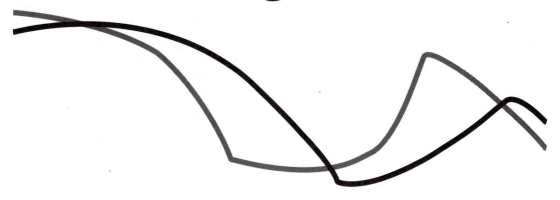

C lients often come to counseling with scattered information surrounding current issues and problems. Sometimes the presenting concerns are somewhat vague and ill defined. The concerns will often be presented in statements such as "I am not getting along with my husband," "The kid won't listen," "I keep making the same dumb mistakes," "I can't stand my job anymore," "I just can't get motivated to do anything," or "She never does her homework and lies." Counselors need to become skilled in taking these vague concerns and identifying relevant issues and problems. Cormier and Cormier (1998) suggest that problems are rarely related to one factor, are usually multi-dimensional, and typically occur in a social context. Therefore, counselors need finely tuned initial assessment skills in order to identify the complex interaction of factors that are related to the client's problems. Sexton et al. (1997) found that counseling outcome research indicates that this initial intake session is critical to the effectiveness of the overall counseling. Counseling tends to be more effective when the counselor is able to quickly conceptualize the relevant issues. Sexton and his colleagues also found that if counselors can build positive expectations about the process during these very early sessions, then the counseling is more likely to be effective. Researchers have found that clients' expectations about counseling before they enter have very little influence on eventual outcome; however, the expectations that clients build during those initial sessions have a significant influence on outcome (Sexton et al., 1997). Hence, the effectiveness of the counselor in assessing the situation in those early sessions is critical to the effectiveness of the counseling.

Initial Intake Interview

Often counselors use interviewing skills to begin the counseling process and gather relevant clinical information. Initial or intake interviews usually gather information about the range and scope of the concerns, pertinent details about the current situation, and relevant background information to the current problems. Nelson (1983) found that the interview was one of the most commonly used assessment strategies. Despite the evidence that the interview is the most popular assessment strategy used, it is not always easy to conduct effectively. There is evidence that guidelines and training are needed to obtain accurate and valid information from an interview (Duley, Cancelli, Kratochwill, Bergan, & Meredith, 1983).

An effective initial interview is a balancing between gathering information and building a therapeutic relationship. The initial assessment and information gathering need not have a detrimental effect on the relationship; a skilled clinician can gather pertinent information while beginning to establish a working alliance. Therefore, this discussion will first address information customarily gathered in an initial interview and then proceed with an overview of therapeutic skills for conducting that interview.

Information Gathered in Initial Interview

The information gathered in an initial counseling interview will vary somewhat depending on the setting (e.g., school or agency) and the services delivered by the organization. There are some important areas that clinicians need to explore before commencing with the treatment phase of counseling, such as:

1. Should this person be counseled?
2. What are the major issues or problems?
3. What is the most effective treatment or counseling approach for this client?
4. Should there be family members or others involved in the counseling?
5. Can I work effectively with this client?
6. What type of relationship should I have with this client?
7. How can I evaluate the effectiveness of the counseling?

In order to gather sufficient information to make good clinical decisions, the initial interview needs to address demographic information, presenting concern, client background information, medical information, and sufficient information to define the problem. A final area that some researchers are encouraging practitioners to assess in the initial stages of counseling is the stage the client is at in the change process (see Prochaska, DiClemente, & Norcross, 1992).

Demographic information. Typically, demographic information is gathered through the intake paperwork of an agency, or it already exists in organizations such as schools. It is important, however, to ensure that the demographic information is current and correct. Accurate telephone numbers and emergency numbers can be critical in crisis situations. There is also pertinent demographic information that needs to be gathered to make clinical decisions. For example, it could be important for the practitioner to have information on the client's marital status, race or ethnicity, employment status, and occupation. Also, in cases where clinicians may need to report suspected child abuse, information on all those living in a household and where the children attend school could prove to be important.

Presenting concern. Many clients enter counseling because of specific issues that are causing them difficulties. It is important for the counselor to understand the issues or problems that brought the client to counseling. Outcome research results indicate there is a connection between attending to a client's presenting concerns and an effective outcome (Sexton et al., 1997). This process involves more than noting the presenting complaint, but also gathering information on when it started and events that were occurring at that same time. The counselor should also explore the frequency of the problem, the degree to which the problem is affecting the client's daily functioning, and methods the client has used to attempt to deal with the problem in the past. More detailed information is needed about the issues before treatment decisions can be made. This subject will be discussed in the later section on defining the problem. Often, however, counselors will need to gather historical or client background information, before further delineating the problems, in order to gain a contextual framework in which to further assess the issues.

Client background information. Once the clinician has gained some initial information about the presenting concern, the counselor needs to elicit background information from the client. Some clinicians will call this gathering of background information a **psychosocial interview**. This gathering of background information is not a detailed exploration of the client's past, but rather an overview of the client's background, particularly as it relates to the presenting problem. Table 6.1 includes the common areas that are addressed in gathering background information. Counselors should explain the reasons for gathering this background information to the client. All of this information does not

TABLE 6.1

Background information to include in initial intake interview

1. **Identifying Information**
   Client name, address, phone number, age, gender, marital status, occupation, workplace or school, work telephone numbers, name of another person to contact in case of an emergency.

2. **Purpose of Counseling/Presenting Problem**
   State presenting concern and gather detailed information on the problem/concern.

3. **Physical Appearance**
   Clothing, grooming, height, weight.

4. **Present Level of functioning In Work/School, Relationships, and Leisure**
   Analysis of present level of function in work, relationships, and leisure activities. Degree presenting concern is affecting activities.

5. **Medical History and Current Status**
   Present health, current health complaints, health history, treatments received for current complaints, date of last physical examination, current medications, other drugs either O-T-C or "street drugs," sleep patterns, appetite level or changes, exercise patterns.

6. **Past Counseling Experiences or Psychiatric History**
   Type of treatment, what were the concerns, how long did it last, what was the outcome, what was positive, what wasn't helpful, were medications prescribed for emotional/psychological problems?

7. **Family Information**
   Current marital status, number and ages of children living at home, other people living in home, any violence or physical abuse, family-of-origin makeup, significant influences of family-of-origin on present problems, history of psychiatric problems on family, history of substance abuse in family.

8. **Social/Developmental History**
   Significant developmental events that may influence present, any irregularities in development, current social situation, religious affiliation and values.

9. **Educational/Occupational History**
   Occupational background, educational background, reasons for terminating previous jobs, military background, overall satisfaction with current job, stresses related to occupation.

need to be collected in the intake interview; some information is better gathered in an easy-to-complete form. In some settings (e.g., schools) or for specific issues (e.g., career counseling), the counselor may not need to gather detailed information on the client's background. Nevertheless, Cormier and Cormier (1998) suggest that counselors in all settings should gather some background information.

Health and medical history. Clinicians need to have knowledge about the client's medical conditions in order to understand the client holistically. This exploration of health issues needs to include an analysis of current health issues, including a listing of current medications. Counselors want to ensure that there is no physiological base to the concerns of a client and, therefore, it is often wise to refer clients to a physician for a physical examination. Even if a client has had a recent physical, it is important to gather medical information and explore the possible side effects of any medications that the client is taking. Certainly with many clients, a thorough assessment needs to include an analysis of drug and alcohol use. Counselors should also gather information on past psychiatric illnesses and treatments.

Defining the client problem. Once the clinician has gathered information about the presenting concern and sufficient background information, the initial interview should also focus on defining the client problem or problems. Problem assessment plays a critical role in counseling, for it is crucial that the counselor have a clear understanding of the issues and problems. Mohr (1995) found that counseling can have a negative outcome for clients, and one of the major reasons for this negative outcome is that clinicians underestimate the severity of the client's problems. Many clients seek counseling for multiple issues rather than one specific problem. Therefore, it is important that counselors investigate the range of problems. Once the counselor has identified the dominant concerns or problems, the counselor should then explore these issues in greater detail. The following are topics to address in the examination of each significant problem.

1. *Explore the problem from multiple perspectives.* The counselor should attempt to view the problem or concern from diverse vantage points. This can be accomplished by having the client describe the problem in terms of affective, behavioral, cognitive, and relational perspectives. If the counselor is working with a family, then having each member describe the problem contributes to a multidimensional perspective. If a counselor is working with a single client, then asking the client how others may describe the problem will also promote a better understanding of the problem.

2. *Gather specific information on each major problem.* The counselor should encourage the client to describe the problem(s) in detail. Included in this description should be information on when the problems began, the history of the problem, what events were occurring when the problem arose, and what factors or people contributed to the situation. Information on the antecedents and consequences of the problem can be particularly helpful later when selecting treatment interventions.

3. *Assess problem intensity.* Counselors need to assess the degree to which the problem or issues are impacting the client. The problem's severity and the frequency or duration of problematic behaviors should be explored. Having clients rate the severity of the problem on a scale from 1 to 10 can provide an indication of the degree of negative impact. In certain situations, like anxiety attacks, the counselor may have the client chart or record the problematic behaviors.

4. *Assess degree to which client believes the problem is changeable.* In the assessment of client problems, it is important to explore the degree to which the client believes the problems are malleable or immutable. Assessment in this area will be helpful later in determining interventions and possible homework assignments.

5. *Identify methods the client has used to solve the problem previously.* Counselors need to explore the methods the client has already used to address the problem. This will provide insight into the client and avoid duplicating efforts that have already been attempted.

Once the counselor has assessed each of the significant problems the client is experiencing, the next step is to prioritize these problems. If the counselor addresses all of the problems at once, the counseling process is likely to be stymied. The prioritizing of the problems is still part of the assessment process, which can serve as a transition into the treatment phase of counseling. Determining which problems to address first in counseling will depend on the situation, the client, and the counseling relationship.

Assessing the change process. Within the counseling field, there appears to be a growing interest in understanding the fundamental principles and process of change (Bandura, 1977; Highlen & Hill, 1984; Lyddon & Alford, 1993). The transtheoretical model of Prochaska et al. (1992) is considered one of the most influential models of behavior change (Morera et al., 1998). Prochaska et al. argue that counselors need to select interventions based on the client's stage in the change process. They studied both people in counseling and self-changers and were able to identify the stages of change. Much of the research has been related to modifying addictions, but these same stages have been found to pertain to clients with diverse problems.

Prochaska and associates (Prochaska & DiClemente, 1992; DiClemente et al., 1991) have found that people progress through five stages as they change and that counseling will be more effective if the interventions are geared toward the individual's stage in the change process. *Precontemplation* is the first stage in the change process. At this stage, the individual has no intention of changing behavior in the foreseeable future. Many clients may be unaware or underaware that there even is a problem. They often enter counseling because they are coerced or pressured by others. They may attempt to demonstrate change because of the pressures, but they will quickly return to old behaviors when the pressure is off.

The second stage is *contemplation*, where individuals become aware that a problem exists and begin to consider the problem. At this stage, however, they have not made a commitment to take action. The contemplation stage is characterized by the serious consideration of the problem, with the client beginning to weigh the pros and cons of seeking solutions to the problem.

In *preparation*, the client begins to make small alterations in behavior with the intention of taking action in the next month. For example, clients will cut down on cigarettes or only drink on the weekends. Their actions may be small, but they intend to take stronger action in the near future.

In the *action* stage, individuals modify their behavior, experiences, or environment in order to address their problems. The action stage involves overt behaviors and the devotion of considerable time and energy to the change process. Counselors often mistakenly equate this stage with actual change and ignore the requisite process that the client needs to go through in order to implement change.

The last stage in the process is *maintenance,* during which the individual works to prevent relapse and consolidate the gains achieved in the action stage. This is not a static stage; rather, maintenance is the continuation of the change.

In general, maintenance lasts for at least six months, during which the client focuses on methods for stabilizing and continuing the change.

Assessing a client's stage and level of change is not a traditional part of the intake interviews. It does, however, dovetail nicely with the developmental perspective of counseling (Lyydon & Alford, 1993) and the contention that the counselor's role is to facilitate positive change. Assessment of the client's stage in the change process is usually accomplished through the interviewing of the client. Responses to questions related to the client's presenting concerns and background will typically reflect his or her stage in the change process. There is also an instrument, the Stages of Change Questionnaire (McConnaughy, DiClemente, Prochaska, & Velicer, 1989; McConnaughy, Prochaska, & Velicer, 1983), that can be used with clients to assess their stage within the change process.

In conclusion, in the content of the initial interview, counselors should consider the major types of information they want to elicit from a client before they begin the initial interview. Initial interviews often provide the foundation for further assessment and, therefore, should cover a spectrum of topics. Typical information gathered in these interviews concerns demographic information, presenting concern, client background information, medical information, and sufficient information to define the problem. The goal in interviewing is to gain valid information, but in order to elicit information from a client, the counselor must establish an atmosphere in which the client feels comfortable in divulging personal information.

Interviewing Skills and Techniques

A sound interview is accomplished by gathering information in a therapeutic manner. Therefore, counselors need to attend to both the content of the initial interview and the skills they use in gathering that information. The initial interview is the first contact with the client and first impressions do have an influence on counseling outcome. Counselors should reflect on how they can appear credible to the client in terms of being perceived as trustworthy, expert, and attractive. LaCrosse (1980) found that initial client perceptions of counselors' expertness accounted for 31 percent of the variance in favorable therapeutic outcome. Clients who perceive their counselors as being trustworthy, expert, and attractive helpers have better outcomes in counseling than clients who do not have these perceptions of their counselors (Heppner & Claiborn, 1989).

Numerous individuals have written about the importance of using effective communication skills in initial interviews (Cormier & Cormier, 1998; Fine & Glasser, 1996; Ivy, 1994; Okun, 1997). Communication skills are needed to communicate that the clients are being heard and understood in their responses to the interview questions. Open-ended questions are often used in interviewing because they are less likely to "lead" or unduly influence the client. In closed-ended questions, there is a set of "closed" responses from which the client can select an answer, such as answering either "yes" or "no" to questions like "Did you come to counseling because you are feeling depressed?" Open-ended questions require a more elaborate answer that the client has to construct. Examples of open-ended questions are "What brought you to counseling?" "Can you describe for me the problems that you are having now?" "What situations are not going as well as you would like them to go?" With interviews that do not have a structured format, the counselor will often use other communication skills to draw the client out. Commonly used techniques are paraphrasing, clarifying, reflecting, interpreting, and summarizing (Okun, 1997).

Both counselors' verbal and nonverbal behaviors impact the effectiveness of the initial interview. The climate the counselor builds during the interviewing process influences the degree to which clients are willing to disclose personal information. Table 6.2 includes some general guidelines for conducting initial counseling interviews. It should be remembered that clients respond to different therapeutic styles and that there is not one correct manner of conducting an initial interview.

Structured and Unstructured Initial Interviews

One of the decisions a counselor needs to make about the initial session is whether to use a structured or unstructured interview. Sometimes this decision will be made for the counselor, for some agencies require that a structured interview be performed with each new client. A **structured interview** is one where the counselor has an established set of questions that he or she asks in

TABLE 6.2

Common guidelines for conducting an initial interview

- Assure the client of confidentiality (clearly state any exceptions such as harm to themselves or someone else).
- Ask questions in a courteous and accepting manner.
- Word questions in an open-ended format rather than a closed format.
- Avoid leading questions.
- Listen attentively.
- Consider the client's cultural and ethnic background in structuring the interview.
- Adjust your approach to the individual client (some clients are more comfortable with a more formal process; others prefer a more warm and friendly approach).
- Avoid "chatting" about unimportant topics.
- Encourage clients to express feelings, thoughts, and behaviors openly.
- Avoid psychological jargon.
- Use voice tones that are warm and inviting, yet professional.
- Allow sufficient time and don't rush clients to finish complex questions.
- If clients' responses drift from pertinent topics, gently direct them back to the appropriate topics.
- Vary posture to avoid appearing static.

the same manner and sequence to each client. In an **unstructured interview** the counselor may have an idea about possible items but gears the interview in a unique and different manner depending on the needs of the client. A **semi-structured interview** is a combination of the structured and the unstructured, where certain questions are always asked but there is room for exploration and additional questions. There are advantages and disadvantages to all three methods of interviewing.

The major advantage of the structured interview is that it is more reliable (Aiken, 1996). Reliability concerns the proportion of error, which counselors will want to minimize. Furthermore, as was addressed earlier, reliability is a prerequisite to validity. So the structured interview may possibly be more valid than an unstructured interview, but this is not guaranteed. Some practitioners believe that structured interviews will have a negative impact on the counseling relationship because the client will feel interrogated. This is not always accurate, because the style of the interviewer has a significant influence on the counseling relationship and the degree of comfort the client feels in disclosing information. The soundness of a structured interview is intimately linked to the questions included in the interview and the counselor's ability to elicit crucial information. It is difficult to assemble a structured interview that can respond to the vast array of problems and situations faced by clients. With structured interviews, it is important to include a question at the end that would encourage the client to disclose any important information that may not have been addressed.

The advantage of unstructured interviews is that they can be easily adapted to respond to the unique needs of the client. Unstructured interviews, however, are less reliable and more prone to error than structured interviews. I have supervised counseling students where the initial interviews focused only on a relatively minor issue and the counselors neglected to gather adequate information. Unstructured interviews tend to take longer to gather information as compared to well-developed structured interviews. The decision to use either a structured or an unstructured interview should be based on the purpose. For example, if the purpose is for screening clients to see if they are appropriate for a clinic, then a structured interview that reduces the amount of error is probably better. If, on the other hand, the purpose is to better understand the specifics of an individual client, then an unstructured interview may allow for more individualized exploration. The unstructured interview requires much more skill on the part of the interviewer than the structured interview.

Interviewing Children

The previous suggestions on interviewing, such as establishing rapport, gearing the vocabulary toward the client's educational level, and asking questions in a warm professional manner apply as well to children. The counselor also needs to gear the initial interview toward the child's developmental level.

Starting with phrases such as "I am going to talk with you for a little while to see if the two of us can figure out some ways to make your life better" or "Your mom told me some problems were going on, but I would like to hear what you think is going on" may help the child understand the purpose of the initial interview. It may also be helpful to provide a statement concerning why you are asking them questions at this stage in the counseling, such as "I really want to understand so I am going to ask you some questions to help me understand." Children particularly need to understand the purpose for the interview and counseling, because they have had little exposure even to the media's representation of counseling. Many children will see a counselor as an adult in a punitive role and will have difficulty trusting the counselor. Therefore, when assessing the problem with child, it is important to define the limits of confidentiality.

Sattler (1993) proposes the following guidelines when interviewing children:

1. Formulate appropriate opening statements.
2. Make descriptive comments.
3. Use reflection.
4. Give praise frequently.
5. Avoid critical statements.
6. Use simple questions and concrete referents.
7. Formulate questions in the subjunctive mood when necessary.
8. Be tactful.
9. Use props, crayons, clay, or toys to help young children communicate.
10. Use special techniques to facilitate the expression of culturally unacceptable responses.
11. Clarify an episode of misbehavior by recounting it.
12. Handle children who are minimally communicative by clarifying the interview procedures.
13. Handle avoidance of a topic by discussing it yourself.
14. Understand silence.
15. Handle resistance and anxiety by giving support and reassurance (pp. 420–424).

If the child becomes involved in disruptive play, begins crying, or misbehaves in some way, Greenspan and Greenspan (1981) recommend not stopping the behavior too quickly. They suggest that observing this behavior may be insightful, and disciplining too quickly may negatively affect the interviewing process. On the other hand, a counselor does not have to sit and watch the child destroy the counseling office. Simple statements like "Can I ask you not to do that," "We don't allow behavior like that in the center" or "Let's talk for just 10 minutes and then we will do something else" can be helpful. Periods of silence or times when the conversation halts is more common in interviewing children than with adults. Silence may be an indication that the child is thinking about what to say or is reflecting on a situation or problem. If the silence becomes extreme then the counselor might intervene with a question like "These questions seem difficult for you to answer, can you tell me about that?"

or "You seem a little quiet, what are thinking about right now?" In assessing children and their problems, counselors need to be more patient and skillful with their interventions.

Strengths and Limitations of Interviewing

In terms of reliability, structured interviews are more reliable than unstructured ones. The validity of the interview will be influenced by the quality of the questions asked. Counselors should also consider the validation evidence and the inferences they make about the client based on the initial interview. The information gathered in an interview must be carefully analyzed and the counselor should consider other evidence that may substantiate or challenge the clinical judgments being made. The strength of interviewing is the ability to directly question the client about issues, problems, and personal information. The limitations of interviews are usually related to the lack of validation evidence and the influences of counselor subjectivity. As Dawes (1994) demonstrated, clinicians tend to be biased in their decision making. Therefore, clinicians need to ensure that they gather and analyze the information gained from interviews using objective and sound methods.

All clients will not respond in the same manner to a clinical interview. Certainly gender and culture need to be considered in determining whether to use this assessment strategy. Some cultures do not encourage immediate self-disclosure to someone outside of the family. Clients may have difficulty relating to the questions and formulating a response. A counselor could perceive this difficulty as resistance when it may be more a matter of unfamiliarity and discomfort. Interviews are a good method for gathering initial information; however, they are not the only method. Counselors may consider supplementing their intake interviews with other information such as checklists or rating scales. These other methods of gathering information may provide information that was not addressed in the interview. Furthermore, the information from checklists or rating scales may complement the interview and aid the counselor in identifying the more pressing and significant issues.

Other Instruments That Can Be Used in Initial Assessment

The counseling process frequently begins with gathering information about the client and his or her concerns. Most practitioners start this process by talking with the client and using a structured, semi-structured, or unstructured interview. Some counselors, however, supplement that information by using other assessment tools. Some of these tools are informal assessment instruments (e.g., checklists or rating scales) that are incorporated into initial paperwork. Other assessment devices that can be used are more formal instruments that provide information on symptoms and issues.

Checklists

A checklist can be a relatively simple and cost-effective method for gathering initial information from clients. Usually in a checklist, individuals are instructed to mark the words or phrases in the list that apply to them. Checklists can be filled out by the client or by an observer (typically a parent or teacher). When multiple individuals complete a checklist on a client, a counselor can acquire a rich body of therapeutic information. For example, clinicians working with children can expand on in-session observations by having children's parents and teachers complete a brief checklist.

Standardized checklists. Counselors can construct their own checklists or use a number of standardized checklists. Some of the standardized checklists focus on clients reporting their current symptoms. The *Symptom Checklist-90-Revised* (SCL-90-R, Derogatis, 1994) and the *Brief Symptoms Inventory* (BSI, Derogatis, 1993) are two popular instruments that are used in many mental health settings at intake. The instruments are related and very similar, except the SCL-90-R contains 90 symptoms whereas the BSI contains 53. The client simply responds to the listed symptoms using a 5-point scale of distress (0–4) ranging from 0 (*not at all*) to 4 (*extremely*). The SCL-90-R takes about 15 minutes to take; the BSI is less time consuming.

There are two methods in which these two symptom inventories can be used as valuable initial screening tools. A clinician can simply scan the results of these instruments and retrieve which symptoms are distressing to the client. Included in these measures are items such as thoughts of ending their life, feelings of worthlessness, feeling afraid in open spaces, and feeling that most people cannot be trusted. The SCL-90-R and the BSI can also be scored providing measures on nine scales: somatization, obsessive-compulsive, interpersonal sensitivity, depression, anxiety, hostility, phobic anxiety, paranoid ideation, and psychoticism. There are also three composite scores that can be particularly helpful to counselors in determining whether to refer the client for psychiatric evaluation: the Global Severity Index, the Positive Symptom Total, and the Positive Symptom Distress Index. Client responses can be compared to nonpatient adults, nonpatient adolescents, psychiatric outpatients, and psychiatric inpatients. The internal consistency measures and test-retest coefficients are quite high over short time periods. Derogatis recommended that the results of either the SCL-90-R or the BSI are good for no more than 7 days. There are many other commercially available checklists that can be used with adults.

There are also a number of checklists developed for use with children and adolescents. A widely used checklist for children is the Child Behavior Checklist, which actually involves five separate rating scales (parent/guardian report, teacher report, self-report, direct observation, and interview). With these instruments, clinicians can gather information from multiple sources. There is version for children 2 to 3, but the most widely used version is for children ages 4 to 18. The *Child Behavior Checklist for Ages 4–18* (Achenbach, 1997) measures behavior problems and competencies, with scores in seven areas: Anxious/Depressed, Withdrawn, Somatic Complaints, Social Problems, Thought Problems, Attention Problems, Aggressive, and Delinquency. There are also three broad scores related to Internalizing, Externalizing, and Total Problems. Although these instruments are labeled checklists, in many ways the instruments are more similar to a rating scale. Another checklist that is used with children is the *Revised Problem Behavior Checklist* (Quay & Peterson, 1987).

Informal checklists. Some counseling centers and agencies have developed informal checklists to be used in their facilities. An example of one of these brief checklists is included in Table 6.3. Some of these settings have performed studies on the reliability and validity of these instruments but many have not. If there is no psychometric information available, then the practitioner should proceed with caution. These informal checklists can provide some preliminary information, but counselors need to be cautious in using these results without reliability and validity information. These informal checklists can only be viewed as *possible* problems, and counselors' clinical decisions should never rest on this information. In using these checklists, clinicians should also be aware that some individuals have a tendency to check numerous items while others check very few. Therefore, a client who has checked numerous problems should not necessarily be viewed as being more disturbed than a client who checked only a few problems.

Rating Scales

A rating scale is slightly more sophisticated than a checklist, for these measures ask the client or an observer to provide some indication of the amount or

TABLE 6.3
Example of an informal checklist

What concerns now bring you to seek counseling service?

_____ Depression	_____ Emotional/physical/sexual abuse	_____ Career issues
_____ Anxiety	_____ Binge eating	_____ Academic concerns
_____ Stress	_____ Self-induced vomiting	_____ Financial pressures
_____ Anger control	_____ Relationship problems	_____ Multicultural issues
_____ Panic attacks	_____ Family conflict	_____ Sleep disturbance
_____ Fears/phobia	_____ Conflict with friends/roommates	_____ Physical complaints
_____ Grief/loss	_____ Conflict with faculty	_____ Obsessive thinking
_____ Suicidal thoughts	_____ Lack of relationship	_____ Alcohol/drug concerns
_____ Unwanted sexual experience	_____ Indecisiveness	_____ Lack of assertiveness
_____ Sexuality issue	_____ Low self-esteem	_____ Trauma/assault/accident

Other: (please specify) _____

TABLE 6.4

Example of an informal rating scale

Calm	— — — — — Nervous	Superior	— — — — — Inferior
Sad	— — — — — Happy	Indecisive	— — — — — Decisive
Outgoing	— — — — — Shy	Strong	— — — — — Weak
Fearful	— — — — — Confident	Compulsive	— — — — — Lackadaisical
Patient	— — — — — Impatient	Trusting	— — — — — Suspicious
Confident	— — — — — Anxious	Competitive	— — — — — Cooperative
Aggressive	— — — — — Submissive	Relaxed	— — — — Tense
Pessimistic	— — — — — Optimistic	Independent	— — — — — Dependent
Adventurous	— — — — — Timid	Irrational	— — — — — Rational
Energetic	— — — — — Lethargic	Confused	— — — — Insightful
Honest	— — — — — Shrewd	Moral	— — — — Wicked
Impulsive	— — — — — Planful	Hopeless	— — — — — Elated
Even-paced	— — — — — Erratic	Abusive	— — — — — Victimized
Sluggish	— — — — — Active	Sick	— — — — Well
Hostile	— — — — — Gentle	Courageous	— — — — — Afraid

degree of the problem, attitude, or personality trait being measured. Table 6.4 provides an example of an informal rating scale. Sometimes rating scales contain a numerical scale, where numbers are assigned to different categories. As an example, clients would rate their level of anxiety from (1) not at all anxious, to (5) extremely anxious. Another common rating scale is the semantic-differential, where like those in Table 6.4, the individuals choose between two bipolar terms.

There are a number of findings related to rating scales that are germane when counselors are interpreting these measures. In general people tend to respond in the middle of the ratings, which is called *central tendency error*. Individuals are less likely to rate themselves or others at either the low or the high extremes. Another finding pertains to *leniency error*, which concerns individuals' reluctance to assign unfavorable ratings. People are more likely to endorse the positive as compared to the negative. Finally, in terms of individuals' ratings of someone else, there often is a *halo effect*. This research indicates that people are influenced by first impressions and these impressions influence subsequent ratings. Thus, there can be either a positive halo or a negative halo effect.

Rating scales can also be incorporated into the initial assessment with clients. For example, clients could be asked to rate on a five- or a seven-point scale the severity of the problem, the degree to which the problem is affecting their daily functioning, their commitment to addressing the problem, and the likelihood that the problem will change. These informal rating scales can be asked verbally or incorporated into an intake form.

There also are standardized rating scales such as the *Conners' Rating Scales–Revised* (Conners, 1996). The *Conners' Rating Scales–Revised* are instruments designed for screening with children ages 3 through 17, with the instrument being completed either by the parent, teacher, or adolescent. There are both long forms and short forms for each of the three versions (parent, teacher, or adolescent). The Conners' ADHD (Attention Deficit Hyperactivity Disorder) Index can be derived from all versions of this scale. Besides this indicator of posssible ADHD, there are other scales (e.g., oppositional, anxious/shy, social problems).

Other Screening Inventories

There are a number of other initial screening instruments that are not checklists or rating scales. An example of these instruments is the *Problem Oriented Screening Instrument for Teenagers (POSIT)*. The POSIT was developed in a recent program initiated by the National Institute on Drug Abuse (NIDA) called the Adolescent Assessment/Referral System (Rahdert, 1997). The aim of the project was to identify an assessment and treatment referral system for troubled youths 12 through 19 years of age. After many years of working, a team of nationally known clinician/researchers developed the POSIT. The purpose of the POSIT is to screen for potential problem areas that should be assessed more thoroughly in order to select appropriate treatment options. There are ten functional areas that the POSIT assesses. The POSIT is composed of 139 yes/no items, with the results indicating whether a problem may exist in one or more of the ten areas. Currently, the POSIT and a personal history questionnaire are used to determine if further problem assessment is necessary. This new screening tool is only beginning to be used, but it has the potential to be very useful.

   In conclusion, there are a number of both formal and informal instruments that can supplement the initial information gathered in an intake interview. Some counselors incorporate these techniques routinely, whereas others will periodically use checklists, rating scales, or other types of inventories. Counselors can improve their effectiveness by using multiple methods for gathering information. No one source of information, such as a test, should be the sole basis of any decision. Multiple sources of information will provide a more comprehensive overview of the client and the client's problems. Sometimes in the process of gathering information, a counselor will determine the need to assess the client more thoroughly on a specific problem. For example, during the initial intake interview, the counselor may see signs of depression and want to gather information specific to depression. Thus far, we have discussed general initial assessment, but counselors also need to consider methods for assessing specific client problems.

Assessing Specific Problems in the Initial Sessions

Certain specific problems should be considered in the initial stages of counseling, because if these specific issues are overlooked there could be negative results, even the death of a client. For example, if the counselor does not assess clients' suicide potential, then a client may commit suicide when intervening would have saved the client's life. Depression is significantly related to suicide and is another factor that counselors should consider during the initial stage of counseling. A third area that counselors should assess in the initial intake is substance abuse because of the psychological and physiological effects of psychoactive substances. Although there are other specific problem areas that clinicians should consider in the initial assessment stage, these three will be discussed in detail because of the ramifications of misdiagnosing these problems.

Assessment of Suicide Potential

In the initial session, a counselor needs to evaluate each client's potential for suicide. Neglecting to identify a client with suicidal ideation could result in an avoidable death. The probability of working with a potentially suicidal client is high. According to the National Institute of Mental Health (NIMH, 1998), suicide is the ninth leading cause of death in the United States. In 1995, 31,284 individuals died as a result of suicide. Although suicide is rare for children before puberty, it does exist. For children ages 5 to 14, suicide is the seventh leading cause of death. Predicting which clients might commit suicide is very difficult because individuals often vary greatly from day to day and even from hour to hour. A counselor may work with a client who appears to be at minimal risk; however, a few hours later something may happen to significantly alter the risk of suicide (e.g., the client's spouse asks for a divorce).

Having information on the demographic factors that research shows are related to suicide can assist counselors in screening clients for potential suicide. In general, men are more likely than women to commit suicide, although some studies show women are more likely to attempt suicide (Garrison, 1992). These results, however, do not indicate that a woman's disclosure of suicidal thoughts is any less serious than a man's disclosure. Adolescent suicide has increased 300% in the last 20 years, but the suicidal rate for the elderly is still higher than the rate for teenagers. The group with the highest suicide rate is white men over 85, with a rate of 68.2/100,000 (NIMH, 1998). White clients are more likely to commit suicide than are minority clients, with white clients being twice as likely to commit suicide as African-American clients. However, suicide rates for certain Native American tribes are higher than the general population (Berlin, 1987). Marital status has also been found to be associated with risk; those who are single, divorced, or widowed are at greater risk than those who are married. Individuals responsible for children under the age of 18 have also been found to be at lower risk than those without those responsibilities.

There are also clinical aspects that should be considered when evaluating clients for the potential of committing suicide. Major depression and alcoholism account for between 57% and 86% of all suicides, with the majority of those being related to depression (Clark & Fawcett, 1992). The relationship between depression and suicide is so significant that all depressed clients should be evaluated for possible suicidal ideation. One of the important signs to look for in suicide assessment is a sense of hopelessness or helplessness. For most suicidal clients, the situation seems hopeless and the only way to end the pain is through death. In addition, those who have attempted suicide before are likely to try again. A client who has a history of a psychiatric disorder is also at greater risk than one who has never suffered from a disorder. For children, adolescents, and adults, a recent loss, divorce, or separation will increase the chances of attempting suicide. Other personality factors found to be related to suicide are impulsivity, inability to express emotions, perfectionism and superresponsibility, sensitivity, pessimism, and dependency (Stelmacher, 1995).

Counselors need to be proficient in detecting suicidal thoughts and assessing the intensity of those thoughts. Counselors must assess accurately in order to determine if clients are in immediate danger of harming themselves. If the client is in immediate danger, then the practitioner must have procedures for responding to this potentially deadly situation. Stelmachers (1995) recommended that clinicians concentrate on seven areas when assessing the risk of suicide.

1. *Verbal Communication.* If a client verbalizes that he or she is considering suicide, then that is a clearly identifiable signal to investigate the lethality of the situation. Counselors need to listen closely because some clients will be very subtle in their disclosures. For example, a client may say in a causal manner, "Sometimes I just want to end it all." Themes of escape, reducing tension, punishing, or self-mutilation can be signs of possible suicidal ideation. Sometimes beginning-level counselors feel uncomfortable asking clients if they are going to commit suicide. A less abrupt approach is to ask clients if they have ever considered harming themselves. Even jokes about suicide should be pursued. A counselor should never be lulled into a false sense of security if a client denies having any suicidal thoughts.

2. *Plan.* If there is any indication of possible suicidal thoughts, then the next step for the counselor is to assess if there is an actual suicide plan. The counselor's concern for the client should increase if a plan exists and if the plan is specific, concrete, and detailed. However, impulsive clients may not have developed a plan but may still commit suicide if the situation deteriorates.

3. *Method.* The counselor should investigate whether a specific method has been selected. In analyzing the method, the counselor needs to evaluate the availability of the method and degree to which the method is lethal. McIntosh (1992) found that firearms accounted for more than half of the suicidal deaths, followed by hanging, strangulation, and suffocation, while taking poisons often did not result in death. A counselor needs to determine the degree to which there is a risk and the feasibility of the suicidal plan. The counselor should also explore if the method includes provisions to avoid being rescued (or the opposite, where the plan facilitates being rescued).

4. *Preparation.* Another area to explore involves whether the client has started the preparation process. For example, some clients will have

secured the gun or pills already or even have written the suicide note. Sometimes the preparation process will be subtle, where the client will be giving away possessions or getting finances in order. The level of danger is proportionally related to the amount of preparation.

5. *Stressors.* One of the areas to assess is the past, present, and future stressors. A client may not be in immediate danger but may quickly become suicidal if certain circumstances occur. Stressors that are commonly associated with suicide are loss (particularly loss of a significant relationship), physical illness, and unemployment. For some clients, anniversaries or special days are difficult and may exacerbate the sense of loss and depression. Identifying the potential stressors will also be helpful in the continual monitoring of suicide potential. If the counselor identifies potential stressors, then the clinician can respond more proactively when the stressors begin to build.

6. *Mental State.* The assessment of the client's mental state is important in determining both the immediate and long-term risks. As covered earlier, certain psychological factors, such as depression, are clearly associated with attempting suicide. Clients reporting being despondent, impotent, angry, guilty, distraught, and tormented should be continually monitored. A client who suddenly improves should not always be viewed positively. Some clients who are in the process of becoming more actively suicidal will have uplifted spirits because they have finally found a solution to ending the pain. In the assessment of mental state, the practitioners would be wise to assess the client's use of alcohol and drugs. These psychoactive substances can affect impulsivity and other emotions, thereby increasing the suicidal risk. Another consideration is possible homicidal behaviors, which are occasionally combined with suicidal behaviors.

7. *Hopelessness.* Most suicidal clients will exhibit a degree of hopelessness. Study after study has documented the prevalence of this affective state with suicidal individuals (Stelmachers, 1995). Often death is seen as the only method for relieving the pain. The degree of hopelessness should be explored with clients who verbalize some suicidal thoughts. In addition, the level of hopelessness is a gauge to determine the risk for clients who do not report any suicidal thoughts.

A counselor does *not* just assess suicide risk once; any assessment of suicide is time limited and pertains only to the risks under current circumstances. Therefore, counselors need to continually reevaluate the suicide potential of clients. Sometimes clinicians may enlist the family in the monitoring of the client. There are also formal instruments that were constructed to assess the risk of suicide. Most clinicians, however, do not use these instruments in isolation but use both interviewing and observation in conjunction with a formal instrument.

Suicide potential instruments. The *Suicide Probability Scale* (Cull & Gill, 1992) is a 36-item instrument that provides an overall measure of suicide risk. For more detailed information, there are subscales that assess hopelessness, suicide ideation, negative self-evaluation, and hostility. An advantage of this instrument is that there are separate norms for normal individuals, psychiatric patients, and lethal suicide attempters (those who attempted suicide using a method that could have been lethal).

Aaron Beck, the noted cognitive therapist, has constructed two scales that are related to suicide potential. The *Beck Scale for Suicide Ideation* (Beck & Steer, 1991) can be used to identify and screen clients who will acknowledge suicidal thoughts. There are five screening items that reduce the amount of time for clients who are not reporting any suicidal ideation. The authors recommended that this instrument not be used alone but in combination with other assessment tools. Another of Beck's instruments, the *Beck Hopelessness Scale* (Beck & Steer, 1993), has been shown to be related to measures of suicidal intent and ideation. This instrument also has norms available for suicidal clients. Another noted contributor in the area of assessment, William Reynolds, has developed three instruments in this area. Two of the instruments screen for suicidal ideation: the *Suicidal Ideation Questionnaire* (Reynolds, 1988) is for adolescents and the *Adult Suicidal Ideation Questionnaire* (Reynolds, 1991) is for adults. The *Suicidal Behavior History Form* (Reynolds & Mazza, 1992) is a semi-structured interview that provides a systematic method of obtaining and documenting a history of suicidal behaviors.

Validating instruments that would assess potential to commit suicide is somewhat problematic. It would not be ethical to give a sample of potentially suicidal individuals an instrument and then simply sit back and collect data on which ones actually committed suicide. Hence, a counselor using an instrument needs to examine the validation information in order to determine what the instrument measures (e.g., suicidal ideation, correlation with depression measures, attempted suicide). None of the instruments designed to specifically identify suicide potential is sufficiently refined to use in isolation. In order to screen for suicide, the counselor needs both astute observational and interviewing skills combined with trained clinical decision making. Some practitioners will also use other instruments in the global assessment of suicide potential, such as measures of depression, personality, or symptom checklists. A counselor should consult with another professional if there are any concerns related to the assessment of suicide risk. Often times with a suicidal client, a counselor may need to ensure that the client receives a psychiatric evaluation.

Depression Assessment

Because of depression's direct connection to suicide, it is important for counselors to begin to assess for depression early in the counseling process. Depression is characterized by feelings of sadness that can range from the common "blues" to severe depression. In order to assess whether a client is depressed, a counselor needs to have understanding of some of the common characteristics of depressed clients. With some clients the symptoms of depression will be easily recognized. With other clients there may be "masked depression," where the client wants to conceal the dysphoric mood or may be denying the depressed feelings. In cases of masked depression, practitioners need to understand the subtle signs of depression and explore the issue further if initial suspicions of depression are confirmed.

According to McNamara (1992), the symptoms of depression usually include a dysphoric mood that is often accompanied by feelings of anxiety, guilt, and resentment. Depression is characterized by difficulties with concentration, decision making, and problem solving. Clients tend to be pessimistic and have negative attitudes toward themselves, others, and the world. Behavioral and physical symptoms are also usually present, particularly if the depression is more serious. Social withdrawal is a symptom, and the clients are often prone to crying, inactivity, and loss of interest in activities that were previously pleasurable. In terms of physical symptoms, fatigue is almost always present. This can be accompanied by loss of appetite and inability to sleep, or the reverse may be true where the appetite and the amount of sleep required increases substantially. Headaches, muscle aches, and decreased libido are other indicators of possible depression. In some cases, there may be a reduction in speech and a slowing of body movements.

The assessment of depression includes determining both the severity of the depression and the type of depression. Chapter 13, which addresses diagnosis, will discuss different types of depression. Many of the symptoms are common to the different types of depression; yet, the practitioner must be skilled in differentiating among the types and assessing the risk of suicide. Sometimes clinicians will employ one of the following standardized instruments to assess the severity of the depression. Included in the clinician's assessment of depression is whether the client should be referred for a psychiatric evaluation and possible medication.

Beck Depression Inventory. Ponterotto, Pace, and Kavan (1989) identified 73 different measures of depression used by researchers or mental health practitioners. Of these different measures, the *Beck Depression Inventory* (BDI) was the most commonly used. In fact, the BDI was used 10 times more often than the second most popular instrument. A new version of the BDI has recently been published, the *Beck Depression Inventory-II* (BDI-II, Beck, Steer, & Brown, 1996). The BDI was revised to align with the *Diagnostic and Statistical Manual of Mental Disorders-Fourth Edition* (DSM-IV) criteria for depression. Like its predecessor, the BDI-II contains only 21 items and usually takes clients about five minutes to complete. With each item, there are four choices that increase in level of severity. Therefore, the BDI-II results provide an index of the severity of the depression. Due to the recent revision, there is limited psychometric information available on the BDI-II. The overall coefficient alpha is higher for the BDI-II (.92) than the BDI. Steer and Clark's (1997) research with college students supported the high reliability of the BDI-II and contributed to the construct validity of the instrument. The BDI-II is based on the BDI, which was extensively researched. Reviews of the BDI (Conoley, 1994; Sundberg, 1994) were generally positive but stressed the BDI should not be used alone in the assessment of depression. In addition, Conoley warned that the items related to suicide could easily be faked.

Other depression instruments. There are other standardized instruments that could be used in the assessment of depression. For children and adolescents, there are the *Children's Depression Inventory* (Kovacs, 1992), *Children's Depression Rating Scale, Revised* (Poznanski & Mokros, 1996), the *Reynolds Adolescent Depression Scale* (Reynolds, 1987), and the *Reynolds Child Depression Scale* (Reynolds, 1989). Other instruments besides the BDI-II for adults are the *Hamilton Depression Inventory* (Reynolds & Kobak, 1995), and the *State Trait-Depression Adjective Check Lists* (Lubin, 1994). The *Revised Hamilton Rating Scale for Depression* (Warren, 1994) is another instrument designed to assess the client's level of depression; however, the clinician rather than the client completes this instrument.

Substance Abuse Assessment

According to Greene and Banken (1995), clinicians frequently fail to recognize clients' symptoms as reflecting substance abuse or dependence. The prevalence of substance abuse in clinical settings is high, with the range of estimates being between 12 and 30 percent (Moore et al., 1989). It has not been determined what precisely constitutes *abuse* of a substance as compared to use of a substance. In Chapter 13, there will be a discussion of the criteria for a diagnosis of Substance Abuse.

In counseling it is important to identify early whether a client has a substance abuse problem. A counselor who does not explore the possibility of substance abuse could easily proceed with addressing issues that are essentially a result of the client's substance abuse. One method for exploring the possibility of substance abuse is to simply ask the client. Oetting and Beauvais (1990) found that self-reports were reasonably reliable. There are, however, some problems with validity because some clients are reluctant to disclose the use of certain substances or the amount of use. Nevertheless, counselors should explore with every client what drugs they are taking and the amount of alcohol they typically consume. In terms of medications, prescription, over-the-counter, and street drugs should all be explored. These should be investigated, first, because heavy use of any of these types of drugs can be problematic. A second reason for exploring all types of drugs is because even some commonly used over-the-counter medications have side effects. Sometimes client's symptoms (e.g., being tired all the time) are a result of the medication; counselors need to consult the *Physician's Desk Reference* in order to be knowledgeable about the side effects of any drug the client is taking. The following are some examples of questions to ask a client, particularly if the clients indicate that they are drinking or taking drugs.

1. Do you take any medications, over-the-counter drugs, or other drugs such as street drugs? If medication or over-the-counter drugs are used, for what and how much? If street drug, what and how much?
2. Do you drink alcohol? If yes, how many drinks in a typical week?
3. How often do you get drunk or high in a typical week?
4. When did you start drinking or taking the drug(s)?
5. Has anyone ever mentioned that this is a problem? Who? Why do you think they see it as a problem?
6. Where and with whom do you usually drink or use drugs?
7. Has drinking or taking the drugs ever caused you any problems (e.g., problems with family, employers, friends, or "the law")?
8. Have you ever tried to quit? What happened? Were there any withdrawal symptoms?
9. Is your drinking or drug use causing you any financial difficulties?
10. Do you ever mix drugs or mix drugs and alcohol? Do you ever substitute one substance with another substance?

Early in the counseling process, the counselor needs to focus on assessing which substances are used, the amount taken, and the problems associated with the substance use. Another topic that should be included in assessment of substance abuse is the social and interpersonal aspects, as this information will be helpful in the treatment phase. Treatment will vary depending on whether the client is alone or drinking or using with friends. Another goal is to identify the external and internal triggers that precede the use of the substance.

Standardized instruments in substance abuse. There are a number of standardized instruments designed specifically to assess substance abuse. Table 6.5 includes a listing of some of the more frequently used instruments in this area. One instrument that is used by practitioners in this area is the *Substance Abuse Subtle Screening Inventory* (SASSI-2, SASSI Institute, 1996). The SASSI Institute purported that the SASSI-2 has an 88 percent rate of accuracy in identifying individuals with substance-related disorders. Because of the newness of the revision of this instrument, there is not sufficient research to see if other researchers support these findings. Another commonly used assessment tool is the CAGE, which is a simple interviewing technique often used in medical settings. The CAGE (Mayfield, McLeod, & Hall, 1974) is a mnemonic device for four questions:

1. Have you ever felt you need to **cut down** on your drinking?
2. Have people **annoyed** you by criticizing your drinking?
3. Have you ever felt bad or **guilty about drinking**?
4. Have you ever had a drink first thing in the morning to steady your nerves or get rid of a hangover (**eye opener**)?

If the answers to these questions indicate a problem, then the clinician should gather more detailed information about the drinking. Sometimes, however, clients will deny that drinking or drug use is a problem. One technique is

TABLE 6.5

Assessment related to substance abuse

Harrell, A. V., & Wirtz, P.W. (1989). *Adolescent Drinking Index.* Port Huron, MI: Sigma Assessment System.

Horn, J. L., Wanberg, K. W., & Foster, F. M. (1987). *Alcohol Use Inventory.* Minneapolis, MN: National Computer Systems.

Miller, G. (1990). *Substance Abuse Screening Form—Adolescent Form.* Bloomington, IN: SASSI Institute.

Miller, G. (1990). *Substance Abuse Screening Form—Adult Version 3.* Bloomington, IN: SASSI Institute.

Miller W. R. (1984). *Comprehensive Drinker Profile.* Odessa, FL: PAR.

Schonfeld, L., Peters, R., & Dolente, A. (1993). *Substance Abuse Relapse Assessment.* Odessa, FL: PAR.

Skinner, H. A. (1982). *The Drug Abuse Screening Test-20: Guidelines for Administering and Scoring.* Toronto: Addiction Research Foundation.

Winter, K. C. (1996). *Personal Experience Inventory for Adults.* Los Angeles: Western Psychological Services.

Winter, K. C., & Henly, G. A. (1989). *Personal Experience Inventory.* Los Angeles: Western Psychological Services.

to have the client self-monitor and record all drinking. Some clients will be surprised by the amount recorded. Another technique, sometimes referred to as the "acid test," is to ask the client to control or limit his drinking. For example, the client would be asked to have no more than three drinks at any one occasion for three months. This will provide an indication if the drinking can be controlled.

In the assessment of substance abuse, the counselor must also assess whether he or she can provide the appropriate services. With some clients, it is necessary to refer them to specialists in this area. There are other times when the appropriate referral would be to an outpatient program or an inpatient facility specializing in substance abuse.

Summary

The initial process of gathering information in counseling usually involves the counselor interviewing the client. The skill with which the counselor performs this initial assessment has an influence on the effectiveness of the counseling. Interviewing is one of the most frequently used counseling assessment tools. Because interviewing is used so frequently, counselors should consider the reliability and validity of their own interviews. Within the initial interview or intake interview, it is important not only to identify the most pressing problems but also to explore the major problems from diverse perspectives. Gathering detailed information about the problems will provide a sound foundation for the selection of interventions and treatment approaches. Prochaska et al. (1992) found that assessing where the clients are in the change process is also important information to gather before determining the treatment strategy. Structured, semi-structured, and unstructured interviews each have strengths and limitations.

Some counselors incorporate formal and informal assessment measures into the initial paperwork completed by the client. Checklists and rating scales can be an efficient method for gathering information. Commonly used instruments are the *Symptom Checklist-90-Revised* or the shorter version of this instrument, the *Brief Symptoms Inventory Symptom Checklist*. These measures of symptoms can also be used through the counseling process to monitor if there are decreases in symptoms (e.g., feeling anxious) as a result of the counseling. An initial screening instrument that shows promise is the POSIT for adolescents that was recently developed by the National Institute on Drug Abuse. With some of the checklists and rating scales for children, a parent or guardian completes them rather than the child. Besides using standardized instruments, counselors can develop informal checklists and rating scales; however, these should be used with extreme caution.

The initial assessment of the client also needs to consider specific issues, such as potential suicide, depression, and/or substance abuse. Assessment of these potential problems should involve a multifaceted approach. Because of the ramification of suicide, counselors should routinely include an investigation of suicide potential in their counseling with clients. An assessment of suicidal risk should include an investigation of possible intent, whether there are plans and a specific method, the progress made in instituting the plan, and an evaluation of the client's mental state, particularly the degree of hopelessness. The evaluation of suicide potential should not be a single process but rather a continual monitoring and evaluating of the potential risk. Depression is a common disorder, and counselors need to be aware of the subtle signs of depression in order to assess the severity of the depression. Substance abuse is another area counselors need to include in their initial assessment. Because many clients deny that either alcohol or drugs are a problem, the counselor should systematically explore both drug and alcohol use with clients. The assessment of substance abuse needs to include inquiry into the amount of the substance used, whether the use can be controlled, and the consequences of the use.

CHAPTER 7

Intelligence and General Ability Testing

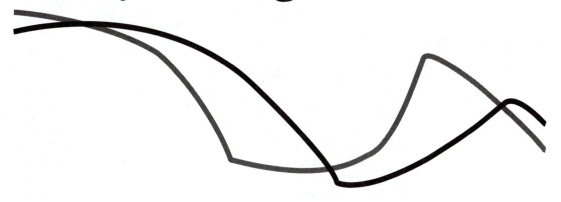

Very few counselors will be involved in the administration of individual intelligence tests; however, many counselors will be involved in activities that require knowledge of intelligence testing. A school counselor is often a regular member of the committee that compiles Individual Educational Plans (IEPs) for students with special educational needs. Mental health counselors frequently work with individuals with learning disabilities or other cognitive impairments that were diagnosed with intelligence testing. Parents often seek the help of a marriage and family counselor when they suspect their child is not achieving in school at a level that is reflective of the child's intellectual level. A rehabilitation counselor may work with a client who has recently experienced a traumatic brain injury. In all of these cases, knowledge of intelligence testing will assist counselors in better serving their clients.

Although terms such as intelligence and IQ are a common part of everyday language, there is no uniformity within the profession on either the definition or the structure of intelligence. Some professionals in the field of assessment prefer the term *general ability* because of the negative connotations associated with intelligence testing. The debate about the meaning of intelligence and intelligence test scores is somewhat emotionally charged. According to Neisser et al. (1996), political agendas rather than scientific knowledge often fuel the debate related to intelligence testing. In order to facilitate the understanding of intelligence testing, this chapter will briefly review several different perspectives on the nature of intelligence. This overview of models will lay a foundation for the discussion of the specific intelligence or general ability tests. Included in the discussion of intelligence tests will be both individually administered and group tests. The chapter will then conclude with a summary of research related to pertinent issues in intelligence testing.

Models of Intelligence

Psychometric Approach to the Study

A major influence since the turn of the century on the study of individual differences in intelligence has been the *psychometric* (or differential) *approach.* Psychometric theories of intelligence are based on the premise that intelligence can be described in terms of *mental factors* (Bjorklund, 1995). Factors are general mental skills that influence mental performance in a variety of situations. The term *factor* is used in this approach because many of the theorists have used the statistical technique of factor analysis as the basis for their assertions. From this theoretical perspective, researchers need to identify one or more factors of intelligence, and intelligence tests would then be developed to measure differences on those identified factors. Theorists, however, are not in total agreement on the number or types of factors that constitute intelligence.

At one extreme in terms of the number of factors in intelligence is *Spearman's* (1927) model. Spearman was one of the first theorists to discuss factors and he postulated a two-factor theory of intelligence. Spearman contended that everyone has *g,* or a *general ability factor,* that influences performance on all intellectual tasks. The second type of factors was specific factors that influence performance in specific areas. Spearman contended that these specific factors were all to some degree correlated with *g* (general ability) and that, in essence, intelligence was a rather homogeneous construct. To put it very simply, smart people were smart and dumb people were dumb. This homogeneous view of intelligence has had considerable influence on peoples' views of intelligence.

On the other end of the continuum concerning the number of factors in intelligence is Guilford's (1967, 1988) structure-of-intelligence theory that includes 180 unique intellectual factors that are organized around three dimensions. Figure 7.1 illustrates this complex model in which the first dimension is *mental operations* and contains six forms. These mental operations can involve five *content areas,* which is the second dimension. Finally, there are six possible *products,* the third dimension, that interact with the combinations of operations and content areas.

Between the extremes of Spearman and Guilford is another early theorist, Thurstone, who also had considerable influence on others' views of intelli-

FIGURE 7.1

Guilford's structure-of-intelligence model

From Educational and Psychological Measurement, *Vol. 48, p. 1–4. Reprinted by permission of Sage Publications, Inc.*

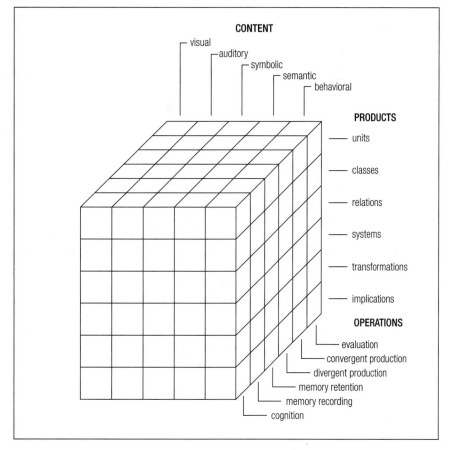

gence. Thurstone (1938) originally proposed a model of seven "primary mental abilities" rather than one solitary factor. Thurstone in several studies demonstrated that seven common factors collectively accounted for most of the individual differences associated with intelligence. These seven primary mental abilities were: (1) *Verbal comprehension,* (2) *Word fluency,* (3) *Number facility,* (4) *Perceptual speed,* (5) *Memory,* (6) *Space,* and (7) *Reasoning.* Thurstone's original theory did not include a general ability factor (*g*), but he did propose that the different factors were somewhat related to each other.

Other factor theorists were primarily hierarchical in their approach. One of these theorists was Vernon (1950), who contended there was a *g* and two second-order factors, "v:ed" representing verbal and educational aptitudes and "k:m" representing spatial, mechanical, and practical aptitudes (see Figure 7.2). Other abilities then branched down from these levels to other levels. Another theorist who proposed second-order factors was Cattell (1971, 1979). In this model, the second-order factors are *fluid abilities* (Gf) and *crystallized abilities* (Gc). Cattell proposed that fluid abilities are biologically determined and

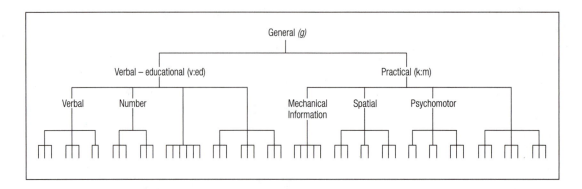

General *(g)*

Verbal – educational (v:ed)

Practical (k:m)

Verbal   Number

Mechanical   Spatial   Psychomotor
Information

FIGURE 7.2

Vernon's hierarchical model of intelligence

affect all fields of relational perception. Fluid abilities are considered to be relatively culturally free and are often reflected in tests of memory span and spatial thinking. Crystallized abilities, on the other hand, include acquired skills and knowledge and are influenced more by cultural, social, and educational experiences. Tests of verbal comprehension and social relations are tapping crystallized abilities. As we will see, Cattell's theory had a direct influence on the development of the Stanford-Binet Intelligence Scale: Fourth Edition. Horn (Horn, 1985; Horn & Noll, 1997) has expanded Cattell's theory and added several other intelligences to the Gf-Gc model.

There are more similarities among the psychometric approaches than what might at first appear. Toward the end of their careers Spearman and Thurstone's views became more similar. Spearman acknowledged that separate group factors (e.g., verbal abilities, mathematical reasoning) do exist and Thurstone concluded that his primary factors are correlated, suggesting the possibility of one general factor. In general, most psychometricians agree that there is one general ability factor (*g*) and a number of lower-level factors that reflect more specific skills. Differences among the theorists are primarily related to the extent to which intelligence can be described by *g* and the make-up of the lower-level factors (Bjorklund, 1995).

Developmental progressions. Rather than focusing solely on the structure of intelligence, developmental theorists suggest that intelligence can be understood better by examining how intelligence develops. The most well known of the developmental theorists is Jean Piaget (1972). Unlike the psychometricians, Piaget had little interest in how individuals might differ in intellectual abilities, for he was interested in children's development. Others have adapted Piaget's concepts to the analysis of individual differences and measuring intelligence. One of the ways in which Piagetian approaches have influenced the measuring of intellectual functioning is through the examination of differences in development.

Piaget suggested a developmental progression, with individuals moving sequentially through the stages of the *sensorimotor* period, *preoperational* period, *concrete* period, and *formal operations* period. Children move through these successively higher stages of intellectual development through the use of two intellectual functions. One of these is *assimilation,* which is the process by which a child incorporates a stimulus into an existing cognitive structure or schema. The second process is *accommodation* and this is the process in which the child creates a new schema or significantly alters an existing schema based on new information. According to Piaget, cognitive development does not occur only through maturation; learning and the environment also influence the process. Piaget's tasks can be modified to serve as measures of individual differences; however, the tasks have not directly influenced the major standardized tests of intelligence.

Another developmental theorist that is having an increasing influence on the field of education is the Russian psychologist Vygotsky. Vygotsky's theories are complex and currently are having an influence on instruction but little influence on intelligence testing.

Some researchers have recently been interested in biological development, particularly the study of the brain as the basis for measuring intelligence (Neisser et al., 1996). With increasing sophistication in brain imaging technology, it soon may be possible to understand more on the influence of biological development and specific characteristics of brain functioning.

Related to biology is Ceci's (1990,1993) bioecological theory, which is a recent theory that also incorporates a developmental perspective in the understanding of intelligence. Ceci believes that biological factors have a major influence on intelligence; however, he contends that there is no single, underlying factor (*g*), nor is human intelligence highly heritable. Ceci, along with others, sees intelligence as being multifaceted, with individuals varying in the domain-general abilities. Therefore, there are not intelligent people, only people who are intelligent in certain domains. *Context* is central to Ceci's theory, for he argued that intellectual abilities are highly influenced by the context in which they are gathered or performed. For example, one of his studies showed that children learned better when the context was a video game versus a laboratory context. The context in which people learn affects the knowledge base individuals possess and this is also central to Ceci's theory. Thus, Ceci argued, some individuals' intelligence might not be reflected in the methods currently used to assess intelligence. He contended that intelligence is reflected in knowledge acquisition and the ability to process, integrate, and elaborate on this knowledge in a complex manner.

Information processing. Rather than studying the structures or development of intelligence, information processing models focus on how individuals process information. Hence, the focus is not on *what* we process (factors of intelligence) but on *how* we process. One information processing approach that has had an influence on intelligence testing is the work of Luria (1966). Luria proposed that intellect could best be described by two methods of processing information: simultaneous processing and sequential processing. **Simultaneous processing** involves the mental ability to integrate input all at once. To solve simultaneous processing items correctly, an individual must mentally integrate fragments of information to "see" the whole. **Sequential processing** involves different processing skills, where the individual must arrange the stimuli in sequential or serial order in order to solve the problem. An example of these processing methods being used in intelligence assessment is the Kaufman Assessment Battery for Children (K-ABC, Kaufman & Kaufman, 1983).

An information processing theory that has recently received some attention is Sternberg's (1985, 1988) triarchic theory. Sternberg's theory of intelligence is quite extensive and incorporates three subtheories: (a) the internal world of the individual or the mental processes that underlie intelligence; (b) the experiential subtheory; and (c) the contextual or external world of the individual. The information processing portion of the theory is part of the first subtheory, which addresses the internal world of the individual. According to Sternberg, individuals' abilities to process information depend on their use of three components: the metacomponents, the performance components, and the knowledge-acquisition components. The *metacomponents* are the higher-order, executive processes that are used to plan what to do, monitor it while it's being done, and then evaluate it after it's done. Consider, for example, the interaction between planning abilities and intellectual capabilities. Sternberg argued that more intelligent people focus on critical issues that need to be solved, while less intelligent people attend to less important situations. The metacomponents influence the *performance components* selected (e.g., encoding, mental comparisons, retrieval of information). Once again individuals vary in their abilities to use these performance skills. According to Sternberg, intelligence is related to selecting the appropriate strategies for processing diverse information. The third component, *knowledge acquisition,* is where we selectively encode, combine, and compare information to add to our knowledge base. Thus, Sternberg argues that differences in intelligence are a reflection of differences in people's abilities to process information at the metacomponent, performance, or knowledge-acquisition levels.

The second subtheory within Sternberg's triarachic theory is related to the relationship between experience and intelligence. This subtheory is related to the ability to process information within existing experience. According to Sternberg, intelligence is best measured when the task is rather novel or when the task is in the process of becoming automatized. In Sternberg's view, the ability to deal with novelty is a good measure of intelligence. In essence, more intelligent people are able to react more quickly and process the information more efficiently. Another of his contentions is that the ability to automatize is also an indicator of intellect. If a person is effective at automatizing information, then the individual will have more resources available for dealing with novelty.

The third subtheory within Sternberg's theory concerns the contextual or external world of the individual. Sternberg contended that intelligence is contextually bound. For example, having an uncanny knowledge of elephants' migratory patterns is not highly valued in many settings in Western society. Thus, people will vary in their abilities to select, adapt, and shape environments, which are also, according to Sternberg, marks of intelligence. Although Sternberg's theory has not had a direct influence on intelligence instruments, his contention that intelligence tests only measure a selective portion of the complex construct of intelligence is having an influence. Most of us probably know someone who would not do particularly well on the instruments we will discuss later in this chapter; however, the person may be "street smart" or "have an uncanny ability to size the situation up." Sternberg is one of the leaders in promoting the expansion of the methods of viewing and measuring intelligence.

Other theories. Another theorist who has also advocated for expanding our views of intelligence is Gardner (1993) and his theory of multiple intelligences. Gardner contended that any set of adult competencies that are valued in a culture merits consideration as a potential intelligence. As the name of his theory implies, he argued that there are *multiple* intelligences rather than one single entity. Gardner's theory is different from others, such as Thurstone, in that he proposes seven relatively independent "frames of mind": (1) linguistic, (2) logical-mathematical, (3) musical, (4) spatial, (5) bodily-kinesthetic, (6) interpersonal, and (7) intrapersonal. Gardner suggested that current psychometric tests only measure linguistic, logical, and some aspects of spatial intelligence, while ignoring the other intelligences. He has argued that measures need to value intellectual capacities in a wide range of domains and that the methods should be appropriate for the domain (e.g., for spatial ability, testing individual's ability to navigate in a new city). There are some difficulties with implementing Gardner's ideas, but his theory has attracted considerable attention in the assessment area.

In conclusion, the different theoretical approaches have had an influence on the assessment of intelligence. The psychometric approach has had the most direct influence on the instruments that are commonly used today. The newer theories, however, provide some important insight into the complexities of intelligence testing and will certainly influence future methods. As we have seen, defining and conceptualizing intelligence is often perplexing, which means the measuring of intelligence is also plagued by many of these same issues.

Individual Intelligence Testing

As stated earlier, counselors are typically not responsible for the administration, scoring, and interpretation of individual intelligence tests. In order to administer an individual intelligence test, a professional must have certain course work and receive specific training and supervision on the use of that instrument. This chapter will not provide the necessary information to become proficient in the administration and interpretation of these instruments. The intent of this chapter, however, is to overview commonly used tests so that counselors can use these results in counseling contexts or participate in multidisciplinary teams involving intelligence assessment. This overview will include a brief description of the most widely used instruments.

Wechsler Scales

David Wechsler has been extraordinarily influential in the testing of intelligence. Wechsler developed a series of three intelligence instruments that are similar in approach but geared toward different age groups. The *Wechsler Preschool and Primary Scale of Intelligence—Revised* (WPPSI-R, Wechsler, 1989) is designed for children 3 through 7 years 3 months old; the *Wechsler Intelligence Scale for Children—Third Edition* (WISC-III, Wechsler, 1991) is for children 6 through 16; and the *Wechsler Adult Intelligence Scale—Third Edition* (WAIS-III, Wechsler, 1997) is for individuals 16 through 89 years old. The Wechsler scales are commonly cited in research, and numerous reports on test usage indicate that the Wechsler instruments are the most frequently used intelligence tests (Archer, Maruish, Imhof, & Piotrowski, 1991; Piotrowski & Keller, 1989). If we examine all types of test results that counselors use, the results from the Wechsler scales are frequently used. Elmore, Ekstrom, Diamond, and Whittaker (1993) found the WISC-R to be the most widely used assessment instruments by school counselors, and Bubenzer, Zimpfer, and Mahrle (1990) found the WAIS-R to be the third most widely used instrument and the WISC-R the fifth most widely used instrument by community mental health counselors. Because of their widespread use, counselors should be familiar with these instruments and the strengths and limitations of the Wechsler scales.

The WPPSI-R, the WISC-III, and the WAIS-III all have 12 to 14 subscales that contribute to a Full Scale IQ, a Verbal IQ, and a Performance IQ (see Figure 7.3). All three of these IQ measures are deviation IQs and have a mean of 100 and a standard deviation of 15. The Full Scale IQ is the global and aggregate measure of cognitive abilities. The Verbal IQ measures intelligence using verbal mechanisms. The Performance IQ is designed to be a nonverbal measure of intelligence and requires the individual to manipulate objects rather than answer questions. The Performance subtests were designed to overcome the biases associated with language and culture. In a psychological assessment report, some psychologists may focus on the differences between an examinee's performance on the Verbal as compared to the Performance scales. There are, however, divergent views on the meanings of the discrepancies between the Verbal and Performance scores and how the discrepant scores should be interpreted.

Due to the similarities of all the Wechsler intelligence instruments, the following information on the *Wechsler Intelligence Scale for Children—Third Edition* (WISC-III) will also acquaint the reader with many aspects of the WPPSI-R and the WAIS-III. Tables 7.1 and 7.2 provide a brief overview of the scales that are mandatory in the WISC-III. There are some minor differences within the subscales among the WISC-III, the WAIS-III, and the WPPSI-R, but this summary provides a good introduction to the subscales. The verbal subtests are: Information, Similarities, Arithmetic, Vocabulary, and Comprehension (see Table 7.1 for brief descriptions of these subscales). Even Arithmetic is considered a Verbal subscale because many of the items are read to the examinee. The subtests in the performance area are: Picture Completion, Coding, Picture

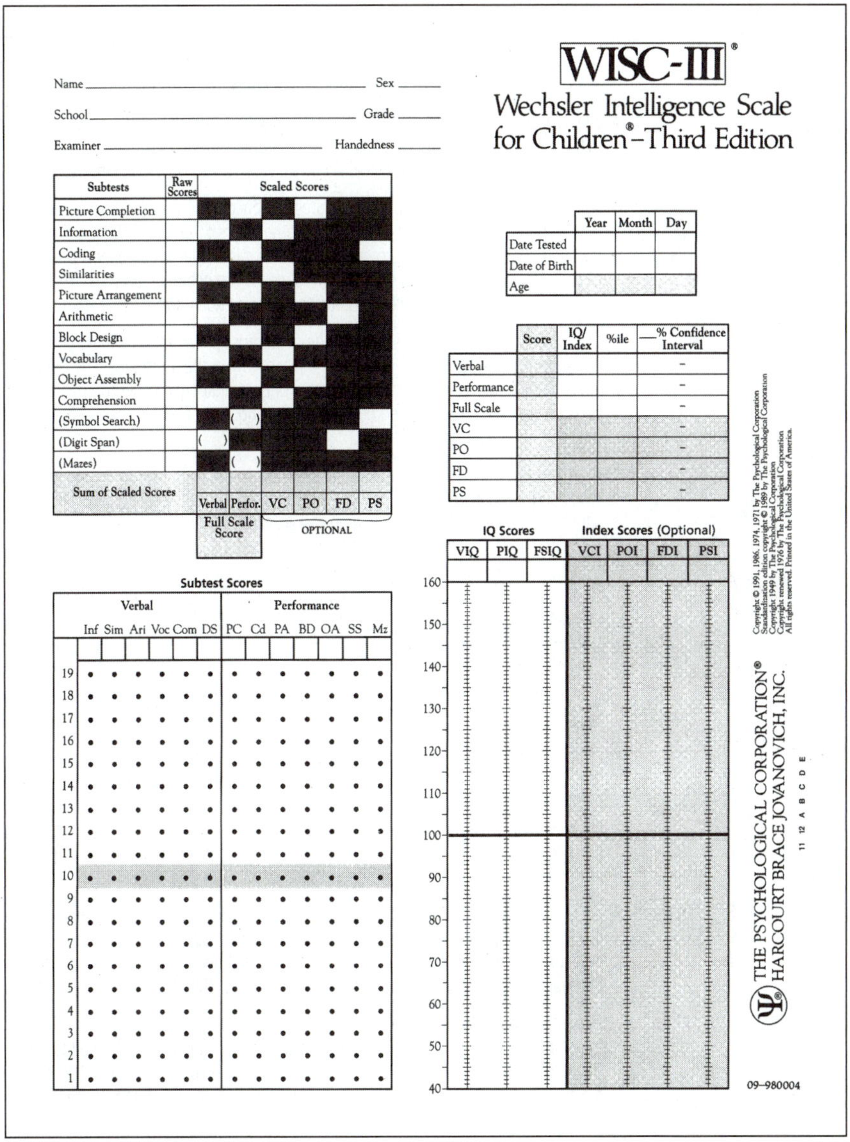

FIGURE 7.3

Profile for the Wechsler Intelligence Scale for Children—Third Edition

Arrangement, Block Design, and Object Assembly (see Table 7.2 for brief descriptions of these subscales). All of these subscales involve the manipulation of objects such as blocks and puzzles. Interested readers should see Kamphaus (1993) for an explanation of the three supplementary scales of the WISC-III, Digit Span, Symbol, and Mazes. It should be noted that a new subtest, Matrix Reasoning, is mandatory in the WAIS-III. All subtests have a mean of 10 and a standard deviation of 3.

TABLE 7.1

*Brief description
of the verbal
subtests of the
WISC-III*

- *Information.* The information subtest taps an individual's general knowledge. The subtest requires the child to answer factual questions (e.g., "Who was the first president of the United States?"). The scale provides an indication of knowledge base, verbal expressive skills, and long-term memory. Educational and cultural background will influence performance on the Information subscale.

- *Similarities.* On this subtest the child has to identify similarity between two verbal concepts. The relationships initially measure learned association, but the items increase in complexity in order to measure higher-order skills. This subtest measures the ability to analyze relationships and the level of logical and abstract reasoning.

- *Arithmetic.* The Arithmetic subtest requires the child to answer mathematical questions that are, for the most part, given to the child orally. It should be remembered that in the Wechsler instruments, the Arithmetic subtest is considered a verbal measure. At the lowest levels the child can simply count to find the answer. The majority of the items are "word problems" and must be solved without calculators or paper and pencils. The subtest measures reasoning, concentration, alertness, and short-term auditory memory.

- *Vocabulary.* In the Vocabulary subtest the child must provide the definition of a given word. This subscale has the strongest relationship with general ability of any of the subscales. The open-ended format often provides information of clinical significance in terms of both academic background and other psychological factors. Performance will be influenced by educational and cultural background and care needs to be taken in interpreting this subscale.

- *Comprehension.* The child is asked questions in which he or she must provide an oral response. There are three types of questions in the Comprehension subtest. The first asks the child what he or she would do in a given situation. The second type of question requires the child to explain some phenomenon or rule. The third type asks the child to explain a proverb. This subtest measures judgment more than previous academic learning. It measures verbal comprehension, verbal expression, and long-term memory. It also provides an indication of response to social convention: some children, with, for example, conduct disorder, may respond in a deviant manner. It is viewed as being a clinically rich subscale.

TABLE 7.2

*Brief description
of the perform-
ance subtests
of the WISC-III*

- *Picture Completion.* In this subtest the child is shown a picture in which some important part is missing (e.g., the cord on a telephone) and the child must identify the missing detail. In order to eliminate verbal influences, respondents can point to the missing part. The subtest, however, is influenced by cultural factors (e.g., if you don't regularly use a telephone it is harder to know the cord is missing). Picture Completion measures visual perception, alertness, memory, concentration, and attention to detail. It also provides an indication of the child's ability to discern essential from nonessential details.

- *Coding.* This subtest is titled Digit Symbol on the WAIS-III and Animal Peg on the WPPSI-R. Coding requires the child to copy symbols according to a specified pattern as quickly as possible. The child needs visual perception skills and short-term memory skills in order to copy the symbols effectively. The subtest also measures degree of persistence, speed of performance, and fine motor skills.

- *Picture Arrangement.* In Picture Arrangement, the child examines a series of related pictures similar to those found in a comic strip. The child must rearrange the series of pictures so that the order tells a logical story. Because the task is to arrange the pictures in a logical sequence, the subscale measures nonverbal reasoning. It also is designed to measure social judgment and knowledge base. There is some concern about which factor this subtest is related to.

- *Block Design.* Materials for the Block Design include nine blocks of which some are all red, some are all white, and others are half red and half white. The child must use these blocks to copy certain designs. Block Design is usually considered the best indicator of nonverbal intelligence. The subtest taps reasoning and analysis of spatial relationship. Furthermore, the subtest analyzes the degree to which visual input is integrated with motor functions.

- *Object Assembly.* Object Assembly consists of cut-up pictures of familiar objects (puzzles). It measures pattern recognition, assembly skills, and psychomotor abilities. Visual analysis and perceptual organization skills are necessary to perform effectively on this subscale. As with Block Design, children who are slow and methodical will not score as well as children who hurry. Object Assembly is an optional subtest in the WAIS-III.

The scoring of the Wechsler subscales is somewhat complex because different points are awarded depending on the quality of the responses. Throughout the administration of the scales, the examiner also gathers anecdotal information such as task-approach skills, level of concentration, and motivation. A qualified examiner can extract rich and important information from the performance on the intelligence tests and also from observing the individual during the testing.

There is some discussion and debate about the factor structure of the WISC-III. There is considerable support for the three factors of the Full Scale IQ, Verbal IQ, and Performance IQ scales (Kamphaus, 1993). There are, however, four other proposed factors of the WISC-III: Verbal Comprehension (VC), Perceptual Organization (PO), Freedom from Distractibility (FD), and Perceptual Speed (PS). The Freedom from Distractibility factor is titled Working Memory in the WAIS-III. In the top left side of Figure 7.3, you can see the subtests that are related to each of the Scaled Scores. Some clinicians have found these indexes helpful in describing the strengths and limitations of children. The Perceptual Speed factor is new and its clinical utility is not as established as the other three factors. Braden (1995) concluded there is considerably more support for the overall factor structure of the WISC-III as compared to the WISC-R. Nonetheless, he further contended that the number, reliability, and composition of the subfactors have not been fully resolved. This information would suggest that counselors can have more confidence in findings related to the Full Scale, Verbal, and Performances IQs, and less confidence in information related to Verbal Comprehension, Perceptual Organization, Freedom from Distractibility, and Perceptual Speed.

The normative sample of the WISC-III is 2,200 and is representative of the 1988 U.S. Census data. In the standardization process, ethnic minority children were oversampled so that the groups would be large enough to perform item analysis studies (Sandoval, 1995). The average internal consistency reliability coefficient for the Full Scale IQ is .96, with a standard error of measurement of 3.20. The average reliability coefficient for the Verbal IQ is .95 and the Performance IQ is .91.

In their reviews of the WISC-III, both Braden (1995) and Sandoval (1995) concluded that the validity of the instrument is well established. The amount of research performed since its publication is 1991 is substantial. Wechsler (1991) reported strong correlations between the WISC-III and other measures of intelligence. Numerous studies have indicated that the WISC-III predicts relevant outcomes, such as academic achievement. Weiss, Prifitera, and Roid (1993) found that WISC-III showed little predictive bias when used with males, females, Caucasians, African-Americans, and Hispanics. They found marginal intercept bias that suggested it might overpredict achievement for African-Americans and underpredict English grades for females (see Chapter 14 for an explanation of intercept bias). Furthermore, there is also substantial support for the WISC-III as a sound tool for clinical diagnosis (e.g., mental retardation, learning disabilities).

In conclusion, the Wechsler instruments are the most widely used individually administered intelligence tests. Spanish versions of the Wechsler scales are also available and have been researched and validated. A skilled psychologist can derive an abundance of useful information from the administration of the WPPSI-R, WISC-III, or WAIS-III. Although most interpretations of the results will focus on cognitive abilities, some psychologists can use these testing results to identify personality factors and learning styles.

Stanford-Binet Intelligence Scale

One of the oldest and most widely used intelligence assessments is the *Stanford-Binet,* which is now in its fourth edition (Thorndike, Hagen & Sattler, 1986a, 1986b). The Stanford-Binet evolved from the Binet-Simon, which was published in 1905 and contained only 30 items. The Binet-Simon was then revised in both 1908 and 1911. The first version of the Stanford-Binet was published in 1916 under the leadership of Terman at Stanford University. This version of the instrument was the first to include an intelligence quotient (IQ), which was a ratio of mental age to chronological age. Major revisions of the Stanford-Binet were performed in 1937, 1960, and 1972. The fourth edition of the Stanford-Binet built on this extensive historical experience and also revised some of the procedures in order to address criticisms of earlier editions. For instance, the content was expanded from a predominately verbal focus to include more quantitative, spatial, and short-term memory tasks. The fourth edition also abandoned the ratio IQ in favor of a deviation IQ.

The current version of the Stanford-Binet was constructed for use with individuals two years of age through adulthood. This version was based on the theoretical model summarized in Figure 7.4. As reflected in this figure, the theoretical model is hierarchical, with g, a general reasoning factor, at the top level. The authors believed that general intelligence could be best measured by assessing diverse cognitive tasks. The development of the fourth edition was influenced by the work of Cattell and includes measures of both crystallized (scholastic and academic abilities) and fluid (primarily abstract/visual reasoning) abilities. The Verbal Reasoning Subtests and the Abstract Reasoning Subtests are considered to be measures of crystallized abilities, while the Abstract/Visual Reasoning Subtests are determined to be measures of fluid abilities. The authors also included a third area, short-term memory, in this second level of the hierarchy. The Stanford-Binet Fourth Edition consists of 15 subtests, with 4 subtests in Verbal Reasoning, Abstract Reasoning, and Short-Term Memory and 3 subtests in Quantitative Reasoning.

The administration of the Stanford-Binet requires that only a portion of the 15 subtests be given at each age level. For each individual, the examiner needs to determine both the basal and ceiling levels. The *basal level* is where the individual gets all items correct on two consecutive levels. The *ceiling level* is reached when the individual misses three out of the four items on two con-

FIGURE 7.4

Theoretical Model for the Stanford-Binet

© 1986 by the Riverside Publishing Company. Reproduced from the Stanford-Binet Intelligence Scale, 4/E, by Robert L. Thorndike, Elizabeth P. Hagen, & Jerome M. Sattler, with permission of the publisher.

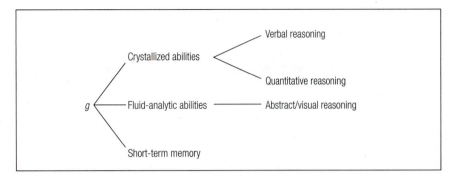

secutive levels. Where to begin on each subtest is determined by the individual's performance on the *routing test*, which is the Vocabulary Subtest. The authors selected Vocabulary because knowledge of words has been found to be highly correlated with overall intellectual abilities. Due to the complexities of administering the Stanford-Binet, it is important that the administrator be highly trained.

Once the basal and ceiling levels have been reached, the raw scores are converted to Standard Age Scores (SAS) (see Figure 7.5). The subtests all have a mean SAS of 50 and a standard deviation of 8. The four content areas (e.g., Verbal Reasoning) have a mean of 100 and a standard deviation of 16. The total composite score reflects general ability and also has a mean of 100 and a standard deviation of 16. The standard deviation of 16 on the Stanford-Binet is different from many other intelligence measures (e.g., the Wechsler scales) that have a standard deviation of 15.

The standardization sample for the current version of the Stanford-Binet is over 5,000 children between the ages of 2 and 23. The sample was stratified on the basis of geographic region, community size, ethnic group, age, and gender, based on the 1980 census. Socioeconomic status was evaluated through parents' occupational and educational level. There is concern that the sample has an overrepresentation of children at the higher SES levels and an underrepresentation of children at the lower levels. The authors attempted to adjust for this imbalance through differential weighting when computing scores, which was positively reviewed by Glutting and Kaplan (1990) in their review of the Standard-Binet.

Reliability of the Stanford-Binet has primarily been investigated using internal consistency and test-retest methods because there is not an alternative form to the fourth edition. The total composite score is the most reliable measure, with reliability coefficients being reported in the .95 to .99 range (Thorndike et al., 1986b). The standard error of measurement for the composite score is about 2 to 3 points. The reliability coefficients for the four content areas range from .80 to .97. The range of reliabilities for the 15 individual subtests are mostly in the .80s and .90s with the exception of Memory for Objects. The validity

FIGURE 7.5
Stanford-Binet Intelligence Scale: Fourth Edition

STANFORD-BINET INTELLIGENCE SCALE

RECORD BOOKLET

Stanford-Binet Intelligence Scale: Fourth Edition

9-74539

Name ______

______ Sex ______

Ethnicity NA H B W/NH O/AA PI Other ______

	YEAR	MONTH	DAY
Date of Testing			
Birth Date			
Age			

School ______

Grade ______

Examiner ______

Father's Occupation: ______

Mother's Occupation: ______

FACTORS AFFECTING TEST PERFORMANCE
Overall Rating of Conditions

Optimal Good Average Detrimental Seriously detrimental

	RAW SCORE	STANDARD AGE SCORE *
Verbal Reasoning		
1 Vocabulary		
6 Comprehension		
7 Absurdities		
14 Verbal Relations		
Sum of Subtest SAS's		
Verbal Reasoning SAS		
Abstract/Visual Reasoning		
5 Pattern Analysis		
9 Copying		
11 Matrices		
13 Paper Folding & Cutting		
Sum of Subtest SAS's		
Abstract/Visual Reasoning SAS		
Quantitative Reasoning		
3 Quantitative		
12 Number Series		
15 Equation Building		
Sum of Subtest SAS's		
Quantitative Reasoning SAS		
Short-Term Memory		
2 Bead Memory		
4 Memory For Sentences		
8 Memory For Digits		
10 Memory For Objects		
Sum of Subtest SAS's		
Short-Term Memory SAS		
Sum of Area SAS's		

	COMPOSITE SCORE *
Test Composite	
Partial Composite	
Partial Composite based on ______	

	1 2 3 4 5	
Attention		
a) Absorbed by task		Easily distracted
Reactions During Test Performance		
a) Normal activity level		Abnormal activity level
b) Initiates activity		Waits to be told
c) Quick to respond		Urging needed
Emotional Independence		
a) Socially confident		Insecure
b) Realistically self-confident		Distrusts own ability
c) Comfortable in adult company		Ill-at-ease
d) Assured		Anxious
Problem-Solving Behavior		
a) Persistent		Gives up easily
b) Reacts to failure realistically		Reacts to failure unrealistically
c) Eager to continue		Seeks to terminate
d) Challenged by hard tasks		Prefers only easy tasks
Independence of Examiner Support		
a) Needs minimum of commendation		Needs constant praise and encouragement
Expressive Language		
a) Excellent articulation		Very poor articulation
Receptive Language		
a) Excellent sound discrimination		Very poor sound discrimination

Was it difficult to establish rapport with this person?
Easy ______ Difficult

***Be sure that all Standard Age Scores (SAS's) are based on the tables in the *Guide* with the number 9-74502 on the cover.**

The Riverside Publishing Company

Robert L. Thorndike
Elizabeth P. Hagen
Jerome M. Sattler

information on the fourth edition of the Stanford-Binet is considerable (see Thorndike et al., 1986b). The Stanford-Binet is highly correlated with other intelligence measures. Glutting and Kaplan (1990) criticized the factor structure of the Stanford-Binet, but others have found support for the factor structure (Boyle, 1990; Thorndike, 1990). Kamphaus (1993) concluded that there is considerable validity support for the Verbal Reasoning and Abstract/Visual Reasoning areas, but less for the Quantitative and Short-Term Memory composites.

Kaufman Instruments

Another prominent name in the field of intellectual assessment is Kaufman. Alan and Nadeen Kaufman are a husband-and-wife team of psychologists with extensive experience in test development. In the 1980s, they published the *Kaufman Assessment Battery for Children* (K-ABC, Kaufman & Kaufman, 1983a, 1983b), which reflected many advances in intelligence testing but, also, has been the focus of controversy. They further went on to publish the *Kaufman Adolescent and Adult Intelligence Test* (KAIT, Kaufman & Kaufman, 1993). The Kaufman instruments are not as widely used as the Wechsler instruments and, therefore, will not be discussed in the same degree of detail.

The Kaufman instruments are an integration of different theoretical approaches, such as Luria's information processing and Horn-Cattell's theory of fluid and crystallized intelligence. The Kaufman Assessment Battery for Children yields five major scores: Sequential Processing, Simultaneous Processing, Mental Processing Composite, Achievement, and Nonverbal. The subtests within the K-ABC can also be used to compute the Nonverbal Scale, which is designed for those with hearing impairments or limited English proficiency. The Mental Processing Composite is intended to measure "the total intelligence in the assessment battery." The Mental Processing Composite is subdivided into Sequential Processing and Simultaneous Processing. Crystallized intelligence is reflected in the Achievement Scale and fluid intelligence is reflected in the process scales. There are 16 subtests in the K-ABC; however, a maximum of 13 of these will be administered to any one child. The subtests use pictorial and diagrammatic materials, with many of the subtests having a game-like quality. The K-ABC was designed to engage children from different ethnicities and include information that diverse children would be acquainted with.

The five scales of the K-ABC have a mean of 100 and a standard deviation of 15. The K-ABC was designed for normal and exceptional children ages 2.5 to 12.5. The sample is ethnically diverse and about 7% of the sample were drawn from children in special education programs. The K-ABC tends to show smaller differences between African-American children and Caucasian children when compared to other intelligence measures. The internal consistency reliability coefficients range from .84 (Simultaneous scores for preschool children) to .97 (Achievement scores for school age children). The subtests vary in terms of reliability.

Some individuals have noted difficulties in interpreting the results of the K-ABC. Page (1985) noted numerous contradictions in the Interpretive Manual. Anastasi (1985) argued that the terms "achievement" and "mental processing" lend themselves to misinterpretation. An achievement test is, by definition, one that measures instructional content to which a child has been exposed. The Achievement subtests of K-ABC, however, were explicitly designed *not* to measure factual knowledge taught in schools. Many teachers, parents, and counselors may not be aware that the Achievement Scale measures crystallized intelligence. Another problem Anastasi noted was that

Simultaneous and Sequential Processing Scales may not be measuring processing, and a more accurate label for these scales was verbal and nonverbal reasoning.

The *Kaufman Adolescent and Adult Intelligence Test* (KAIT, Kaufman & Kaufman, 1993) is designed for individuals ages 11 to 85+. The Core Battery can be given in 60 minutes, while the Expanded Battery with a neurological focus can be administered in 90 minutes. The KAIT only includes three intelligence scales: Fluid (Gf), Crystallized (Gc), and Composite Intelligence. There are six subtests in the KAIT, three for fluid intelligence and three that assess crystallized intelligence. Flanagan (1995) criticized the KAIT for having a dichotomous view of fluid and crystallized intelligence that is not supported by current theorists in the area nor by research. The instrument appears well standardized with a national sample of 2,000. The reliability information provided is acceptable. Although the manual provides extensive validity information, there is some concern about the KAIT, particularly related to the instrument's ability to assess fluid intelligence (Flanagan, 1995).

Other Individual Instruments

A few other individually administered intelligence tests are used sufficiently to merit a brief overview. A comparatively new instrument is the *Differential Ability Scales* (DAS, Elliot, 1990). The DAS is based on the British Ability Scales, which has been used in England since 1983. The DAS has been standardized in the United States. As the name implies, the focus of the DAS is on identifying specific abilities. The instrument does provide a measure of General Conceptual Ability, a special Nonverbal Composite, and "cluster scores."

Another frequently used instrument is the *Slosson Intelligence Test—Revised* (SIT-R, Nicholson & Hibpshman, 1990). The Slosson provides a relatively quick assessment of cognitive abilities for children and adults. The SIT-R consists of 187 items that are given orally; the examinee's language skills will influence performance. This shorter assessment is not quite as reliable as the longer individually administered intelligence assessments. On the positive side, the SIT-R is highly correlated with the Verbal Scale and Full Scale IQ scores of the Wechsler instruments.

There are individually administered intelligence tests that have focused on trying to eliminate some of the cultural biases and influences of language proficiency on intelligence. For example, the *Raven's Progressive Matrices* (Raven, Court, & Raven, 1983) contains matrices that have a logical pattern or design with a missing part. The examinee then selects the appropriate item that progresses the pattern. Hence, progressive matrices are nonverbal; however, some researchers contend that culture also influences these skills. Another attempt to reduce cultural bias is the *Peabody Picture Vocabulary Test—III* (Dunn & Dunn, 1997), which measures receptive vocabulary knowledge. There is both an English and a Spanish version, where the individual is given a word and asked to simply point to the appropriate picture. The *Test of Nonverbal Intelli-*

gence—3 (TONI-3, Brown, Sherbenou, & Johnsen, 1997) provides a language-free measure of intelligence, where the instructions can be given in pantomime and examinees point to the answers.

Conclusion

In conclusion, the information gained for individually administered intelligence tests can be helpful to counselors. The amount of useful information depends on the expertise of the individual administering and interpreting the results. Counselors need to become proficient consumers of psychological reports that include intelligence assessment. This involves having sufficient information about the instruments used to be able to evaluate the psychologist's report. For example, a counselor who receives a psychological report for a Hispanic 9-year-old boy with limited English proficiency needs to understand the cultural influences on the intelligence test used. Instrument manuals, critiques and reviews of instruments, journal articles, and books can aid the counselor in becoming an informed professional in this area of intelligence assessment.

Group Intelligence Testing

Group intelligence tests are used more than individual tests, particularly in school settings. While individual intelligence tests can provide detailed information about an individual, group intelligence tests are frequently used to supply information about a group. School boards, administrators, and parents who want to evaluate a school's performance will often examine the differences between ability levels—as measured by group intelligence test results—with performance level—as measured by group achievement test results. Group intelligence test results are also frequently used in working with individuals. In some cases, group intelligence tests serve as screening tools for children who may need additional testing to identify possible learning or cognitive limitations or disorders. Sometimes group intelligence test results can be helpful in sorting out the issues that are germane to a child experiencing academic problems. The case of Alice illustrates this use of group intelligence test results.

Alice is an eleven-year-old student in fifth grade, whose parents sought counseling for her because she was doing "poorly" in school. The parents reported that Alice was getting mostly Cs and an occasional B. The parents were both in professional occupations and both had graduate degrees. They reported that Alice was not performing up to her abilities and they wanted the counselor to identify methods to motivate her. Alice, on the other hand, told the counselor that she was trying hard to do well in school. The counselor asked about homework and, once again, received discrepant information from Alice and her parents. Alice contended that she worked diligently for hours on homework, while her parents reported that she dawdled the hours away. The counselor secured a release of information from the parents to talk with Alice's teacher and review Alice's school records. Children in Alice's school took an annual standardized group achievement test that also included a measure of intelligence or general ability. The counselor found that Alice consistently scored below average in terms of intellectual abilities compared to both national and local norms. In fact, the results consistently indicated that Alice's IQ was around the 40th to 44th percentile even though instruments from different publishers had been used in this school district. Alice's teacher concurred with the group intelligence tests' results and voiced that she believed Alice was probably overachieving rather than underachieving.

Group intelligence or ability tests can provide certain information, but they also have certain limitations. With individually administered intelligence tests, it is possible to observe behaviors that often reflect the level of motivation. In a group setting, it is impossible to document the behaviors of the entire group and sometimes individuals are not motivated to perform at their highest level. Many of us have heard of children who have taken group-administered tests and bubbled the answer sheets into attractive patterns rather than reading the questions! Furthermore, group intelligence tests require more reading than individually administered tests and are, therefore, more problematic for individuals with limited reading skills. Cultural considerations and language usage also need to be considered in group intelligence tests. The results of any instrument should never be interpreted in isolation, and the results of a group intelligence test particularly need to be interpreted in the context of other information.

The *Cognitive Abilities Test* (CogAT) is a revision and extension of the Lorge-Thorndike Intelligence Test. The instrument is designed to assess the pattern and level of cognitive development for children in kindergarten through grade 12. The current form of the instrument, Form 5, provides separate scores for verbal, quantitative, and nonverbal reasoning, and a composite score can also be provided. The time allotted to take the CogAT is between 90 and 98 minutes depending on the level. The CogAT was constructed with overlapping items at the different age levels. The item overlap allows for a continuous scale score for kindergarten through grade 12. The CogAT can be machine scored and purchasers can choose from the following scoring options: raw scores, standard age scores, national grade and age percentile ranks, and grade and age stanines. The CogAT can also be scored locally by hand or by computer. For schools interested in administering combined ability and achievement testing, the CogAT is concurrently normed with the Iowa Tests of Basic Skills, the Tests of Achievement and Proficiency, and the Iowa Tests of Educational Development. There is an *Interpretive Guide for Teachers and Counselors* to assist in the interpretation of the results.

Another frequently used group intelligence test is the *Otis-Lennon School Ability Test*, Seventh Edition (OLSAT7). The OLSAT is also for students in kindergarten through grade 12. The scores provided are a total, verbal, and nonverbal score, plus certain cluster scores (e.g., verbal comprehension, pictorial reasoning) depending on the level. The time required for this assessment is a maximum of 75 minutes. The current version of the OLSAT was standardized with the *Stanford Achievement Test, Ninth Edition* (Stanford 9). A previous edition was standardized with the *Metropolitan Achievement Test, Seventh Edition.* The *Test of Cognitive Skills* (TCS) is another group intelligence test; however, it is for use with students between the second and twelfth grades. The subscales are somewhat different from other group measures and include: analogies, sequences, memory, and verbal reasoning. The TCS is standardized with an achievement test titled the Comprehensive Test of Basic Skills.

The *Multidimensional Aptitude Battery* (MAB) is another group intelligence test; however, it is not designed for use in schools. The MAB was designed to be a convenient alternative to the WAIS-R. The MAB is for either adolescents or adults and can be given either individually or in groups. Like the WAIS-R, it provides a Full Scale IQ, a Verbal IQ, and a Performance IQ. There are five verbal subtests and five performance subtests, with each subtest having a time limit of seven minutes.

Another group intelligence test that is mostly used in industrial settings is the *Wonderlic Personnel Test* (WPT, Wonderlic Personnel Test, Inc., 1992). The WPT is a 50-item test, with a 12-minute time limit. There is a PC version of the Wonderlic Personnel Test and a paper and pencil version. There are also four alternative formats of the WPT that were constructed to comply with the Americans with Disabilities Act (ADA). The WPT was designed to measure general cognitive ability and correlates very highly with the WAIS-R.

Issues in Intelligence Testing

Controversy and debate about intelligence testing are certainly not new phenomena. A recent book by Hernstein and Murray (1994), *The Bell Curve: Intelligence and Class Structure in American Life,* received enormous media attention and revived some of the debate surrounding the nature of intelligence and the meaning of intelligence test scores. The third section of this chapter will examine some of the issues related to intelligence testing and summarize the research findings related to the specific issues.

Is Intelligence Stable?

The interest in this topic concerns whether intelligence scores tend to vary due to various influences or remain stable as individuals develop and age. Infants and preschool children have the least stable intelligence test scores, which is reflected in the reliability coefficients of the instruments for these younger children. The answer to whether intelligence is stable from childhood through old age depends on what research is examined. Early research in this area indicated that intelligence tended to gradually decline after the age of 20, with the decline becoming more apparent for individuals in their 50s through 70s.

There is a commonly held notion that as we age, our memory, speed of processing, and mental agility decrease. You have probably heard someone cite their age as the reason for forgetting some detail. The findings of these early studies, however, have not been supported by more sophisticated research methodologies. Early research on intellectual stability involved *cross-sectional studies,* where people at different age levels were tested and their intelligence scores compared. What these early findings did not take into account were the cultural differences that affected the scores of different generations of individuals. For example in these cross-sectional studies, many of the older individuals did not have the same educational experiences as the younger individuals. The assessment field is in general agreement that these early results indicating decreases in intellectual function were the result of cultural differences among the different generations (Anastasi & Urbina, 1997). Later researchers were able to complete *longitudinal studies,* in which the same people were tested repeatedly at different ages in their lives. Some of the more prominent longitudinal studies (e.g., Bayley & Oden, 1955; Tuddenham, Blumemkrantz, & Wilken, 1968) indicated that intelligence gradually increases from childhood into middle age and then levels off.

Probably the best indicators of the stability of intelligence come from those studies that employed cross-sectional and longitudinal designs, following same-aged individuals over time as well as comparing 30-year-olds in 1950 with 30-year-olds in 1980 (e.g., Schaie & Strother, 1968). These well-designed studies indicate intelligence is mostly steady through adulthood with slight declines that occur after the age of around 65. The intellectual declines that do occur tend to be in the areas of fluid intelligence as compared to crystallized (Kaufman, 1990). Whether there is a decline in intelligence, however, appears to be related to a complex interaction of variables, such as physical health, mental activities performed in the later ages, and the degree that education is continued throughout the lifespan.

What Do Intelligence Test Scores Predict?

Earlier in this chapter, the different views concerning what constitutes intelligence and different methods for measuring it were overviewed. The conclusion is that there is no generally agreed upon definition of intelligence, nor is there consensus on the most appropriate methods for assessing this somewhat illusive construct. Yet, intelligence tests continue to be used in our society; therefore, it is important for counselors to understand the research findings related to what these tests actually measure. The following discussion is not going to address findings related to any specific instrument, but rather general trends in intelligence testing.

Intelligence tests appear to be related to academic performance. The correlation between intelligence and school performance is consistently around .50 (Neisser et al., 1996). Although this is often considered a substantial coefficient, we also need to remember that only 25% of the variance is explained by the relationship between intelligence and school performance. Therefore, success in school is related to many other factors in addition to intelligence (e.g., motivation). We do find, however, that children with higher intelligence test scores are less likely to drop out of school as compared to children with lower scores.

The relationship between IQ scores and occupational success and income is not as simple. The degree to which intelligence scores are related to occupational prestige, and to a lesser amount income, is partly due to the connection between education and intelligence. Higher prestige occupations, such as doctor and lawyer, typically require a college education or more. Admissions scores for college (e.g., SAT) and post-degree work (e.g., GRE, MCAT) are highly correlated with intelligence tests. Although Hernstein and Murray (1994) contended that intelligence scores predicted occupational attainment, a Task Force appointed by the American Psychological Association (Neisser et al., 1996) did not reach that same conclusion. At most, they concluded that intelligence accounts for about one-fourth of the social status variance and one-sixth of the income variance. This relationship further decreased when the parents' socio-economic status was taken into consideration.

Hunter and Schmidt (Hunter, 1986; Hunter & Schmidt, 1983) have studied the effects of abilities and aptitudes on job performance. Their findings, which they term **validity generalization**, are primarily related to aptitude testing and the *General Aptitude Test Battery* (GATB), which will be discussed in detail in Chapter 8. The GATB does include a measure that some professionals contend is synonymous with intelligence and, thus, Hunter and Schmidt's findings do have some relevance in regard to the predictive ability of intelligence tests. To put it succinctly, Hunter and Schmidt have shown that cognitive ability is highly related to job performance. In fact, they contended that employers should hire the individual with the highest cognitive ability in the pool of applicants.

Some researchers have been interested in the relationship between mental processing speed and intelligence. The hypothesis is that those of higher intelligence can perceive, retrieve, and respond to information more quickly than those who are less intelligent. The results vary a little depending on the tasks used, but in general we find that individuals with higher intelligence test scores tend to perform simple perceptual and cognitive tasks quicker than those people with lower scores (Deary, 1995).

Is Intelligence Hereditary?

This is one of the most controversial issues in intelligence testing, for the question essentially is asking how much of measured intellectual ability is innate and how much is due to environmental factors. There are many traits that vary among people (e.g., weight, propensity for some diseases, or aspects of personality), and scientists have attempted to discern the amount of variation that is attributable to genetics and the amount that is due to environmental factors.

A *heritability index* (h^2) is intended to provide an estimate of proportion of variance associated with genetic differences. The reverse then applies, where $1 - h^2$ is an indicator of the amount of variance due to environmental factors. Determining estimates of the genetic contribution to intelligence is, at this point, difficult. Some of the studies have examined the differences between monozygotic (MZ) twins and dizygotic (DZ) twins who have been raised together and those who were adopted and raised apart. Monozygotic twins have the same genetic makeup, while dizygotic twins have half of their genes in common. Other studies involved several kinds of kinship and the influences of genetics on intelligence.

In general, the heritability indexes for intelligence tend to be around .50 (Chipuser, Rovine, & Plomin, 1990; Loehlin, 1989). This h^2 figure would probably be larger (i.e., around .80) if we only included studies with adult samples (McGue, Bouchard, Iacono, & Lykken, 1993). Although genes appear to have a substantial influence on performance on intelligence tests, this effect is not sufficiently large enough to indicate that intelligence is inexorably set at conception. Environmental factors also have a significant effect on intellectual development. Neisser et al. (1996), in their extensive review of research in this area, concluded that variation in the unique environments of individuals and between-family factors significantly influences IQ scores of children. IQ scores seemed to be most related to the interaction between an individual's genetic makeup and environmental influences. A child is born with certain capabilities, but the degree to which those capabilities are realized is significantly influenced by the environment surrounding that child.

What Environmental Factors Influence Intelligence?

Many environmental factors influence the intellectual development of an individual, but it is clear that the cultural environment in which a person matures has a significant influence on that person's intellectual development. Postmodern philosophy has stressed the influences of culture and language in the overall development of an individual (Gergen, 1985). A child of Indian descent growing up in rural Malaysia has different experiences than an upper-middle-class Caucasian child growing up in San Francisco. Cultures differ in a multitude of ways that are both overt and subtle; therefore, we are unable to directly identify all the cultural factors that influence performance on intelligence tests. Even within a population, there are subgroups where there are cultural variations. For instance, in the United States there are different tribes of Native Americans. The culture of Arapahos is different from the culture of Shoshones, even though the two tribes share a reservation in Wyoming.

Although intelligence tests try to eliminate the effects of schooling, attendance at school does influence performance on intelligence tests (Ceci, 1991). Children who attend school regularly have higher test scores than children who attend intermittently. If we examine differences between children who are the same age but because of birthday deadline vary in the number of years attending school, those who have attended longer will have higher IQ scores. Precisely how schooling influences intelligence test performance is difficult to determine. Certainly, many intelligence tests incorporate information items, such as "Who is Madame Curie?" The probability of being exposed to this information increases with attendance at school. Children in school are also more likely to be exposed to manipulation of objects and puzzles. Furthermore, schools promote problem-solving skills and abstract thinking. It must be noted that not all schooling is alike and that the quality of the school experience also influences IQ scores. Those who attend poor-quality schools will not receive the same instruction and their intelligence scores will reflect this deficiency (Neisser et al., 1996).

Family environments have an influence on many aspects of development, including cognitive development. Early research indicated that intelligence scores were directly influenced by parents' interest in achievement (Honzik, 1967) and methods of disciplining (Baldwin, Kalhorn, & Breese, 1945; Kent & Davis, 1957). Recent research, however, has questioned these early findings about the degree to which family factors influence intelligence (Scarr, 1992, 1993). Severely neglectful or abusive environments, however, can affect children's cognitive development. For example, prolonged malnutrition in childhood affects cognitive development. After a child is provided a minimally nurturing environment, it is difficult to determine what other factors may contribute to performance on intelligence tests.

Environmental factors that can affect intelligence also include exposure to certain toxins. The negative consequences of exposure to lead have been well documented (Baghurst et al., 1992; McMichael et al., 1988). Prenatal exposure to large amounts of alcohol can produce effects on the child called fetal alcohol syndrome (Stratton, Howey, & Battaglia, 1996). Mental retardation is often associated with fetal alcohol syndrome. There is conflicting research about the effects on cognitive development related to prenatal exposure to small amounts of alcohol, caffeine, over-the-counter pain medication, and antibiotics.

Are There Group Differences in Intelligence?

Probably the most controversial issue related to the testing of intelligence concerns ethnic and gender group differences. Before we begin a discussion of these group differences in intelligence it is important to remember that research has continually shown that within-group variance is greater than between-group variance. This means that within any ethnic group the variation in scores is quite large; in fact, the variation *within* the group is greater than *between* groups. Hence, there is overlap among the groups that challenges the conclusions about the superiority or inferiority of one group compared to another. Furthermore, because of the large variation in intelligence scores, it is inappropriate to stereotype any individual based on group performance scores.

Gender differences. Although there do not appear to be general intellectual differences between males and females, there are some differences on specific tasks or abilities. Men appear to be better in visual-spatial ability, which involves tasks that require the individual to visualize and mentally rotate objects. In fact, a recent meta-analysis (Masters & Sanders, 1993) found an effect size of .90, indicating that men in general score almost a standard deviation higher than females on visual-spatial tests. On the other hand, females appear to have the advantage over males in terms of some verbal tasks. On synonym generation and verbal fluency, females score higher than males, with the effect sizes ranging from .50 to 1.20 (Gordon & Lee, 1986, Hines, 1990). Thus, females' scores on these tests of verbal tasks tend to be between a half of a standard deviation to over a full standard deviation higher than males'.

An interesting phenomenon occurs in terms of gender differences concerning some quantitative abilities. Females show superior quantitative abilities in elementary school, but around the time of puberty, males then start achieving higher scores (Hyde, Fennema & Lamon, 1990). Males' superiority in quantitative abilities continues through adulthood and into old age. These differences in abilities between males and females can probably best be explained by a combination of social, cultural, and biological factors.

Ethnic group differences. In general, African-Americans, Hispanics, and Native Americans tend to score lower on intelligence tests than European-Americans (Whites) or Asian-Americans. African-Americans tend to score about one standard deviation (15 points) below Whites (Jensen, 1980; Reynolds, Chastain, Kaufman, & McLean, 1987). African-Americans tend to do poorly on both the verbal and nonverbal subtests that have a high correlation with general intelligence (Jensen, 1985). Socioeconomic factors seem to have some influence on test scores; however, Black/White differences are reduced, but not eliminated, when socioeconomic factors are controlled for (Loehlin, Lindzey, & Spuhler, 1975). Chapter 14 in this book will address questions of test bias, which some researchers have argued contributes to the disparity in IQ means between African-Americans and Whites. There is some research that indicates the difference between African-Americans and Whites on IQ scores is decreasing, but more definitive studies are needed before this can be considered an established finding (Neisser et al., 1996).

Hispanic-Americans' average intelligence test scores typically are between those of African-Americans and Whites (Neisser et al., 1996). Counselors need to be aware that linguistic factors may influence Hispanic individuals' performance on intelligence tests. Hispanic children often score higher on the performance subtests than on the verbal subtests (Kaufman, 1994). For many Hispanic children, English is not their first language, which may partially explain the discrepancy between performance and verbal scores. Dana (1993) contended that translation of standard intelligence tests into Spanish does not resolve these problems. On the positive side, there are reasonably high correlations among general intelligence test scores and school achievement for Hispanic children (McShane & Cook, 1985).

Concerning Native Americans' performance on intelligence tests, we have to be careful not to generalize due to the multitude of distinct tribes within this general population. The traditions and cultures of these various Native American tribes vary and, thus, performance on aspects of intelligence tests also tends to vary. A general finding is that Native American children, like Hispanic children, seem to score lower on the verbal scales as compared to the performance scales (Neisser et al., 1996). Besides cultural differences, McShane and Plas (1984) suggested that Native American children are plagued by chronic middle-ear infections that can negatively affect their development in the verbal area. The behavior during testing of Native Americans may also be misperceived by examiners. Native Americans tend to be deferential to a White examiner, and examiners may perceive these behaviors as a lack of motivation.

There is some debate concerning the average intelligence scores for Asian-American children, with studies reporting averages from around 100 to 111. A general finding is that Asian-Americans achieve substantially more both academically and occupationally than their intelligence scores would predict (Flynn, 1991). Asian-Americans tend to do well in school and a high proportion of them are employed in managerial, professional, and technical occupations than would be expected based on their intelligence scores. This "overachievement" demonstrates some of the problems with IQ-based predictions (Neisser et al., 1996). It should also be noted that there is great diversity among Asian-Americans (e.g., Chinese, Filipino, and Vietnamese) and that stereotypes concerning Asians can also be detrimental.

The ethnic-group difference in intelligence test performance does not appear to be related to any one factor, such as heredity or language differences. Neisser et al. (1996) concluded that researchers have not yet been able to explain these differences. Therefore, simple conclusions about the differences in intelligence among ethnic groups by individuals are probably based more on political or social views rather than scientific evidence. In counseling individuals, counselors need to remember that there is great variation in intelligence within all ethnic groups and that a counselor cannot predict a client's level of cognitive abilities based on his or her ethnicity.

What Is the Flynn Effect?

As this section of the chapter is devoted to issues in intelligence testing, it is important to note the steady rise of intelligence scores in recent years. This rise in intelligence score is often called the "Flynn effect" after James Flynn (1984, 1987), who was one of the first researchers to identify this trend. In the last fifty years, the average IQ score has increased more than a full standard deviation. The average gain is about three IQ points each decade. Interestingly, these gains in IQ scores are not reflected in gains in achievement, for scores on the Scholastic Aptitude Tests (SAT) declined between the mid-1960s and early 1980s (Neisser et al., 1996). There are numerous possible explanations for the Flynn effect, such as improvement in nutrition, more test sophistication, changes in education and educational opportunities, and changes in parenting practices. Although the increases in intelligence scores are well documented, the reasons for this rise are debated within the field. There are also differing opinions on whether this trend will continue or if there will be a leveling-off of average IQ scores.

Summary

Intelligence is a word commonly used in everyday conversation (e.g., "John" is intelligent or "someone" is not very intelligent). In addition, intelligence testing has a rich and substantial history, where certain instruments have been used extensively in a variety of settings. Given these factors, one might expect more agreement on the definition and theoretical basis for intelligence. Numerous theorists contend that a psychometric or factorial approach best explains the construct of intelligence. These individuals suggest that intelligence is composed of one or more factors. There is some debate about whether intelligence can best be described as one general factor (*g*) that affects all cognitive performance. Many intelligence tests have a composite score or a full scale IQ score that represents a measure of *g*. Other factor theorists contend that intelligence can be better explained by focusing on lower-order factors, such as the differences between fluid and crystallized intelligence. Developmental theorists suggest that intelligence can be better understood by examining how the structure of intelligence develops. Certainly, the most influential theorist in this developmental area is Piaget. Rather than studying the structures or development of intelligence, information processing models study how information is processed. These theorists hope that by analyzing how the brain works, they will understand the phenomenon of intelligence. The Kaufman Assessment Battery for Children (K-ABC) was influenced by the work of Luria, who proposed that individuals process information both simultaneously and sequentially. Finally, there are new models of intelligence that propose expanding the methods of testing intelligence. The models of Sternberg and Gardner are influencing how the field considers and conceptualizes intelligence.

Theories of intelligence have influenced the development of some of the most commonly used intelligence tests. Examinees are given an individual intelligence instrument in order to thoroughly assess their cognitive capabilities. The most frequently used instruments are those developed by Wechsler, which Kamphaus (1993) criticized for not having a theoretical base. The Wechsler intelligence tests are similar in content but geared toward different age groups. The Wechsler Adult Intelligence Scale—III (WAIS-III) is for adults, the Wechsler Intelligence Scale for Children—III (WISC-III) is for children ages 6 through 16, and the Wechsler Preschool and Primary Scale of Intelligence—Revised (WPPSI-R) is for children 3 through 7 years old. The Wechsler instruments provide an indication of Full Scale IQ and measures of Verbal IQ and Performance IQ. Another commonly used instrument is the Stanford-Binet—Fourth Edition. General intelligence is measured by an aggregate of second-level factors influenced by the work of Cattell (i.e., crystallized ability and fluid ability). The authors also included a third area, short-term memory, in this second level of the hierarchy. The authors of the Kaufman Assessment Battery for Children (K-ABC) designed it to be appropriate for children from diverse ethnic groups. Although some reviewers criticized the K-ABC, this instrument does represent some innovative methods of assessing intelligence. Group intelligence tests are easier to administer; however, these instruments cannot provide the degree of information individually administered intelligence tests provide. Furthermore, performance on group intelligence tests will be highly dependent on the reading abilities of the test takers.

There are numerous issues related to the use of intelligence tests. Information from intelligence tests can be helpful in counseling clients, particularly in terms of educational and career decisions. A skilled clinician, however, must be aware of the strengths and limitations of these measures. Multicultural factors are particularly important to consider when results from intelligence tests are used in decision making. Intelligence test results can provide information about a client's cognitive abilities, but that information needs to be integrated with other information in order to have a more thorough understanding of the client.

CHAPTER 8

Measuring Achievement and Aptitude: Applications for Counseling

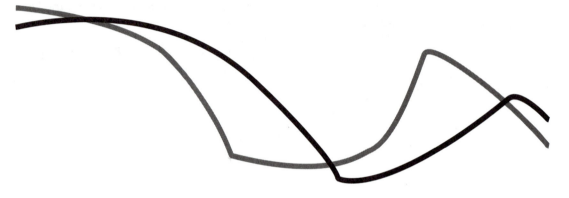

When I teach a course on appraisal and say to my class of counseling students, "today we are going to start talking about achievement and aptitude assessment," the students look as if they would rather be in any other classroom in the entire university. In fact, a few students have been tempted to fake a sudden illness, just to be able to leave class. Yet, many of the students in my class will work with families where the children are having difficulties in school. Knowledge about achievement testing will help these future counselors work more effectively with those families.

As you will remember from the first chapter, **achievement tests** provide information about what an individual has learned or acquired. A student may have a deficit in only one academic area, but that may cloud the parent's entire view of his or her child. As an example, I once had a client whose parents were very disappointed in the academic performance of their second-grade daughter. The parents perceived the child to be an "academic failure" and provided evidence of poor spelling in stories and letters the daughter had written to relatives. These parents, however, were not particularly knowledgeable about child development and had unrealistic expectations concerning what a second grader should be able to spell. The results of an achievement test the daughter had taken in school helped the parents to understand that their child was not an academic failure. The daughter's lowest achievement score was in spelling but it was at the 62nd percentile. Hence, a counselor who understands and can interpret achievement tests can help parents understand their child's academic strengths and limitations.

Knowledge of aptitude assessment can also be useful to counselors. **Aptitude tests** *predict* future performance or ability to learn. Often clients come to counseling because they are trying to make a decision about their futures (e.g., seek a new job, go back to school, decide on a career) and aptitude tests can provide useful information in these decisions. In fact, many of us have probably wondered at some point in our lives if we had the aptitude for a particular task. Many aptitude tests are used for selection purposes, such as employers selecting employees and colleges accepting students. Some of these same instruments, however, can be used in counseling situations in order to assist clients in making better decisions about their futures.

In general, achievement tests measure acquired learning and aptitude tests measure potential or ability to learn new tasks. While there are a number of different types of both achievement and aptitude tests, sometimes the difference between them is somewhat ambiguous. The contrast between achievement and aptitude tests is one of purpose more than of content. For example, the same math problems might be used to see if someone has learned a mathematical concept (achievement) or those same problems could be used to predict future performance in jobs requiring some mathematical knowledge (aptitude). The following chapter briefly discusses some of the achievement and aptitude tests commonly used by counselors.

Assessment of Achievement

The assessment of achievement can take many forms. Drummond (1996) categorized achievement tests into the following six areas:

1. *Survey achievement batteries* These are instruments that assess individuals over a wide range of subjects. These instruments often measure knowledge in the areas of reading, mathematics, language arts, science, and social studies. Survey achievement batteries can be norm-referenced or a combination of norm-referenced and criterion-referenced instruments.

2. *Individual achievement tests* These are achievement instruments that are administered individually. Many of these instruments can be administered to both children and adults, and typically cover the areas of reading, mathematics, and spelling.

3. *Diagnostic tests* These tests are used to diagnose learning difficulties, particularly learning disabilities. The diagnostic tests also assess achievement strengths and limitations of the individual.

4. *Criterion-referenced tests* These instruments measure knowledge or comprehension and determine if a certain criterion or standard has been met. A wide variety of academic areas can be assessed with criterion-referenced tests.

5. *Minimum-level skills test* This type of assessment measures the skills necessary for promotion to another grade, to enter an occupation, or to graduate from high school. A minimum level of performance is established before individuals complete these instruments.

6. *Subject area tests* Many achievement tests measure knowledge in a certain subject matter. An example of subject area assessment would be a test that covered knowledge of assessment strategies in counseling.

Survey Achievement Tests

Survey achievement tests are administered to thousands of students in multiple school districts throughout the nation and are frequently designed for kindergarten through twelfth grade. These batteries of achievement tests typically have a number of subtests that measure achievement in certain academic areas (e.g., reading, mathematics, and language arts). These survey achievement tests can help a counselor understand where a child's or adolescent's strengths and limitations are within the different achievement areas. Furthermore, the results from these tests can provide information about a student's progress from year to year. For instance, school counselors may want to intervene with students when their performance is generally consistent for a couple of years and then the scores begin to decrease.

There are numerous achievement batteries that can be purchased. Table 8.1 provides a sample of some of the commonly used ones and the appropriate grade levels for those instruments. These achievement batteries cover multiple achievement areas so that a counselor can identify strengths and limitations.

TABLE 8.1

Achievement batteries and grade ranges

Instruments	Grades
California Achievement Tests	K–12
Iowa Tests of Basic Skills[a]	K–9
Iowa Tests of Educational development[a]	9–12
Tests of Achievement and Proficiency[a]	9–12
Metropolitan Achievement Tests	K–12
Stanford Achievement Test Series	K–13
TerraNova	K–12

Note: [a] signifies these instruments are related.

Many of these batteries are constructed so that a child's progress can be continually charted from kindergarten through twelfth grade.

Another advantage of these achievement batteries is that many of them are concurrently normed with tests of academic intelligence or general ability. For example, the Stanford Achievement Test Series can be given simultaneously with the Otis-Lennon School Ability Test in order to get estimates of ability/achievement comparisons. The Iowa Tests series can be given with the Cognitive Abilities Test and the California Achievement Tests, and the Comprehensive Tests of Basic Skills are coordinated with the Tests of Cognitive Skills. If major discrepancies are identified between ability and achievement with one of these achievement batteries, then additional testing that is more thorough and individually administered may be warranted.

There are also achievement batteries for adults because some adults seek information about their current level of achievement in order to upgrade their skills. For example, a high school dropout may want to know where his or her academic deficiencies are in order to learn those skills that were missed. An example of an adult achievement battery is the Test of Adult Basic Education (TABE), which is a test of basic skills in reading, mathematics, and language. The current version of the TABE offers both a Survey Version and a Complete Battery. The Survey Version can be used for screening and placing, while the Complete Battery provides more complete information for determining educational interventions. Either version of the TABE could be used in programs assisting adults in earning a GED or in JTPA and School-To-Careers programs. There are also expanded forms of the TABE that measure work-related basic skills and work-related problem-solving skills.

TerraNova. The following discussion of the *TerraNova* is designed to provide a detailed example of a current achievement battery. The TerraNova serves as a good example because it evolved from the Comprehensive Tests of Basic Skills (CTBS), a widely used and positively evaluated achievement battery. The TerraNova is also a good example because it incorporates both norm-referenced interpretation and criterion-referenced interpretation based on item response theory. The TerraNova is for children between kindergarten and twelfth grade. The publishers designed the TerraNova to measure concepts, processes, and skills taught throughout the nation.

The TerraNova is a new, modular series that offers multiple measures of achievement. The modular system offers a variety of assessment choices from which a school or program can choose. Schools can select from a basic battery that assesses Reading/Language Arts (tested together but scored separately) and Mathematics to a more comprehensive assessment that assesses: Reading/Language Arts (scored separately), Mathematics, Science, Social Studies, Word Analysis, Vocabulary, Language Mechanics, Spelling, and Mathematics Computation. Figure 8.1 and Figure 8.2 provide an example of an Individual Profile Report that would be kept in the student's school file and an example of the Home Report that would be sent to parents (CTB/McGraw-Hill, 1997a).

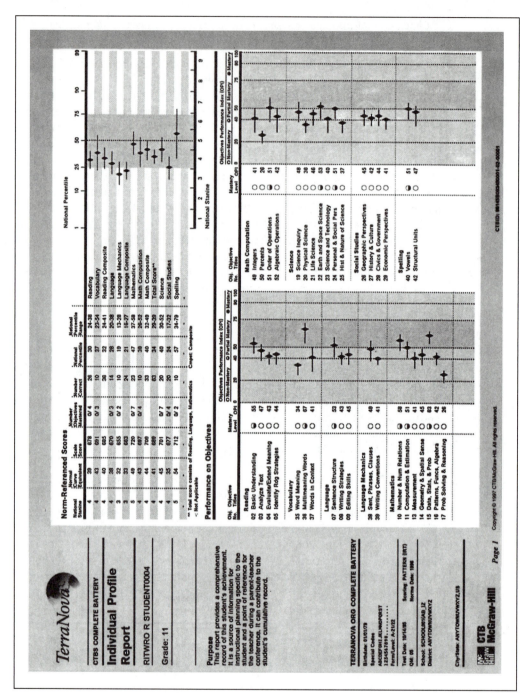

FIGURE 8.1 *Example of TerraNova Individual Profile Report*

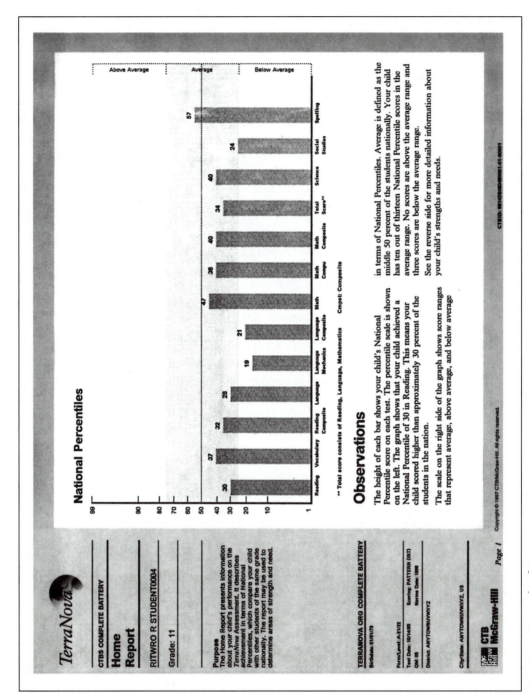

FIGURE 8.2 *Example of TerraNova Home Report*

© 1997 CTB/McGraw-Hill. All rights reserved. Reprinted by permission.

The TerraNova's modular approach also allows for different testing formats. A school may choose either a format with all selected-response items (i.e., multiple-choice format) or one with some constructed-response items. With constructed-response items the students must create a short response. Selected-response items are scored by machine, while the constructed-response items are scored by readers using assessment scoring guides. The developers of TerraNova have been influenced by the authentic assessment movement and are in the process of developing the "Performance Assessment" edition. With this edition, students will move through a series of activities cumulating in a final product that will be assessed (CTB/McGraw-Hill, 1997b). There is also a Spanish version of the TerraNova called the SUPERA, which compares Spanish-speaking students with a national sample of Spanish-speaking students (CTB/McGraw-Hill, 1996).

The construction of the TerraNova involved item-response theory. Because the Terra Nova includes both selected-response and constructed-response items, different models of item-response theory were employed. Each item was evaluated in terms of its content and its psychometric specifications. Readers interested in the implementation of item-response theory should see the *Technical Bulletin* (CTB-McGraw-Hill, 1996). As you will remember from the discussion of item response theory in Chapter 5, often items are selected so that 50% of the students at that grade level can answer the question correctly. Rather than selecting items that 50% of the sample from each grade level got correct, the developers of TerraNova selected items with a range of difficulties for each of the targeted grade levels. In addition, each item was also evaluated for possible bias.

Each of the options within the TerraNova provides norm-referenced, criterion-referenced, objective mastery, and performance level information. Figure 8.1 is an example of the Individual Profile Report, which would be seen by school personnel. The section labeled Norm-Referenced scores compares the individual to individuals at the same grade level, with different norms being available for the first third of the school year, the second third, and the last third of the school year. Information was not available on the size, geographic representation, and ethnic makeup of the norming group. Schools may choose from a variety of derived scores, such as national percentiles, national percentile ranges, stanines, and grade equivalents. The Performance on Objectives section (see bottom half of Figure 8.1) provides the criterion-referenced and objective mastery information. The Performance Objectives are based on curricula, standards, and the National Assessment of Educational Standards. The Objective Performance Index (OPI) scores indicate the projected number of items a student would get correct if there were 100 items in this specific area. The circles that are completely darkened, half darkened, or blank indicate the level of mastery. Nonmastery is indicated by a blank circle and is given if the OPI is less than 50. This would mean the student would be expected to get fewer than 50 items correct on a 100-item test in that area. Partial mastery is indicated by a half-darkened circle for OPI scores between 50 and 74. Mastery is indicated by a fully darkened circle, which means the student had an OPI higher than 75. The information in this section of the profile is deigned to help teachers and parents identify specific content areas that need remediation. It should be noted that some OPI scores are based on only four questions and, thus, there are questions about adequately representing the specific academic area.

Preliminary reliability information on the TerraNova reflected coefficient alphas mostly in the mid .80 to mid .90 range (CTB/McGraw Hill, 1996). Standard error of measurement information is provided on each scale. Further, as reflected in Figure 8.1, the Individual Profile Report can provide percentile scores using standard error of measurement so that individuals can see the range of expected scores. The TerraNova has only recently been published and, hence, there is not as much construct validity information as found in other instruments. This is not as disturbing because the TerraNova is an extension of the Comprehensive Test of Basic Skills and there is substantial evidence for the CTBS. In addition, there is considerable content validation evidence, and the use of item-response theory and the thorough analysis of all items supports the content validity of the TerraNova. In conclusion, the TerraNova is a new instrument that appears to hold promise. There are other sound achievement batteries on the market and this discussion merely provides an example of one survey achievement battery.

Individual Achievement Tests

The second type of achievement test concerns those instruments that are administered individually. These individually administered achievement tests often are used in psychoeducational evaluations, where children are screened for learning disabilities, mental handicaps, behavioral disorders, or for other academic referrals (Sattler, 1993). For example, frequently an individual achievement test is given in conjunction with a general abilities measure to diagnose learning disabilities. In addition, some of these achievement instruments are appropriate for adults and could be used in settings providing retraining for adults (e.g., vocational rehabilitation) in order to assess the academic skills the person has retained.

A commonly used individual achievement test is the *Wide Range Achievement Test 3* (WRAT3, Wilkinson, 1993), which is appropriate for persons ages 5 through 75. The WRAT assesses achievement in the areas of reading, spelling, and arithmetic. Although the WRAT3 usually is administered individually, the Spelling and Arithmetic subtests can be given to a group. There are two equivalent forms of the WRAT that can be used for pre- and postintervention testing. The developer claims that the WRAT3 can be given in 15 to 30 minutes but many examinees take longer.

The Reading subtest of the WRAT3 consists of the examinee reading 42 words aloud. Mabry (1995) suggested that this subtest is not a comprehensive assessment of reading because it only measures pronunciation. The Spelling subtest requires the examinee to spell 40 words, unless the individual is younger than 7, for which age group the requirements are easier. The Arithmetic subtest consists of 40 items, which Mabry also criticized for its inadequate coverage of the arithmetic domain. She further argued that the two forms of the Arithmetic subtest are not equivalent in content or difficulty. Another reviewer, Ward (1995), has been critical of the WRAT3 and suggested caution in using the instrument. Even the WRAT3 manual suggested caution with the use of grade scores.

Another individually administered achievement test is the *Kaufman Test of Educational Achievement* (K-TEA, Kaufman & Kaufman, 1985). There are two forms of the K-TEA: the Brief Form and the Comprehensive Form. The Brief Form covers the areas of Reading, Spelling, and Mathematics. The K-TEA Comprehensive Form is more extensive and contains five subtests: Reading Decoding, Reading Comprehension, Mathematics Applications, Mathematics Computation, and Spelling. The K-TEA, however, is only for children ages 6 through 18. The K-TEA takes about one hour to administer for older children and less time for younger children. Both Doll (1989) and Sattler (1993) contended that the K-TEA is a useful instrument for the assessment of children's academic skills.

A comparatively new instrument is the *Wechsler Individual Achievement Test* (WIAT, Wechsler, 1992) that was first published in 1992. The WIAT is standardized with the widely used *Wechsler Intelligence Scale for Children—Third Edition.* The publishers contend that the WIAT is designed to assist with the regulatory requirement of the Individuals with Disabilities Education Act (IDEA) and the need to assess and reevaluate children and adolescents. The WIAT Screener is a shortened version of the WIAT and contains three subtests: Basic Reading, Mathematics Reasoning, and Spelling. The WIAT contains eight subtests: Basic Reading, Mathematics Reasoning, Spelling, Reading Comprehension, Numerical Operations, Listening Comprehension, Oral Expression, and Written Expression. The WIAT does not have the history of extensive use that either the WRAT3 or even the K-TEA have, but its relationship to the WISC-III is certainly an advantage.

Diagnostic Tests

Many of the different types of achievement tests can be used for diagnostic purposes. For example, some of the individually administered achievement tests previously mentioned are used to "diagnose" academic strengths and limitations. There are, however, instruments designed specifically for the purpose of diagnosing academic difficulties. Examples of diagnostic reading instruments are the Stanford Diagnostic Reading Test, Fourth Edition, Nelson-Denny Reading Test, and the Classroom Reading Inventory. In the mathematics areas, counselors may see a report where the KeyMath-Revised, the Sequential Assessment of Mathematics Inventories, or the MAT6 Mathematics Diagnostic Tests were used.

Many times testing is performed not to diagnose limitations within a specific subject area but to diagnose a **learning disability**. Most counselors will not be the clinicians performing the testing and diagnosing the disability; however, an understanding of the common diagnostic procedures may be helpful when working with specific clients. Although there are numerous definitions of learning disability, there appear to be four factors that are common within the definitions (Hallahan & Kauffman, 1997). The first factor is an IQ-achievement discrepancy. In the diagnosis of a learning disability, an individual will often be given an individual intelligence test and an achievement test, with the intent of examining discrepancy. Some states and school districts have even specified a precise amount (e.g., two standard deviations) by which the intelligence score must exceed the achievement. The use of discrepancy formulas as the sole diagnostic tool has been criticized by many in the field (Fletcher et al., 1994; Kavale, 1995). The discrepancy between IQ and achievement, however, continues to be relied on heavily in the diagnosis of a learning disability. The second factor, according to Hallahan and Kauffman, is the presumption of central nervous dysfunction, with some clinicians incorporating neurological evaluation into their assessment of a possible learning disability. The third factor is psychological processing disorders, and a thorough assessment of possible learning disabilities will also assess the information processing area. The last factor is that learning problems should be screened to determine if the problems are due to environmental disadvantage, mental retardation, or emotional disturbance. It is assumed that learning disabilities are related to central nervous system and psychological processing dysfunction and not to these other factors.

A comprehensive diagnostic instrument is the *Woodcock-Johnson Psycho-Educational Battery—Revised* (WJ-R, Woodcock & Johnson, 1989,1990). This psychoeductional battery consists of two individually administered instruments: the Woodcock-Johnson Tests of Cognitive Ability and the Woodcock-Johnson Tests of Achievement. Learning problems often are diagnosed using the WJ-R by examining the discrepancies between the cognitive ability scores and the scores on the achievement section. The WJ-R is designed to assess both cognitive and various academic achievement abilities for individuals ages 2 through 95. Even though there is some debate about interpreting discrepancies, the authors of the Woodcock-Johnson have incorporated tables providing their suggestions for evaluating an individual's ability/achievement discrepancy. The WJ-R is not designed to be administered in its entirety; rather, the examiner typically gives the standard battery and then chooses from supplemental tests depending on the situation.

The revision of the Woodcock-Johnson used the Horn-Cattell model as the foundation for the assessment of cognitive ability. The cognitive factors assessed are Fluid Reasoning, Gf; Comprehensive-Knowledge, Gc; Quantitative Ability, Gq; Visual Processing, Gv; Auditory Processing, Ga; Processing Speed, Gs; Short-Term Memory, Gsm; and Long-Term Retrieval, Glr. On the WJ-R Tests of Achievement the standard battery yields six cluster scores: Broad Reading, Broad Mathematics, Mathematics Reasoning, Broad Written Language, and Broad Knowledge and Skills. Supplemental tests can be given to gather more detailed achievement information. An examiner can choose from many different derived scores. Consequently, a counselor could read a report that might include one or more of the following: age equivalents, grade equivalents, relative master indices, percentile ranks, extended percentile ranks, standard scores, and extended standard scores. There is also a newly developed instrument for bilingual assessment, the *Bilingual Verbal Ability Tests* (Munoz-Sandoval, Cummins, Alvarado, & Ruef, 1998), that uses subtests from the WJ-R.

Both Cummings (1995) and Lee and Steffany (1995) evaluated the Woodcock-Johnson Psycho-Educational Battery—Revised positively. The internal consistency reliability coefficients for the WJ-R for the major ability and achievement clusters fall in the .90s and most of the subtests have reliability coefficients higher than .80. The normative sample was 6,359 and is representative of the U.S. population as described by the 1980 census report. The WJ-R is often used to assess college students with possible learning disabilities because the norming group is appropriate for that age group. The validity information is quite extensive, which contributes to the use of this diagnostic instrument.

Criterion-Referenced Tests

Criterion-referenced achievement tests are instruments designed to determine if a certain academic standard is met. Many tests you have taken for academic courses are criterion-referenced where certain performance merits an "A," at another level to get a "B," and so on. These tests are only criterion-referenced if the criterion or standard is set before taking the test. Many times criterion-referenced tests are equated with mastery tests. In mastery tests, the person has to reach a certain level of mastery before he or she can proceed. For example, the child must be able to add one-digit numbers together before advancing to a test that measures his or her ability to add two-digit numbers together.

The distinction between a criterion-referenced achievement test and a diagnostic or subject area test is sometimes quite gray, and the reader should not view these categories as being mutually exclusive. A number of existing criterion-referenced tests were developed by school districts or State Departments of Education; however, some publishers have developed criterion-referenced achievement tests. For example in 1997, Harcourt Brace Educational Measurement published the *New Standards Reference Examination: English Language Arts* and the *New Standards Reference Examination: Mathematics*. These are quite interesting assessments because the New Standards instruments incorporate some recent trends in achievement assessment. First, the assessments are based on national and international benchmarked performance standards. The developers used content standards developed by professional organizations such as the National Council of Teachers of Mathematics, the National Council of Teachers of English, and the International Reading Association. The elementary version measures performance level expected at the end of fourth grade; the middle school version measures expected performance at the end of eighth grade; and, finally, the high school version measures expected performance at the end of tenth grade. The second recent development in assessment that is incorporated into these New Standards assessments is the use of performance tasks and portfolio assessment. As you will remember, portfolio assessment involves an accumulation of materials rather than one brief examination. With the exception of some multiple-choice items, the students are required in the New Standards to perform multiple tasks that are scored holistically by trained professionals. The scoring is criterion-referenced and provides information on the student's level of performance.

Minimum-Level Skills Tests

Some authorities in the area of assessment will make a distinction between criterion-referenced tests and minimum-level skills tests, although it could be argued that all minimum-level tests are criterion-referenced tests where the minimum level is the "criterion" for passing. The minimum-level achievement tests that have received the most attention and discussion are those that many states require for high school graduation. Over the years there has been concern about students graduating from high school without minimum competencies. These concerns led many states to require students to pass a minimum competency examination before a high school diploma could be awarded. The states, however, vary widely in what is required and at what grade level the students are tested. Another issue concerns the relationship between the instrument and the curriculum. Because these are achievement tests, minimum competency examinations need to be related to the curriculum. This is not always easy because even students within the same high school can take very different academic course work. There is also some controversy concerning the minimum competencies expected of high school graduates. For example, there are diverse views on the minimum reading level for a high school graduate. In addition, some students have learning disabilities that might affect their performances on a portion of the tests while they can do very well in other academic areas. Consequently, there are numerous difficulties in developing and implementing minimum competency examinations.

Subject Area Tests

The largest number of achievement tests are the single subject tests developed by teachers. These instruments vary in quality, with some teachers developing quite refined assessments and other teachers designing instruments with major flaws. In addition, many textbooks now provide test item banks for which the publishers develop numerous test questions that assess material covered in the text. Whether a teacher develops his or her own items or incorporates items from a test bank, content validity must be considered. Teachers need to ensure that the test adequately reflects the behavior domain being measured. The steps toward ensuring content validity discussed in Chapter 4 need to be incorporated in developing a subject area test. For example, teachers who develop a test specifications table before the items are written are more likely to develop a sound examination because the test will follow this framework rather than being randomly assembled.

As mentioned earlier, advocates of **authentic assessment** and **performance assessment** have had a major influence on teacher-developed subject area tests (Oosterhof, 1994). Authentic and performance assessment strives for greater realism of tasks and greater complexity of tasks. The belief is that simplistic assessments with one correct answer are not adequate measures since real-life problems often can be solved in multiple ways. Hence, in performance assessment there are often multiple solutions. In addition, those arguing for changing achievement testing argue that one short test cannot adequately measure an individual's abilities. They suggest that multiple measures gathered over a period of time provide a more authentic assessment of the individual's achievement level or ability to perform. Therefore, there is a move toward portfolio assessment in which teachers systematically collect multiple indicators of performance. The assessment then focuses on the total evaluation of the products in the portfolio. The rationale is that with the evidence of performance on multiple tasks, better evaluation of the student's strengths and limitations can occur (Gronlund, 1998). Authentic or performance assessment, however, is not simple to implement, and implementing it appropriately requires a substantial commitment of time.

Aptitude Assessment

The purpose of **aptitude assessment** is quite different from achievement testing. Achievement testing provides information on where an individual is, while aptitude testing provides an indication of how the individual will perform in the future. Clients often seek counseling in order to make decisions about the future. Some aptitude instruments predict the ability to acquire a specific type of skill or knowledge, while other aptitude assessments predict performance in a certain job or career. Aptitude instruments are frequently used to predict either academic or vocational performance. The pertinent issue with any aptitude instrument is the degree to which it predicts relative to the criterion of interest.

Scholastic Aptitude Tests

Hood and Johnson (1997) argued that counselors in a variety of fields (e.g., mental health counselors, elementary school counselors) need to be knowledgeable about the predominant scholastic aptitude tests. They contended that counselors in most settings will be consulted by friends, relatives, and colleagues' children who are applying to colleges and universities. Traditionally, the public has expected counselors to be knowledgeable of these prevalent instruments. Hence, counselors who do not have at least a working knowledge of these instruments may not be viewed as credible by some individuals.

Scholastic Assessment Test (SAT). The *Scholastic Assessment Test* (SAT) is a very widely used predictor of college performance. The Scholastic Aptitude Tests has been around since 1926; in 1994 it was revised and renamed the Scholastic Assessment Test. Part of the reason for changing the name of the SAT was to move away from any reference that might imply that the instrument measures innate aptitudes. The SAT program is designed to assist students, high schools, colleges, and scholarship programs with postsecondary educational planning and decision making (College Entrance Examination Board, 1995). The instrument originated to provide a common standard to which students could be compared since subject matter of high school courses and grading procedures varied widely.

The Scholastic Assessment Test consists of the SAT I: Reasoning Test and the SAT II: Subject Tests. The SAT I: Reasoning Test is a three-hour test that measures verbal and mathematical reasoning abilities. Some postsecondary institutions will require applicants to take only the SAT I, while other institutions will require certain subject tests within the SAT II. The SAT II consists of single subject tests, such as Writing, Math Level I, Biology, and French. The individual tests within the SAT II are used for both admissions and course placement.

Students receive scores that range from 200 to 800 on both the Verbal and Mathematical sections of the SAT I (see Figure 8.3). The mean is 500 and the standard deviation is 100. SAT scores after April 1, 1995, have been "recentered" in order to make the Verbal and Mathematics sections comparable. Furthermore, Educational Testing Service (ETS) uses a complex equating process that adjusts for variation in difficulty from one edition to another. The College Entrance Examination Board (1995) recommended that counselors use the range of expected scores calculated using standard error of measurement when interpreting SAT I results. The profile can also help students understand their strengths and limitations within the Verbal and Mathematics areas. Counseling individuals can also be assisted by the Personal and College Profiles (see Figure 8.3), which is sent to the students and high schools. This report provides information about the institutions to which the student requested his or her SAT scores be sent and matches that information with information the student reported (e.g., grade point average, desired size of school).

An instrument related to the SAT is the Preliminary SAT/National Merit Scholarship Qualifying Test (PSAT/NMSQT). The PSAT/NMSQT provides students with an estimate of how they will perform on the SAT and also is used for national scholarship and recognition programs. Students typically take the PSAT/NMSQT during their junior year in high school. Scores on the PSAT/NMSQT range from 20 to 80 and are designed to be comparable to the SAT by adding a zero (e.g., a score of 55 on the Verbal section of the PSAT/NMSQT would be predictive of a SAT I Verbal score of 550). The PSAT/NMSQT can be an effective tool in counseling students facing decisions about college.

FIGURE 8.3

Sample SAT Student Score Report form

SAT materials from 1998–1999 Admission Staff Handbook, College Entrance Examination Board, 1997. Reprinted by permission of Educational Testing Service and the College Entrance Exam Board, the copyright owners. Permission to reprint SAT materials does not constitute review or endorsement by ETS or the College Board of this publication as a whole or of any other questions or testing information it may contain.

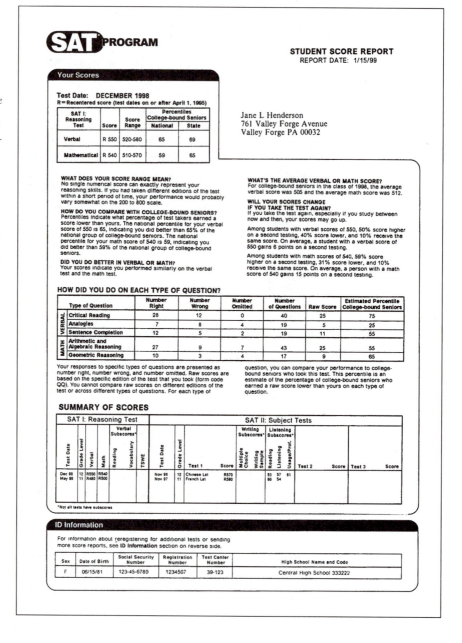

For instance, a counselor would want to work with a student who is planning to attend a very selective college but has low scores on the PSAT/NMSQT.

American College Testing (ACT). The other predominate nationally administered college admissions testing program is the *American College Testing* (ACT) Assessment. The ACT contains four sections that can be useful in counseling in-

FIGURE 8.4

Sample of ACT Assessment High School Report

Reprinted by permission of American College Testing.

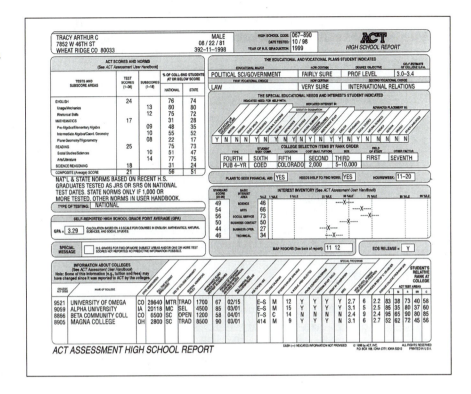

ACT ASSESSMENT HIGH SCHOOL REPORT

dividuals: (1) the results from four academic tests; (2) the High School Course/Grade information questionnaire; (3) the Student Profile section; and (4) the ACT Interest Inventory. First, the ACT Assessment includes four tests of educational development that are the tests used by postsecondary institutions for admissions and placement decisions (see Figure 8.4). These scores are in the upper left portion of the High School Report and cover the areas of English, mathematics, reading, and science reasoning. Individuals receive scores in the four test areas and for seven subscore areas, along with a composite score. The scores for the four academic tests and the composite score range from 1 to 36; however, it should be remembered that the standard deviation for these tests varies. Furthermore, there is some variation in the standard errors of measurement depending on the test and where the score falls in the range of scores. ACT, however, recommended using 2 points to estimate the range for the four academic tests and 1 point for standard error of measurement for the Composite score (ACT, 1997). The average scores for the ACT will vary from year to year, but in general the average composite score for college-bound students is 21 (Hood & Johnson, 1997). The English, Mathematics, and Reading tests all have subscore areas where the scores range from 1 to 18.

Although clients may primarily focus on the scores on the academic tests of the ACT, a counselor can utilize additional information for counseling, particularly career counseling. ACT research indicated that individuals are quite accurate in reporting grade information on the High School Course/Grade information questionnaire (ACT, 1997). In addition, the Student Profile section can provide the counselor with a summary of the client's academic needs and interests. Many college students seek help with career planning (Herr & Cramer, 1992) and the ACT Interest Inventory can be especially helpful. The inventory measures individuals' interests in six areas that were designed to parallel Holland's (1985, 1997) six types. The student's interests are compared to the same nationally representative sample as the academic portions of the ACT. The reporting of percentile ranks uses a band indicating the range based on standard error of measurement. In addition, a counselor can use the World-of-Work Map that is printed on the back of the profile to further explore a client's interests (see *User Handbook* for more information on using the World-of-Work Map).

The ACT Assessment is not the only assessment tool published by ACT. ACT has developed the Educational Planning and Assessment System (EPAS), which provides a series of assessment programs for students in grades 8 through 12. Students in the 8th grade would take EXPLORE, which includes achievement tests in English, Mathematics, Reading, and Science Reasoning. EXPLORE also includes an interest inventory, a study skills checklist, and a course work planner. PLAN is a similar instrument designed for 10th grade students, which tests academic achievement and facilitates postsecondary planning. The tool for 12th graders is the ACT Assessment that was discussed previously. ACT's EPAS also includes Work Keys, which is an instrument designed to assess workplace skills rather than more traditional academic skills. Work Keys can be used by schools or businesses and can be helpful in Tech-Prep, school-to-careers, and workforce development initiatives.

Graduate Record Examination (GRE). Another scholastic aptitude test is the *Graduate Record Examination* (GRE). The GRE, however, is designed to predict performance in graduate school as compared to the previously discussed instruments that predict undergraduate college performance. The Graduate Record Examination Aptitude Test is usually just called the GRE and is a general test for selecting graduate students. Some disciplines will require testing on that specific academic area and will use one of the GRE (Advanced) Tests. There are also other tests that have been developed in specific disciplines for selection of students into professional schools, such as the *Medical College Admissions Test* (MCAT), the *Dental Admission Test* (DAT), the *Law School Admission Test* (LSAT), and the *Graduate Management Admission Test* (GMAT).

This discussion is going to cover only the Graduate Record Examination Aptitude Test, which will be referred to as the GRE. The GRE consists of three sections: the Verbal (GRE-V), the Quantitative (GRE-Q), and the Analytical (GRE-A). The GRE-V covers reasoning, analogies, antonyms, and reading comprehension. The Quantitative (GRE-Q) tests mathematical reasoning, algebra, and geometry. The Analytical portion examines logical and abstract reasoning. With each of these three areas, the mean is 500 and the standard deviation is 100 (Graduate Record Examination Board, 1997).

There also is a computer-based version of the GRE that can be taken at numerous testing sites throughout the country. Individuals can schedule to take the computer version at convenient times and, therefore, do not need to wait until the scheduled testing dates. The GRE was one of the first assessments to utilize computer-adaptive assessment. In the computer-based version, the computer *adapts* the test to the individual taking the GRE. At the beginning of the test the individual is presented with questions of average ability. As the individual answers questions, the computer analyzes the answers to determine the difficulty of the next question. The scoring of the test takes into consideration the number of correct responses and the difficulty of the items. Educational Testing Service, which publishes the GRE, has performed extensive research that indicates the paper-and-pencil version and the computer-based version of the GRE are equivalent (Graduate Record Examination Board, 1997). The advantages and disadvantages of computer assessment will be discussed in Chapter 16.

Validity of Scholastic Aptitude Tests

The most pertinent questions are related to how well these scholastic aptitude tests predict collegiate performance. These tests are used to make decisions that often have a significant influence on people's lives and, therefore, the validity of these instruments deserves analysis. In general, research indicates that the validity of the SAT and the ACT are about the same. Most of the studies indicate that the correlation between scores on these tests and freshman grade point average (GPA) is in the .30 to .50 range. Many studies have found that high school grades are as good as or a slightly better predictor of college GPA than scholastic aptitude tests (College Entrance Examination Board, 1995). The best predictor is a combination of high school grades and a scholastic aptitude test. These two measures seem to balance each other; grades take into consideration persistence and hard work, while the scholastic aptitudes tests are measures that are not influenced by partiality or teacher bias.

The same trend applies to predicting graduate school performance, where multiple predictors are better than any one single predictor. According to ETS (Graduate Record Examination Board, 1997), combining the GRE-Verbal, GRE-Quantitative, and GRE-Analytical scores is a better predictor than using just one score. The combined GRE scores have validity coefficients in the .31 to .37 range, while undergraduate grade point average has validity coefficients in the .35 to .39 range. A better predictor is to combine the GRE scores with undergraduate grade point average. Adding the appropriate single subject test to the combined GRE scores and undergraduate grade point average produced the highest range of validity coefficients (.49 to .63).

Institutions vary in the degree to which scholastic aptitude tests' scores influence admissions decisions. Counselors working with college-bound individuals need to have knowledge about the admissions requirements and typical test score performance in order to counsel these individuals effectively. The following sources can be helpful in providing information to college-bound clients: *The College Handbook, Peterson's Guide to Four-Year Colleges, Peterson's Guide to Two-Year Colleges,* and *Ludden's Adult Guide to Colleges and Universities.* In addition, some of the computer-assisted career information systems contain information on college admissions.

For counselors working with scholastic aptitude tests, it is important to remember that these instruments provide some information but that the information provided should be evaluated in a broader context. Publishers of these instruments suggest that scores from scholastic aptitude assessments be combined with other information (College Entrance Examination Board, 1995; Graduate Record Examination Board, 1997). Counselors need to help clients sort out the meaning of their scores, which can be facilitated by incorporating other germane information into the counseling process. For example, take some time and read the summary of the client in Figure 8.5 and consider what other information you would need to help this client.

Vocational/Career Aptitude Tests

As mentioned earlier, aptitude tests are often used to predict academic or vocational/career performance. Besides the scholastic aptitude tests we have discussed, there are numerous vocational aptitude tests that are used in career counseling to predict job or occupational performance. These vocational or career aptitude instruments will be discussed in this chapter rather than the chapter related to career assessment, but these instruments should be considered when selecting tools for career counseling.

A number of the instruments summarized in this section are used for selection purposes. Employers want to select individuals who can perform the job duties, and employees want to be hired into positions in which they can be effective. Effective selection requires that an instrument accurately predict successful performance of job duties. This is a difficult task since job duties within an occupation will vary depending on the organization and the setting. In addition, if the instrument is to predict performance in an occupation, then the test needs to be validated with information from people who are performing suc-

FIGURE 8.5
The case of Anna

Anna is a 17-year-old high school senior who is undecided about her college plans. She has decided to go to college and major in a field related to business. Her parents both graduated from Ivy League schools and want Anna to attend one of those institutions. Anna had planned on going to one of those schools but is now wondering if she is smart enough. Anna and her parents are in counseling because of recent problems between them. Anna was involved in many school activities in her freshman, sophomore, and junior years but has dropped out of these activities her senior year. Also, Anna and her mother have been arguing about Anna's "lack of motivation." Anna's grades continue to be mostly As with some Bs. Recently, Anna received her SAT scores, which were a Verbal score of 570 and a Mathematical score of 590. She and her parents want the counselor to tell them if she is "bright enough" to go to a selective college.

What other information would it be helpful for the counselor to gather in order to interpret these SAT scores?

cessfully in that occupation. This necessitates a precise definition of what constitutes performing "successfully" in that occupation, because just being employed in a job does not guarantee that the person is successful or competent. The matter is further complicated because job performance cannot be adequately measured in a unidimensional manner. Most of today's occupations cannot be evaluated simply in terms of whether the person does the job or doesn't do the job. Most current occupations are complex and some current authorities in the field contend that multifaceted methods of evaluating job performance are needed (Borman, 1991; Campbell, 1994). Therefore, all of these factors make validating an instrument designed to predict job performance a difficult and time-consuming task. Because it is difficult to gather the information on job performance, it is difficult to get large norming groups. This problem is magnified when test developers want to develop an instrument that predicts performance in a number of occupations. A test developer would need a sufficient number of individuals in each occupation to have an adequate norming group.

There are some vocational aptitude tests designed to measure one aptitude or to predict performance in a single occupational area. For example, psychomotor tests are single-purpose aptitude tests, which were originally thought to be predictive of many occupations. These instruments, however, are predictive of lower-level manual skills but not good predictors of high-order abilities (Anastasi, 1988). Clerical aptitude and mechanical aptitude tests are examples of single-purpose vocational aptitude tests that can predict to certain occupations. Clients, however, frequently want to know their strengths and limitations and how they might perform in multiple occupations. Most clients would not want to spend the time to take numerous single-purpose aptitude tests and, hence, aptitude batteries are used with many clients. Aptitude batteries assess multiple aptitudes and predict performance in various occupations. These aptitude batteries can assist clients in examining their strengths and limitations and, also, assess their potential in a variety of career areas.

Armed Services Vocational Aptitude Test Battery. The *Armed Services Vocational Aptitude Test Battery* (ASVAB), a part of the Armed Services Vocational Aptitude Battery Career Exploration Program, is the most widely used aptitude test in the United States. The ASVAB Career Exploration Program is offered, without cost, by the Department of Defense (DoD) to students in secondary and postsecondary schools. This program includes an interest inventory and other materials to supplement the ASVAB. The ASVAB is designed to predict both educational and occupational successes (U.S. Department of Defense, 1995).

The ASVAB contains ten short tests (Word Knowledge, Paragraph Comprehension, Arithmetic Reasoning, Mathematics Knowledge, General Science, Auto & Shop Information, Mechanical Comprehension, Electronic Information, Numerical Operations, and Coding Speed). Students receive scores on these ten tests and composite scores for Academic Ability, Verbal Ability, and Mathematical Ability. As seen in Figure 8.6, the ASVAB Student Results Sheet

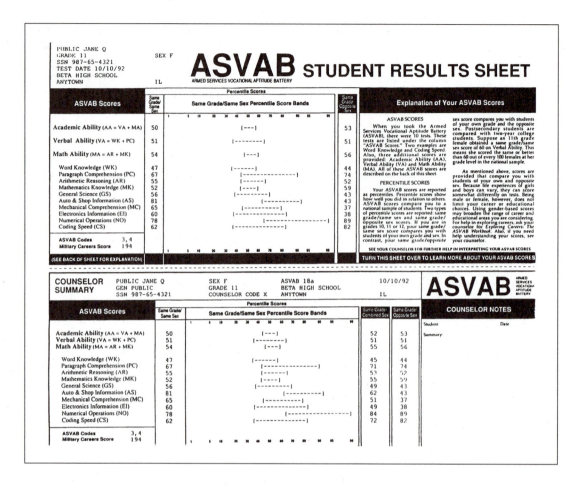

FIGURE 8.6
*Sample ASVAB
Student Results
Sheet*

provides scores in percentile ranks and percentile bands for the same grade/
same sex norms. A percentile rank score is also provided for the same grade/
opposite sex norms. Another composite score is the Armed Forces Qualification Test (AFQT) that is used for screening potential recruits by all of the services. A student can use the booklet *Exploring Careers: The ASVAB Workbook* to
explore the relationship between his or her scores and different occupations.

The current version is the ASVAB 18/19; however, DoD is in the process
of renorming this instrument. The current norming information was gathered
in 1980 from a stratified sample of 12,000 men and women between the ages
of 16 and 23. The reliability coefficients provided are in the .92 to .96 range
for the composite scores and range between .67 and .92 for the ten tests.

Elmore and Bradley (1994) recommend the ASVAB 18/19 for individuals
planning on entering the military within the next two years. They do not recommend the ASVAB for general use by school counselors due to lack of validation studies on the ASVAB Career Exploration Program. Wigdor and Green

(1991a, 1991b) are involved in a massive study of the ASVAB and found it to be a good predictor of performance-based indicators of job proficiency. The majority of the validation studies of the ASVAB, however, have been with military occupations or military training programs. There is also some concern about the average-score differences between minority and nonminority examinees (Prediger & Swaney, 1992; Widgor & Green, 1991a,1991b). The ASVAB is evolving and numerous studies of job performance are continuing to be performed on this widely used instrument. In addition, the DoD is in the process of developing a computer-adapted version that will shorten the time necessary to take the ASVAB.

General Aptitude Test Battery. The *General Aptitude Test Battery* (GATB) was developed by the United States Employment Service (USES) for use in state employment services (U.S. Department of Labor, 1970). A version of the GATB can also be purchased by nonprofit organizations, such as vocational rehabilitation centers, prisons, and schools. The GATB is worthy of discussion because it is the most extensively researched occupational aptitude test. There also is an interest inventory, the USES Interest Inventory (USES-II), that can be administered concurrently with the GATB. The instrument is designed for work applicants ages 16 through retirement.

The GATB consists of 12 tests of which 8 are paper-and-pencil and 4 are apparatus tests. The entire battery can be administered in two and one-half hours. These 12 tests result in scores in nine areas and three composite scores that are listed in Table 8.2. The GATB scores are derived scores that have a mean of 100 and a standard deviation of 20. Bolton (1994) evaluated the GATB as being quite reliable, particularly for adults. The standard errors of measurement for the composite scores are: 3 points for Cognitive, 7 points for Perceptual, and 10 points for Psychomotor. It is not unusual for psychomotor tests to show more variation than other areas.

TABLE 8.2
GATB aptitude scores and composite scores

Aptitude Scores	Composite Scores
General Learning Ability (**G**)	Cognitive = G + V + N
Verbal Aptitude (**V**)	Perceptual = S + P + Q
Numerical Aptitude (**N**)	Psychomotor = K + F + M
Spatial Aptitude (**S**)	
Form Perception (**P**)	
Clerical Perception (**Q**)	
Motor Coordination (**K**)	
Finger Dexterity (**F**)	
Manual Dexterity (**M**)	

There are two major approaches to interpreting and using the scores from the GATB (Bolton, 1994). The first is the more traditional method and involves the 66 **Occupational Aptitude Patterns** (OAPs). The selective aptitude scores are used to derive indicators of success in 66 occupational areas. Examinees receive suitability rating of high, medium, or low in each of the 66 OAP. Selection of the aptitudes to be used in calculating each OAP and cutoff scores for the high, medium, and low designations are based on validity coefficients, test scores of workers, and recommendations from job analysts. These OAP designations and results of the interest inventory can be used together to explore occupations that correspond with the individual's aptitudes and interests. There are, however, some limitations that counselors need to be aware of with the OAP method of interpretation. The amount of research and the strength of the validity coefficients vary among the OAPs and, thus, counselors need to understand which areas should be interpreted cautiously. Another problem is the determination of cutoff scores because the high, medium, and low ratings are quite broad. For example, someone could be very close to a high but still get a medium rating and another person could almost get a low rating and receive the same medium designation. These cutoff scores are also based on only two to four aptitudes and do not take into consideration compensating factors.

Another method of translating GATB scores addresses some of the problems associated with the OAP method but it also has some limitations. This second method is based on the **validity generalization** approach to test validation. Validity generalization stems from the work of two researchers, Hunter and Schmidt, and their associates. These researchers were primarily interested in studying which variables predicted successful personnel selection. In studying the effectiveness of tests in employment selection, they focused on the GATB because there was an abundance of validation studies that had been performed. Other researchers contended that the GATB was fine at predicting performance in some jobs but not good at predicting performance in other occupations. They examined the variations in validity coefficients of job performance tests, which primarily involved the GATB and performance in different occupations. They found that differences in validity coefficients were mainly due to measurement and sampling error (Pearlman, Schmidt, & Hunter, 1980; Schmidt & Hunter, 1977; Schmidt, Hunter, & Caplan, 1981). In a large meta-analysis, Hunter (1980) found that the three composite scores of the GATB were valid predictors of success in all jobs. He found that the relationship between the aptitudes and job performance was linear, indicating that as test scores increased so did ratings of job performance. Hence, the best workers had the highest test scores. Thus, the term *validity generalization* refers to the findings that the same test score data may be predictive for all jobs. The implication is that if a test is valid for a few occupations, the test is valid for all jobs in that cluster. Therefore, these researchers found evidence that validity coefficients could be generalized to other occupations. They also argued that the validity generalization results showed that separate validation studies for every occupation in the United States economy was not necessary with the GATB.

Hunter (1982) demonstrated that the GATB composites could be weighted to predict to five job families that included all occupations listed by the Department of Labor. For example, Job Family 1 was 59% Cognitive, 30% Perceptual, and 11% Psychomotor, while the other four job families had different weighting on these same three factors. Hunter went on to suggest that these weighted scores should be used for top-down hiring. Top-down hiring means an employer should hire the applicant with the highest weighted score because he or she would be the most proficient worker out of the applicant pool.

Many local employment service offices began using the Job Family method and provided employers with a rank ordering of applicants based on the weighted scores for the five Job Families. Previous research, however, had shown that African-Americans, Hispanics, and Native Americans tend to get lower scores than others on the GATB. Some argued that using validity generalization adversely impacted these groups, and so GATB scores were calculated comparing individuals of the same ethnic group. Thus, the rankings provided to the employer would be for different ethnic groups. Hartigan and Wigdor (1989) along with others were very critical of validity generalization and the GATB. The issues were intensely debated, particularly the use of separate ethnic-group norms. The Civil Rights Act of 1991, however, banned the use of separate ethic-group norming and the United States Employment Security returned to the OAP method of scoring the GATB. Research on validity generalization is ongoing, so these methods are likely continue to have an impact on personnel selection and testing.

Differential Aptitude Test. The last aptitude test that will be discussed as an example of assessments in this area is the *Differential Aptitude Test* (DAT) (Bennett, Seashore, & Wesman, 1990). In my opinion, the DAT frequently was used in the past but has decreased somewhat in popularity in recent years. The Differential Aptitude Test is designed for students in grades 7 through 12 but can also be used with adults. The DAT can be used alone or in conjunction with the Career Interest Inventory. There is a computer-adaptive version of the DAT that takes about 90 minutes, whereas the paper-and-pencil version takes about 3 hours. The aptitudes measured are similar to other instruments and include: Verbal Reasoning, Numerical Reasoning, Abstract Reasoning, Perceptual Speed and Accuracy, Mechanical Reasoning, Space Relations, Spelling, and Language Usage. The Verbal Reasoning and Numerical Reasoning scores are combined to produce the Scholastic Aptitude score.

Separate norms are used for males and females on the Differential Aptitude Test. The use of separate gender norms is related to the findings that males and females tend to score differently on a few of the DAT scales. The norming groups for the DAT are large and were stratified to match the 1980 census information. The reliability coefficients are in the .80 to .90 range (The Psychological Corporation, 1991). When the results are computer scored, as compared to hand scored, then the individual's scores appear with confidence bands.

The criticisms of the Differential Aptitude Tests center on the validity of the instrument. Willson and Stone (1994) pointed out that predictive validity information is conspicuously absent. In addition, there is very little differential validity evidence. The term used in the composite score, Scholastic Aptitude, is important since the DAT has been found to be highly correlated with achievement tests and high school and college grade point average (The Psychological Corporation, 1991). A counselor can use the DAT to predict academic performance, but should be very cautious in using the instrument to predict vocational or occupational performance.

Work Samples Assessment

Another method of assessing vocational/career aptitudes is through the use of work samples. Work sample assessments have a different philosophical base, with the contention that work performance can best be assessed by using a sample of the actual work the individual would perform. Thus, work sample assessments attempt to replicate the job activities as closely as possible and then individuals are evaluated on how they perform those "work samples." A variety of settings use work samples, but they are most often used in vocational training, placement, or rehabilitation settings.

An example of a work sample assessment is the *Valpar Component Work Sample* (VCWS). There are currently 23 individual work samples in this system that can be used to assess various cognitive and physical tasks. Each of these work samples has distinct materials that are used in that assessment. For example, the Small Tools (mechanical) Work Sample requires the individual to use various small tools, such as screwdriver, pliers, and wrenches. The Drafting Work Sample has the examinees use drafting tools in activities involving reaching, handling, fingering, and visual acuity. The instrument is scored using a criterion-referenced method, with activities having to be completed correctly and in a certain period of time. There are also norm-referenced data for both nondisabled workers and special disability groups. In addition, Valpar offers a software package that scores the VCWS and interfaces the scores with other vocational material.

Another work sample program has evolved into a computer system. Pesco's SAGE system can still be used without the computer, and it measures a broad spectrum of skills and aptitudes using lightweight units. The SAGE, however, has been adapted to the computer in the Pesco 2001. The SAGE units are taken at the computer with special manipulation units being connected. The computers then score the units and relevant career information and descriptions are provided based on the scores. The system also includes an on-line system that searches various employer databases.

In conclusion, work sample assessment can often provide insights into "real-world" skills that some of the more traditional methods have difficulty measuring. Sound work sample assessments, however, are difficult to design and develop. For many occupations the work tasks are varied and diverse and it is difficult to extract simple tasks that replicate those duties. For example, try to think of work sample tasks for being a counselor. Some might suggest a work sample in which examinees listen to another person and are tested on the amount of information they retain. Counseling, however, involves more than just listening, because good counselors need to be able to conceptualize and use a variety of interventions. Work samples also need to be reliable; often the closer an activity gets to the real world, the more likely it is that extraneous factors are being introduced. Another problem is that some work samples can be quite expensive and not all settings have the facilities to perform these kinds of assessments.

Test Preparation and Performance

Before we conclude with our discussion of achievement and aptitude testing, it is important to examine the research related to the effects of test preparation. You have probably seen advertisements claiming that if an individual purchases a set of workbooks or a CD-ROM or attends a workshop, then the individual is guaranteed a higher score on a test (e.g., the Scholastic Assessment or the Medical College Admissions Test). You may question whether these programs or products actually improve scores significantly. The answer to that question is that it depends on the program. Before we explore which types of training programs have an impact on scores, we need to define some terms. *Test sophistication* is a term applied to the individual's level of sophistication in test taking skills. Test sophistication is not related to knowledge of the content but is related to the format of the tests and skills for maneuvering through that format. A distinction needs to be made between the terms *coaching* and *education*, which are both related to instruction in the content of the examination. Coaching involves training or practice on questions that are the same or similar to the items on the test. Education occurs when the domain or area is covered more broadly and the intent is for the test taker to learn the content or information. With coaching, the intent of the instruction is to do well on the test, not necessarily to teach the content.

Test Sophistication

The question here is "Do programs that provide practice on the testing format make a significant difference?" There is some research that indicates that test scores do improve when individuals retake an alternate form of the test (Donlon, 1984). Furthermore, individuals with extensive experience in taking standardized tests have an advantage. However, short orientation and practice sessions tend to bring individuals without extensive experience equal to those who have had more exposure to tests (Anastasi, 1981). These findings indicate that those who can afford to receive test sophistication training have an advantage over those who cannot afford it. In the last few years, a number of tests (e.g., SAT, GRE) have incorporated into their registration materials booklets that address test-taking strategies, explanation of item formats, and sample test questions. These booklets are designed to provide those who cannot afford to pay for test sophistication training the same sort of experiences as those who can, thus producing "a more level playing field." In addition, many schools provide instruction related to test-taking skills so that all students have the advantage of that information.

Coaching

If a program involves coaching, then it involves more than just test sophistication skills. The effects of coaching have been investigated for many years. Some research findings have found that coaching programs can make a significant difference in scores. Some of these studies, however, have methodological flaws, particularly related to the equivalence of the treatment and control groups (Bond, 1989). There can be significant differences in scores if a researcher simply compares those who participated in these expensive coaching programs with those who did not. There are other significant differences between these two groups, as the members of the group that can afford the coaching program are probably more affluent and have access to other resources that may increase their scores (e.g., tutoring, travel experiences, trips to museums). In general, the studies on coaching have found mixed and inconsistent results concerning the effectiveness of these programs.

One consistent finding is that the closer the resemblance between the coaching material and the actual test content, the greater the improvement in test scores. A "teaching to the test" approach is one in which the focus is on learning the correct answer to individual questions rather than teaching the broader area the test is attempting to measure. Teaching to the test becomes more difficult with instruments like the SAT; because of the truth in testing legislation many of the questions are new for each administration. Powers (1993) has found that programs that claim to increase SAT scores by 100 points are questionable and that their claims are probably not accurate. There are also some indications that longer coaching programs result in higher gains as compared to shorter programs. Once again this make sense, as the more time individuals spend reviewing the material, the more likely it is that they will cover material that will be on the test. The general conclusions are that coaching programs may increase scores slightly, but significant changes only occur if the programs are longer and the content is closely aligned with the material on the test. For many clients, reviewing material on their own can be as effective as these programs and significantly less expensive.

Summary

At some point in their professional life, counselors can expect to be called upon to have knowledge of both achievement and aptitude assessment. The distinction between an achievement and an aptitude test is that an achievement test measures past learning, while an aptitude test predicts potential ability to learn or perform. In order to interpret the results of any achievement test, a counselor first needs to understand whether the instrument is criterion-referenced or norm-referenced. Achievement tests can be developed in many forms: survey achievement batteries, individual achievement tests, diagnostic tests, criterion-referenced tests, minimum-level skills tests, and subject area tests. Any achievement assessment is measuring whether the individuals have learned some content; therefore, evaluation of the content validity of the instrument is paramount. As achievement tests measure learning, it is not appropriate to assess achievement unless the individual has been exposed to the relevant content.

Aptitude assessment is performed to make predictions about the future. Often aptitude assessments are making predictions about educational or vocational/career performance. In the educational area, scholastic aptitude assessment frequently involves predicting performance in college, such as the Scholastic Assessment Test and the American College Testing program. These instruments are often used for selection and placement decisions. Scholastic aptitude instruments can also serve as an effective counseling tool. There are also numerous vocational/career aptitude assessments. The professional counselor needs to understand the strengths and limitations of any aptitude tool he or she is using. It is particularly important to know how good a predictor the instrument is and what precisely is being predicted (e.g., freshman grade point, success in a training program, job performance). A counselor cannot help a client understand the results of an aptitude test without understanding the norming and the validation information on that instrument.

CHAPTER 9

Assessment in Career Counseling

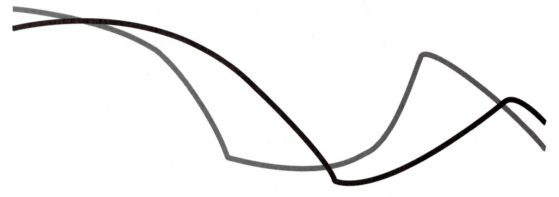

A ssessment has historically been considered an integral part of career counseling. There is a long history to career assessment; many trace the origins back to Frank Parsons. Parsons (1909) encouraged career assessment in his three-step model of career counseling. In fact, the first step was to study or measure the individual—which was essentially testing the individual. Some individuals still view career counseling as only consisting of testing and then providing occupational information. This "test and tell" approach is not reflective of the current status of this counseling area, for research has shown that career counseling is not separate from personal counseling (Swanson, 1995). Assessment, however, is often involved in career counseling, and there are numerous instruments that are routinely used to help individuals explore career directions and make effective career decisions. Spokane (1991) proposed that the purposes of career assessments are to unearth congruent career possibilities, to assess conflicts and problems, to motivate constructive behavior, to acquire a cognitive structure for evaluating career alternatives, to clarify expectations and plan interventions, and to establish the range of abilities. As reflected in Spokane's description, career assessment has diverse goals and covers a wide variety of areas.

Following the lead of Betz (1992), this chapter will divide career assessment into two major categories: tools used to assess individual differences and instruments used in assessing the process of career development. Many career assessment devices are designed to measure different aspects of individuals, such as interests, abilities, values, and needs. These measures of individual differences are used in career counseling because of their relationship to effective career choices or decisions. The other category of instruments is related to the process of career choice. The focus here is not on individual attributes of the client, but rather on where the individual is in the process of selecting a career. In terms of the career choice process, most of the instruments are related to either the level of indecision or the client's stage of career maturity.

Computers have had a significant influence on career assessment and the dissemination of career information. As personal computers have increased in sophistication, it has become possible for clients to complete career assessments on the computer and then immediately have access to information on occupations and preparation based on their results. Some of these computerized programs are interactive and incorporate assessment of clients' interests, values, and skills or abilities. This chapter includes an overview of the two major computer-assisted career assessment programs.

The fourth major topic of this chapter is related to issues in career assessment. One issue is related to structuring inventories so that gender stereotypes are minimized. Research indicates counselors need to interpret career measures with a sensitivity to sex-role socialization and encourage clients to explore nontraditional occupations that may correspond to their attributes. There are also ethnic and racial issues related to career assessments. Racial differences on general ability and aptitude assessments must also be reexamined because many of the instruments discussed in previous chapters are used in career counseling. Furthermore, racial and ethnic issues are also pertinent to other types of career assessments used by counselors.

Assessing Individual Differences

Interests

Interest inventories are often used in career counseling because they can be helpful in describing an individual's general occupational interests. Interest inventories are not the only method of assessing interests; simply asking clients about their interests can also be very useful. Early research indicated that expressed interests were not as good a predictor of occupational choice as interest inventories. Later research, however, found that expressed and measured interests are equally good at predicting occupational choice (Betsworth & Fouad, 1997). The relationship between expressed and measured interests is significant, with the average correlation being around .46 (Athanasou & Cooksey, 1993). Although expressed interests is a good measure, there are some advantages to using interest inventories. Interest inventories have been found to promote career exploration (Herr & Cramer, 1992). In addition, many interest inventories connect the client's interests to specific occupations. Some clients will have a general idea of their interests but will not know which occupations are related to those general interest areas.

In assessing interests, it is important for the counselor to understand the relationship between interests and certain career variables. For example, some individuals believe that if a client is highly interested in a field, he or she will be successful in that career area. Strong interests do not guarantee occupational success (Betsworth & Fouad, 1997). When explaining the results of an interest inventory, the counselor should stress that these instruments are only measuring interests and do not provide an indication of ability. In summarizing existing research on the relationship between interests and abilities, Lent, Brown, and Hackett (1994) reported a small but significant relationship between them. The relationships between interests and occupational satisfaction have also been found to be small (Transberg, Slane, & Ekeberg, 1993). The small relationship is probably because work satisfaction may involve multiple variables (e.g., monetary rewards, and colleagues). Interests are, however, good predictors of career direction (Pryor & Taylor, 1986). Interest inventories have been found to be good predictors of future academic and career choices, but interest alone does not guarantee that once people are in an occupation, they will find it satisfying.

Strong Interest Inventory. The *Strong Interest Inventory*® (SII®, Harmon, Hansen, Borgen, & Hammer, 1994) can trace its roots to the 1927 publication of the Strong Vocational Interest Blank®. The Strong Interest Inventory assessment, often just called the Strong, was also called the Strong–Campbell Interest Inventory prior to 1985. The evolution of this instrument over the past 50 years has resulted in a widely used and respected instrument. Not only is the Strong Interest Inventory commonly used in career counseling (Watkins, Campbell, & Nieberding, 1994), but it is often cited as one of the most widely used instruments in counseling in general (Bubenzer et al., 1990; Elmore et al., 1993). In addition, the Strong inventory is one of the most researched instruments in counseling, with hundreds of studies having been performed. The Strong Interest Inventory uses individuals' responses to items to compare their responses to the response patterns of people in different occupations. It is appropriate for high school students, college students, and adults.

The 1994 version (Form T317) of the Strong Interest Inventory contains 317 items, which are at the eighth to ninth grade reading level. The individuals rate whether they Like, are Indifferent to, or Dislike certain occupations, school subjects, activities, leisure activities, and types of people. They are also asked to choose a preference between two activities and to answer some questions about their character. A new section comprises six pairs in which they choose their preference between the pair. These pairs are all the possible com-

---

®Strong Interest Inventory is a registered trademark of Stanford University Press.

binations of ideas, data, people, and things, and these items are scored for one of the Personal Style Scales.

The results of the Strong Interest Inventory are presented in a six-page profile. Before interpreting a Strong, a counselor should examine the checks of validity of the profile. This can be accomplished by checking some indices on the last page of the profile (see Figure 9.1). Harmon et al. (1994) suggested that the clinician first check the client's total number of responses. As a general rule of thumb, they suggest that at least 300 items need to be answered in order for the profile to be valid. The second check of a profile's validity would be to examine the infrequent responses, which measure the number of unusual responses given by the client. A negative number would indicate that the counselor should explore a possible explanation for the large number of unusual responses. If an explanation cannot be identified, then the counselor should be cautious in interpreting the results. The third check on the profile's validity involves examining the Administrative Indexes. The Administrative Indexes provide the distribution for the sections on the "Like, "Indifferent to," and "Dislike"; the "Yes," "?," and the "No"; and the left, middle, or right choices. Extreme response percentages can be very useful in interpreting the results and in providing clinical information.

The information on the Strong profile is designed so that interpretation moves from general to more specific information. Harmon et al. (1994) suggested explaining the purpose of the Strong to the client before interpreting the results, so that the client understands that it explores general interests, occupational interests, and lifestyle. The interpretation should focus on three areas: the General Occupational Scales (GOTs), the Basic Interest Scales (BISs), and the Occupational Scale (OSs). A summary of the highest scores on these three scales is provided in the Snapshot, which is on the first page of the profile (see Figure 9.1). Additional client information is also provided in the Personal Style Scales, which were introduced in the 1994 version of the Strong.

The General Occupational Themes (GOTs) are measures of general interests and the scales are based on the six personality themes of John Holland (Realistic, Investigative, Artistic, Social, Enterprising, and Conventional). When interpreting the Strong, Harmon et al. (1994) suggested beginning with an overview of Holland's (1985) theory. While describing each GOT theme, the counselor should relate the information to the Basic Interest Scales (BISs) under each theme. There are 25 Basic Interest Scales that can be viewed as subdivisions of the General Occupational Themes. For example, under the Social theme, which is related to helping, instructing, and caregiving, the BISs are: Teaching, Social Service, Medical Service, and Religious Activities. The BISs can help clients understand their underlying interests as related to the six themes of the GOTs. Both the GOTs and BISs are scored for men and women separately. The issues related to scoring and gender differences will be discussed later in this chapter.

In the spirit of going from general to specific, after interpreting the more general interest measures the counselor can then begin to explore the specific Occupational Scales (OSs). These scales reflect the similarity of the client's

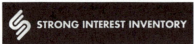

STRONG INTEREST INVENTORY

Profile report for **PAT MICHAELS**
ID:
Age: **24**
Gender: **Female**

Date tested: **03/15/95**
Date scored: **03/15/95**

SNAPSHOT: A SUMMARY OF RESULTS FOR PAT MICHAELS

GENERAL OCCUPATIONAL THEMES

The General Occupational Themes describe interests in six very broad areas, including interest in work and leisure activities, kinds of people, and work settings. Your interests in each area are shown at the right in rank order. Note that each Theme has a code, represented by the first letter of the Theme name.

You can use your Theme code, printed below your results, to identify school subjects, part-time jobs, college majors, leisure activities, or careers that you might find interesting. See the back of this Profile for suggestions on how to use your Theme code.

THEME CODE	THEME	VERY LITTLE INTEREST	LITTLE INTEREST	AVERAGE INTEREST	HIGH INTEREST	VERY HIGH INTEREST	TYPICAL INTERESTS
A	ARTISTIC	☐	☐	☐	☑	☐	Creating or enjoying art
C	CONVENTIONAL	☐	☐	☑	☐	☐	Accounting, processing data
S	SOCIAL	☐	☐	☑	☐	☐	Helping, instructing
R	REALISTIC	☐	☐	☑	☐	☐	Building, repairing
I	INVESTIGATIVE	☐	☑	☐	☐	☐	Researching, analyzing
E	ENTERPRISING	☐	☑	☐	☐	☐	Selling, managing

Your Theme code is ACS—(see explanation at left).
You might explore occupations with codes that contain any combination of these letters.

BASIC INTEREST SCALES

The Basic Interest Scales measure your interests in 25 specific areas or activities. Only those 5 areas in which you show the *most* interest are listed at the right in rank order. Your results on all 25 Basic Interest Scales are found on page 2.

To the left of each scale is a letter that shows which of the six General Occupational Themes this activity is most closely related to. These codes can help you to identify other activities that you may enjoy.

THEME CODE	BASIC INTEREST	VERY LITTLE INTEREST	LITTLE INTEREST	AVERAGE INTEREST	HIGH INTEREST	VERY HIGH INTEREST	TYPICAL ACTIVITIES
A	WRITING	☐	☐	☐	☐	☑	Reading or writing
S	RELIGIOUS ACTIVITIES	☐	☐	☐	☑	☐	Participating in spiritual activities
A	ART	☐	☐	☐	☑	☐	Appreciating or creating art
A	CULINARY ARTS	☐	☐	☐	☑	☐	Cooking or entertaining
R	AGRICULTURE	☐	☐	☐	☑	☐	Working outdoors

OCCUPATIONAL SCALES

The Occupational Scales measure how similar your interests are to the interests of people who are satisfied working in those occupations. Only the 10 scales on which your interests are *most* similar to those of these people are listed at the right in rank order. Your results on all 211 of the Occupational Scales are found on pages 3, 4, and 5.

The letters to the left of each scale identify the Theme or Themes that most closely describe the interests of people working in that occupation. You can use these letters to find additional, related occupations that you might find interesting. After reviewing your results on all six pages of this Profile, see the back of page 5 for tips on finding other occupations in the Theme or Themes that interest you the most.

THEME CODE	OCCUPATION	VERY DISSIMILAR	DISSIMILAR	MID-RANGE	SIMILAR	VERY SIMILAR
A	LIBRARIAN	☐	☐	☐	☐	☑
AIR	TECHNICAL WRITER	☐	☐	☐	☐	☑
A	LAWYER	☐	☐	☐	☑	☐
A	TRANSLATOR	☐	☐	☐	☑	☐
CE	PARALEGAL	☐	☐	☐	☑	☐
SA	SOCIAL WORKER	☐	☐	☐	☑	☐
AES	CORPORATE TRAINER	☐	☐	☐	☑	☐
AE	ADVERTISING EXECUTIVE	☐	☐	☑	☐	☐
ASE	ENGLISH TEACHER	☐	☐	☑	☐	☐
SEA	SOCIAL SCIENCE TEACHER	☐	☐	☑	☐	☐

PERSONAL STYLE SCALES measure your levels of comfort regarding Work Style, Learning Environment, Leadership Style, and Risk Taking/Adventure. This information may help you make decisions about particular work environments, educational settings, and types of activities you would find satisfying. Your results on these four scales are on page 6.

CPP CONSULTING PSYCHOLOGISTS PRESS, INC. • 3803 E. Bayshore Road, Palo Alto, CA 94303

FIGURE 9.1 *Strong Interest Inventory profile*

Modified and reproduced by special permission of the Publisher, Consulting Psychologists Press, Inc., Palo Alto, CA 94303 from **Strong Profile, Standard Edition** *by Allen L. Hammer and Judith Grutter. Copyright 1994 by Stanford University Press. All rights reserved. Further reproduction is prohibited without the Publisher's written consent.*

The test user, in selecting or interpreting a test, should know the purposes of the testing and the probable consequences. The user should know the procedures necessary to facilitate effectiveness and to reduce bias in test use. Although the test developer and publisher should provide information on the strengths and weaknesses of the test, the ultimate responsibility for appropriate test use lies with the test user. The user should become knowledgeable about the test and its appropriate use and also communicate this information, as appropriate, to others.

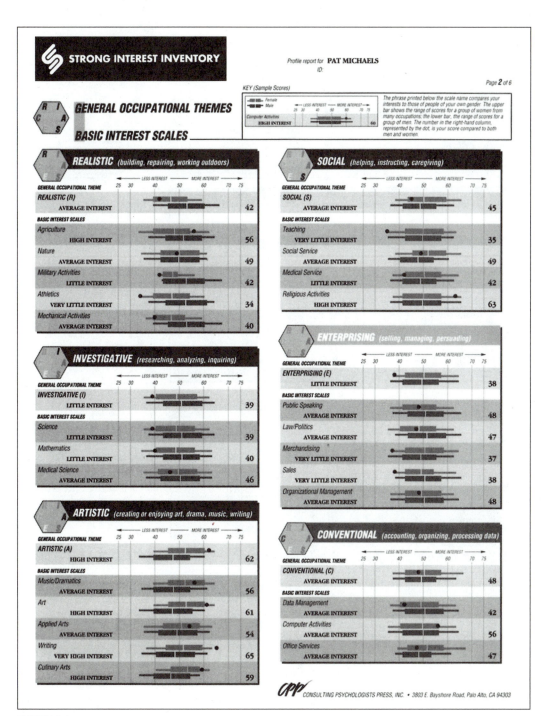

FIGURE 9.1
(continued)

STRONG INTEREST INVENTORY

Profile report for **PAT MICHAELS**
ID:

Page **3** of 6

KEY (Sample Scores)

THEME CODES FEMALE MALE	YOUR SCORES FEMALE MALE	← DISSIMILAR INTERESTS SIMILAR INTERESTS →
RIS (SEC) Dietitian	25 (SEC)	15 20 30 - MID-RANGE - 40 50 55
* 8 Plumber	* 35	

( ) You can find your score compared to this gender under the Theme represented by the first letter of this code. For example, your score compared to male dietitians is shown under the S or Social Theme.

* The position of the dot shows how similar your interests are to those of individuals of your gender who say they are satisfied in their occupation.

* Not enough people of this gender who work in this occupation could be found to make a good comparison.

OCCUPATIONAL SCALES

NOTES

REALISTIC (building, repairing, working outdoors)

THEME CODES FEMALE	MALE		YOUR SCORES FEMALE	MALE	← DISSIMILAR INTERESTS SIMILAR INTERESTS → 15 20 30 - MID-RANGE - 40 50 55
RIS	(SIR)	Athletic Trainer	−1	(SIR)	
R	R	Auto Mechanic	16	−4	
RIA	REA	Carpenter	9	1	
RIA	RIC	Electrician	11	−13	
RCI	RI	Emergency Medical Technician	12	11	
RI	RI	Engineer	17	7	
(CSE)	RC	Farmer	(CSE)	14	
RI	RI	Forester	34	24	
RC	RE	Gardener/Groundskeeper	32	30	
REI	REI	Horticultural Worker	18	8	
(CRE)	RCE	Military Enlisted Personnel	(CRE)	11	
REI	REC	Military Officer	31	15	
*	R	Plumber	*	19	
RE	R	Police Officer	27	10	
RIS	RI	Radiologic Technologist	26	26	
(CE)	RE	Small Business Owner	(CE)	20	
RSI	RSE	Vocational Agriculture Teacher	5	6	

INVESTIGATIVE (researching, analyzing, inquiring)

THEME CODES FEMALE	MALE		YOUR SCORES FEMALE	MALE	← DISSIMILAR INTERESTS SIMILAR INTERESTS → 15 20 30 - MID-RANGE - 40 50 55
IS	IA	Audiologist	32	35	
IRA	IA	Biologist	20	25	
IR	IR	Chemist	18	13	
IR	IRA	Chiropractor	20	22	
IAR	IAS	College Professor	34	31	
IR	IAR	Computer Programmer/Systems Analyst	26	24	
IRA	IR	Dentist	14	15	
IES	(SEC)	Dietitian	23	(SEC)	
IRA	IA	Geographer	28	23	
IRA	IRA	Geologist	12	7	
IRC	ICA	Mathematician	0	−3	
IRC	IRE	Medical Technician	16	6	
IRC	IRC	Medical Technologist	12	15	
IR	IR	Optometrist	17	5	
ICR	ICE	Pharmacist	18	22	
IAR	IAR	Physician	18	5	
IRA	IRA	Physicist	7	9	
IA	IA	Psychologist	27	39	
IR	IRC	Research & Development Manager	4	−1	
IRA	IRS	Respiratory Therapist	12	12	
IRS	IRS	Science Teacher	4	6	
IAR	(AI)	Sociologist	29	(AI)	
IRA	IR	Veterinarian	23	14	

CPP CONSULTING PSYCHOLOGISTS PRESS, INC. • 3803 E. Bayshore Road, Palo Alto, CA 94303

FIGURE 9.1
(continued)

STRONG INTEREST INVENTORY

Profile report for **PAT MICHAELS**
ID:

Page **4** of 6

KEY (Sample Scores)

R I
C A
S

OCCUPATIONAL SCALES (continued)

( ) You can find your score compared to this gender under the Theme represented by the first letter of this code. For example, your score compared to female sociologists is shown under the I or Investigative Theme.

* The position of the dot shows how similar your interests are to those of individuals of your gender who say they are satisfied in their occupation.

* Not enough people of this gender who work in this occupation could be found to make a good comparison.

ARTISTIC (creating or enjoying art, drama, music, writing)

NOTES

THEME CODES FEMALE	MALE		YOUR SCORES FEMALE	MALE
AE	AE	Advertising Executive	39	55
ARI	ARI	Architect	28	37
ARI	A	Artist, Commercial	15	35
AR	A	Artist, Fine	28	38
ASE	AS	Art Teacher	14	29
AE	AE	Broadcaster	38	46
AES	AES	Corporate Trainer	41	43
ASE	ASE	English Teacher	39	46
(EA)	AE	Interior Decorator	(EA)	37
A	A	Lawyer	47	51
A	A	Librarian	58	62
AIR	AIR	Medical Illustrator	11	15
A	A	Musician	34	47
ARE	ARE	Photographer	34	32
AER	ASE	Public Administrator	35	37
AE	AE	Public Relations Director	37	46
A	A	Reporter	38	50
(IAR)	AI	Sociologist	(IAR)	39
AIR	AI	Technical Writer	50	51
A	AI	Translator	47	51

SOCIAL (helping, instructing, caregiving)

THEME CODES FEMALE	MALE		YOUR SCORES FEMALE	MALE
(RIS)	SIR	Athletic Trainer	(RIS)	-5
S	*	Child Care Provider	26	*
SE	SE	Community Service Organization Director	35	27
(IES)	SEC	Dietitian	(IES)	30
S	S	Elementary School Teacher	22	21
SAE	SA	Foreign Language Teacher	25	37
SE	SE	High School Counselor	32	35
SE	*	Home Economics Teacher	6	*
SAR	SA	Minister	32	40
SCE	SCE	Nurse, LPN	10	20
SI	SAI	Nurse, RN	24	33
SAR	SA	Occupational Therapist	26	35
SE	SE	Parks and Recreation Coordinator	22	27
SRC	SR	Physical Education Teacher	-8	-10
SIR	SIR	Physical Therapist	18	20
SEA	SEC	School Administrator	29	25
SEA	SEA	Social Science Teacher	39	37
SA	SA	Social Worker	43	51
SE	SEA	Special Education Teacher	26	36
SA	SA	Speech Pathologist	38	49

CPP CONSULTING PSYCHOLOGISTS PRESS, INC. • 3803 E. Bayshore Road, Palo Alto, CA 94303

FIGURE 9.1
(continued)

STRONG INTEREST INVENTORY

Profile report for **PAT MICHAELS**
ID:

Page **5** of 6

R I
C A
E S

OCCUPATIONAL SCALES (continued)

KEY (Sample Scores)

THEME CODES		YOUR SCORES		←DISSIMILAR INTERESTS				SIMILAR INTERESTS	
FEMALE	MALE			FEMALE	MALE	15	20	30 MID-RANGE 40	50 55
EA	(AE)	Interior Decorator		46	(AE)				•
CSE	*	Dental Assistant		15	*	•			

( ) You can find your score compared to this gender under the Theme represented by the first letter of this code. For example, your score compared to male interior decorators is shown under the A or Artistic Theme.

• The position of the dot shows how similar your interests are to those of individuals of your gender who say they are satisfied in their occupation.

* Not enough people of this gender who work in this occupation could be found to make a good comparison.

NOTES

ENTERPRISING (selling, managing, persuading)

THEME CODES			YOUR SCORES		←DISSIMILAR INTERESTS				SIMILAR INTERESTS		
FEMALE	MALE		FEMALE	MALE	15	20	30	MID-RANGE	40	50	55
*	ECR	Agribusiness Manager	*	0							
EC	EC	Buyer	3	11							
ERA	ER	Chef	15	25							
EIS	*	Dental Hygienist	8	*							
EAS	ESA	Elected Public Official	33	25							
EAS	EAS	Flight Attendant	24	41							
EAC	EAC	Florist	11	20							
EC	EA	Hair Stylist	14	21							
ECS	ECS	Housekeeping & Maintenance Supervisor	28	25							
EAS	ES	Human Resources Director	37	33							
EA	(AE)	Interior Decorator	16	(AE)							
EIR	ECI	Investments Manager	23	15							
E	E	Life Insurance Agent	25	22							
EA	EA	Marketing Executive	34	38							
ECR	ER	Optician	11	12							
ECR	ECR	Purchasing Agent	17	19							
E	E	Realtor	7	18							
ECR	ECR	Restaurant Manager	17	21							
ECA	ECS	Store Manager	23	19							
ECA	ECA	Travel Agent	20	32							

CONVENTIONAL (accounting, organizing, processing data)

THEME CODES			YOUR SCORES		←DISSIMILAR INTERESTS				SIMILAR INTERESTS		
FEMALE	MALE		FEMALE	MALE	15	20	30	MID-RANGE	40	50	55
CE	CE	Accountant	25	15							
CI	CI	Actuary	13	16							
CE	CE	Banker	34	21							
C	C	Bookkeeper	30	24							
CES	CES	Business Education Teacher	23	30							
CE	CE	Credit Manager	35	23							
CSE	*	Dental Assistant	14	*							
CSE	(RC)	Farmer	23	(RC)							
CES	CES	Food Service Manager	27	34							
CIR	CIS	Mathematics Teacher	4	−3							
C	C	Medical Records Technician	29	41							
CRE	(RCE)	Military Enlisted Personnel	23	(RCE)							
CES	CES	Nursing Home Administrator	32	47							
CE	CA	Paralegal	45	44							
CES	*	Secretary	23	*							
CE	(RE)	Small Business Owner	28	(RE)							

CPP CONSULTING PSYCHOLOGISTS PRESS, INC. • 3803 E. Bayshore Road, Palo Alto, CA 94303

FIGURE 9.1

(continued)

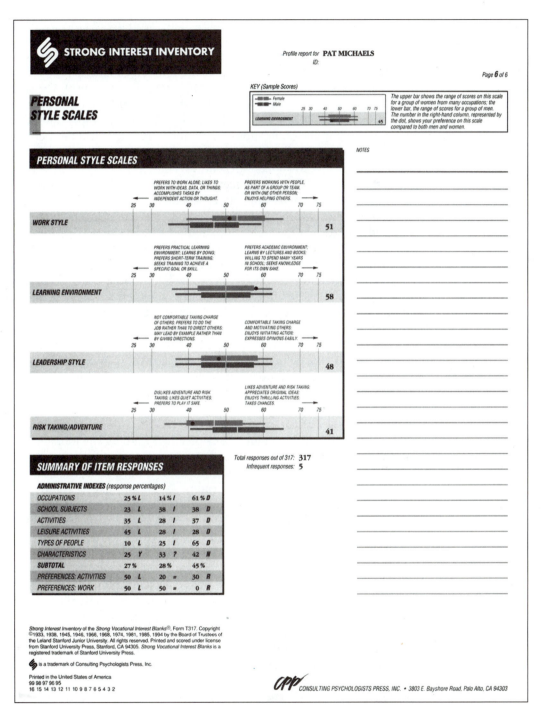

FIGURE 9.1

interest with the interest of individuals actually working in different occupations. Using people actually working in the occupations is one of the strengths of the Strong (Busch, 1995). The Strong Interest Inventory includes a total of 211 Occupational Scales, of which 107 are for women and 104 are for men. The occupations are also grouped by GOTs (Holland's six themes). The scoring of the 211 OSs is quite complicated, but the score for each occupation provides an indication of how closely the client's interests correspond to those of people working in the occupations. The Strong previously had been criticized for focusing on professional occupations, and so additional nonprofessional occupations have been added in recent revisions. The occupations where the client's interests are "Similar" (T-score of 40 or higher) are commonly identified and explored in counseling, but counselors are also encouraged to examine occupations for which there is very low interest. If there are no occupations of 40 and above, then the counselor should focus on the occupations where there is the highest interest. The counselor should work with the client to identify patterns within Holland codes. Harmon et al. (1994) suggested examining areas of high interest and areas of low interest in order to facilitate the identification of interest patterns. In addition, the client's scores on the opposite gender-normed Occupational Scale need to be examined in order to confirm interest patterns (Harmon et al., 1994).

The newly added Personal Style Scales of the Strong Interest Inventory help individuals explore how they go about learning, working, playing, or living in general. These are broad measures with the scales being Work Style, Learning Environment, Leadership Style, and Risk Taking/Adventure. The Work Style scale indicates preferences regarding working with people as compared to working with ideas, data, or things. The Learning Environment scale provides an indication of an individual's preferred learning environment on the continuum from a preference for academic learning to a preference for more practically oriented, hands-on environments. The third scale, the Leadership Style, reflects whether people like to lead by example or like to lead by directing and persuading others. The last scale is the Risk Taking/Adventure scale. This scale indicates whether the client prefers to play it safe or seeks risk-taking and adventurous activities. These scales need to be interpreted cautiously because of their recent development.

The *Strong Interest Inventory: Application and Technical Guide* (Harmon et al., 1994) is a superb resource that can aid counselors in interpreting results. This guide can be particularly helpful in sorting out the unusual results (e.g., where there may appear to be a slight discrepancy between the Basic Interest Scales and the Occupational Scales). This resource also has a chapter devoted to gender issues in interpretation and another separate chapter on using the Strong with special populations.

Scoring, norms, and psychometric information. The scoring of the Strong Interest Inventory is somewhat complex; however, the means on all scales are always 50 and the standard deviations are 10. For both the General Occupational

Scales and the Basic Interest Scales, each individual's responses are compared to a combined General Reference Sample of 18,951 (9,467 women and 9,484 men). The items that measure the six GOTs and the 25 BISs were determined by their content and factor analysis. The profile allows for examining the score in terms of separate distributions for men and women with two different bars that are printed on the profile. In terms of reliability, the test-retest coefficients for a three- to six-month gap for adults ranged from .84 to .92 for the six General Occupational Themes. The coefficients for this same sample varied from .80 to .94 on the Basic Interest Scales. In addition, there is substantial validation evidence for these two scales.

The Occupational Scales were developed using a different norming procedure and a different method of item selection. For the Occupational Scales, items were not selected because of their similarity in content to other items, but rather items were selected because of their ability to differentiate the interests of those in an occupation from the general sample (i.e., General Reference Sample). Thus, the scoring of the Occupational Scales is based on comparing the interests of people in certain occupations to a broadly based group of the same gender. Items that differentiate between the occupation and the General Reference Sample were identified, then weights were assigned based on further analyses. This process results in the Occupational Scales scores being converted to T-scores with means of 50 and standard deviations of 10. Separate-sex norms are used, with the profile containing scores for both females and males. The plotting of the score on the profile, however, is only for the same gender as the client.

There are at least 200 individuals in each occupational sample for all the occupations, except where it was difficult to identify 200 people (e.g., female auto mechanics, male paralegals). In order to be eligible to be a part of the sample the person must (1) be satisfied with his or her work, (2) have at least three years of work experience in the occupation, (3) perform the job duties that are typical and that clearly represent the occupation, and (4) be between 25 and 60 years old. There has been criticism of previous norming groups used in the Strong Interest Inventory concerning the overrepresentation of individuals with postsecondary education (Worthen, 1995). This same criticism seems to apply to the recent edition of the Strong, considering that the modal education level for each occupation is a bachelor's degree (Harmon et al., 1994).

The reliability coefficients for the Occupational Scales varied, with the range for three- to six-month coefficients being from .80 to .99. In terms of the validity of the Occupational Scales, a counselor should be more cautious with these scales than with the General Occupational Themes and the Basic Interest Scales (Worthen, 1995). The scales vary in terms of evidence of concurrent validity, and the predictive validity of the scales is less established.

The Personal Style Scales, which were added in the 1994 version of the Strong, have many features similar to the General Occupational Themes and the Basic Interests Scales. For example, the scores are based on the large sample of 18,951 men and women. The Risk Taking/Adventure scale of the

Personal Style Scale, with a coefficient of .78, has the lowest reliability of the scales on the Strong. Although there is validity information for these scales, it is less than the General Occupational Themes and the Basic Interest Scales.

The Strong Interest Inventory is often considered a model for other interest inventories in terms of its psychometric characteristics. Certainly it is the most researched of the interest inventories. Its long history has resulted in a well-developed inventory. There are, however, certain limitations to the Strong and the counselor needs to consider if it is appropriate for the individual client.

Career Assessment Inventory. In the past the *Career Assessment Inventory* (CAI) was often considered the "working man's Strong." Past editions of the Strong Interest Inventory focused primarily on professional occupations, and the original version of the Career Assessment Inventory (CAI-Vocational Version) focused on careers requiring two years or less of postsecondary training. The newer version, the CAI-Enhanced Version, focuses on careers requiring various levels of postsecondary education. Both versions of the CAI (Johansson 1984, 1986) continue to be published. The profiles of both the CAI-EV and the CAI-VV are patterned after the Strong. Clients receive scores on the General Themes (Holland's six personality types), Basic Interests, and Occupational Scales. There are also Administrative indexes and Nonoccupational scales (similar to the Personal Style scales).

Vacc and Hinkle (1994) voiced some concerns about the two versions of the Career Assessment Inventory. First, they concluded that some psychometric information was missing from the manuals, which made evaluation difficult. They were also concerned about the small samples for some of the Occupational Scales. In addition, they were troubled by the lack of empirical analyses of the items in the General Themes Scales. They suggested that neither version should be used with large groups of clients. They did, however, conclude that the CAI-VV does fill a need for a large population and the CAI-EV has added features that make it more attractive.

Kuder instruments. The interest inventories developed by Fredrick Kuder have almost as long a history as the Strong Interest Inventory. The *Kuder Occupational Interest Survey*, Form DD (KOIS, Kuder & Zytowski, 1991) assesses the interest of high school students, college students, and adults. KOIS consists of 100 items, in which a triad of activities are presented and the client selects the one they would most like to do and the one they would least like. In contrast to the Strong Interest Inventory, the Kuder Occupational Interest Survey does not use a general reference sample; rather, the individual's answers are compared to persons in a college major or working in an occupation. The scoring is related to the amount of correlation between the individual's answers and those of each reference group. Zytowski (1992) suggested that this method provides more verification for conclusions, such as the client's interests are more typical of physicians as compared to chemists. The KOIS provides scores on 65 male occupations and 44 female occupations and 22 male college majors and 18 female college majors. The scoring of the KOIS also includes a V-score, which is a verification scale indicating the validity of the profile.

Most reviewers of the KOIS have contended that the instrument has adequate reliability (Hackett & Watkins, 1995; Herr & Ashby, 1994). Criticisms have focused on the limited research related to predictive validity, particularly studies investigating job satisfaction. Hackett and Lonborg (1993) criticized the inclusion of more male occupations than female occupations and the message this may be sending to female clients. A computer version of the KOIS was recently published, but limited research is currently available on the equivalence of the computer version to the paper-and-pencil version.

Another interest inventory developed by Kuder is the *Kuder General Interest Survey* (KGIS). The KGIS is somewhat unique in that it is geared toward younger adolescents, for it can be used with individuals as young as grade 6. The purpose of the KGIS is not for career decision making, but rather to stimulate career exploration. The item format is the same as KOIS, where clients select from a triad of activities the ones that they would most like and least like. There are 168 items on the KGIS that produce scores in 10 general interest areas. Holland codes can also be retrieved from the KGIS results. The results are based on comparing the individual's interests to a sample of students in grades 6 through 12. Mehrens (1994) evaluated the validity evidence for this inventory as being quite scant. The Kuder General Interest Survey, however, continues to be a popular instrument. The dearth of instruments available for the middle or junior high school population probably contributes to the KGIS's popularity. For high school students, there are probably better interest inventories that provide more sound information.

Self-Directed Search. The *Self-Directed Search* (SDS, Holland, Fritzsche, & Powell, 1994) is another inventory that is usually designated as an interest inventory, but its focus is not exclusively interest and it includes analyses of abilities and competencies. The instrument's conceptual base is Holland's theory; the Self-Directed Search measures the six basic personality types he proposed. There are four versions of the Self-Directed Search that are designed for different groups of individuals. Form R is for high school students, college students, and adults; Form E is for adults and older adolescents with limited reading skills; Form CP (Career Planning) is for employees who aspire to greater levels of professional responsibility; and the Career Explorer version is for middle or junior high school students. All of these versions are self-administered and self-scored. The assessment book is accompanied by an *Occupational Finder* that facilitates the exploration of occupations related to the three-letter summary code produced as a result of taking the Self-Directed Search. There is also a computer version and computerized interpretative reports for Form R.

Unlike most instruments, Holland uses raw scores in determining results (i.e., the individual counts the responses related to the six personality types and the three areas with the most responses produce the three-letter summary code). Daniels (1994) criticized the use of raw data because the four sections of the instruments (i.e., Activities, Competencies, Occupations, and Self-Estimates) vary in the number of items that contribute to the raw scores. In addition, there does not seem to be a theoretical or psychometric reason for the disproportionate contributions to the three-letter summary codes. Although percentiles can be calculated for the SDS, this is not a part of the self-scoring instructions.

In conclusion, the Self-Directed Search can be an inexpensive and relatively easy assessment device to use. Manuele-Adkins (1989) recommended that counselors be more involved than the manual recommends when using the Self-Directed Search. As the manual documents, there are problems with the self-scoring and errors do commonly occur (Holland et al., 1994). There are also differences between how occupations are coded between the Occupational Finder of the SDS and those on the Strong Interest Inventory, which can be confusing for clients who may receive the results from both instruments. The SDS scoring is also criticized because it does not provide any consideration of gender differences, so nontraditional interests may be underrepresented. Finally, in my opinion, the validation information on the SDS is supportive of using the instrument for career exploration activities, but other assessment tools and information should be incorporated into the counseling process if the goal is career selection or decision making.

Other interest inventories. There are many other interest inventories that counselors use. One of the more popular ones that has not been mentioned is the *Jackson Vocational Interest Survey* (JVIS, Jackson, 1996b). The JVIS is a relatively recent contribution to interest assessments and is for adolescents and adults. The JVIS is unique in that it measures preferences in both Work Styles and Work Roles. Work styles concern preferences for work environments and include scales such as Dominant Leadership, Job Security, and Stamina. Jepsen (1994) judged that the JVIS is time consuming but worth the extra time and effort. Another interest inventory that is commonly mentioned is the *Ohio Vocational Interest Survey, Second Edition,* which can be used with students in grades 7 through 12. Very few interest assessments are published for elementary students. Examples of inventories geared for these younger students are: the *Career Finder,* the *Judgment of Occupational Behavior-Orientation* (JOB-O), and the *What I Like To Do* (WILD).

Another method of assessing career interests is through the use of card sort techniques. There are many commercially available card sorts, and practitioners have also developed their own (Slaney & MacKinnon-Slaney, 1990). Often card sorts have occupations listed on cards in which the client sorts the cards into three piles: Would Choose, Would Not Choose, and No Opinion. As Williams (1978) contended, card sorts have the advantage of providing immediate feedback and a creative way of extracting meaningful information from clients. Card sorts allow for an interactive process between the client and counselor, where the counselor can inquire into the reasons for sorting the cards into specific piles. Slaney and MacKinnon-Slaney (1990) maintained that the research on vocational card sorts suggests that they are as effective as other career interventions. The number of research studies on which this conclusion is based is quite small. It may be better to consider card sorts as a supplement to other career assessments. The research does indicate that card sorts should not be self-administered and that the interactive quality between the client and counselor contributes to the usefulness of the technique.

Some counselors work with clients with disabilities and special needs, for whom the more traditional interest inventories may not always be appropriate. The *Wide Range Interest-Opinion Tests* (WRIOT, Jastak & Jastak, 1979) is a widely used interest inventory in this area. The WRIOT is a pictorial inventory, where out of a series of three pictures, the client selects the one liked the most and the one liked the least. Therefore, the instrument does not involve reading and is appropriate for clients where reading may be a problem. There are, however, some technical limitations with the WRIOT. Other instruments geared for this population are the *Pictorial Inventory of Careers*, the *Reading-Free Vocational Interest Inventory,* and the *Ashland Interest Assessment.*

Abilities/Skills

Many of the instruments discussed in Chapter 8 relate to the assessment of aptitude and achievement can be used in career counseling. Certainly the General Aptitude Test Battery (GATB), the Armed Services Vocational Aptitude Battery (ASVAB), and the Differential Aptitude Test (DAT) are customarily used for career exploration and decision making. In addition, all three of these instruments have the option of being used in combination with an interest inventory. Therefore, in considering career assessments, counselors should include those measures mentioned in the previous chapter. Aptitude tests are often used in career counseling because they are good predictors of occupational success (Hunter & Schmidt, 1983). This does not mean that aptitude test results should be examined in isolation as the sole determinant of a client's potential in an occupation. Counselors need to gather information about the "whole client" when assisting clients in the career planning process.

In interpreting aptitude assessment in career counseling, it is important to verify the results with other information. Verifying the results entails asking the clients if the scores are consistent with other information such as grades, work performance, self-perceptions of abilities, and other types of evaluations. This verification of the results accomplishes two goals: first, it provides a method to identify any problems that might have occurred (e.g., client's ability to read may have influenced performance, or the client was ill when taking the instrument and the results don't reflect his or her ability). The second goal the verification process accomplishes is bringing more client information into the interpretative process. Thus, the verification process can also assist in providing a more holistic view of the client's abilities and provide information on other facets of the client's life. Some aptitude publishers have responded to counselors' needs to gather more complete client information by combining an aptitude test with an interest inventory. An example of this is the Unisex Addition of the ACT Interest Inventory (UNIACT) that can either be taken with the ACT or by itself. The combination of aptitude and interests facilitates the combined exploration and leads to a more comprehensive view of the client.

Campbell Interest and Skills Survey. A different method of combining interests and skills or ability assessment is available through the *Campbell Interest and Skills Survey* (CISS, Campbell, 1992). The author of this instrument, Campbell, has a long and distinguished career in vocational assessment, as he was instrumental in the development of the Strong Interest Inventory's predecessor, the Strong–Campbell Interest Inventory. The CISS combines the self-assessment of skills with an exploration of interest. This combination encourages the client to examine the interaction between interest and skills and examine career areas where the two interconnect.

The 320 items of the CISS result in scores on 7 Orientation Scales, 29 Basic Interest and Skills Scales, and 58 Occupational Scales. The Orientation Scales roughly correspond to Holland's six themes, except that the Realistic theme is broken down into two categories, the Producing and the Adventuring orientations. The Basic Scales are subcategories of the Orientation Scales and represent various occupational activities. Unlike the Strong, the norms for these two scales and the Occupation Scales are unisex rather than reporting scores for men and women separately.

Based on the scores on interests and self-assessment of skill level, the profile provides four categories: *Pursue*—high interest and high skills; *Develop*—high interest and lower skills; *Explore*—lower interest and high skills; and *Avoid*—lower interest and lower skills. Fuqua and Newman (1994) evaluated the reference sample of 5,225 as being more than adequate for the average client. The median coefficient alpha is .87 for the Orientation Scales and .86 for the Basic Scales. There is more variability in the Occupational Scales, and the skills assessments on the Occupational Scales tend to be less reliable than the interest scores. This is a comparatively new instrument and, thus, there is not as much validation information as some of the more developed interest inventories. The interest assessment has a strong empirical base coming from the work on the Strong–Campbell Interest Inventory. There is also other research that supports the validity of self-report as a sound method of skills or ability assessment.

Self-estimates of abilities. In considering methods for assessing skills and abilities, counselors may want to consider the use of self-estimates. Westbrook, Sanford, Gilleland, Fleenor, and Merwin (1988) found a significant relationship between self-appraisal estimates of abilities and measured abilities. They found, however, that adolescents generally tended to overestimate their abilities. Their research, however, indicates that counselors can use self-appraisals in career counseling. When utilizing self-estimates of abilities, counselors need to consider the client's self-efficacy beliefs. Self-efficacy concerns one's belief about his or her ability to perform a specific task or behavior. Substantial research has shown that self-efficacy beliefs mitigate tasks approached, academic pursuits, and career choice. Women often have low self-efficacy beliefs, particularly in areas such as mathematics (Lent & Hackett, 1987). Thus, an evaluation of the accuracy of the self-efficacy is necessary if counselors are using self-estimates of abilities. Moreover, it is judicious to investigate self-efficacy beliefs of clients in the interpretation of any standardized aptitude or ability assessment.

Values

In the area of career assessment, the exploration of values is sometimes neglected even though it is often a critical aspect of the career counseling process. As Osborne, Brown, Niles, and Miner (1997) indicated, "The understanding of an individual's values is, perhaps, the most important element of the decision-making process. Values serve as the basis for which life goals are established, and provide a guide for individuals in making personally consistent and meaningful decisions about the future" (p. 82). Work values are more highly correlated than interest with work satisfaction (Rounds, 1990). Some of the instruments that are typically associated with the assessment of values in the career area use terms such as needs or preferences. Even though there are some discrepancies in the definitions of these dimensions, Betz (1992) indicated that they seem to measure an overlapping set of variables.

If a counselor is using a values inventory, the practitioner should remember that no inventory is inclusive of all possible values. Therefore, a client may value something that is not assessed on the instrument being used. Chartrand and Walsh (in press) argue that those career assessments in which the focus is only on work values are insufficient because many people want to examine their values across multiple life roles. Counselors need to supplement the use of a values inventory with an exploration of other possible values. This can be accomplished by asking the client questions about his or her personal values not assessed and by exploring the lifestyle of the client.

Values Scale.   The *Values Scale* (Nevill & Super, 1989) is a measure of both work-related values and general values. The 106 items produce scores on 21 values (e.g., Ability Utilization, Achievement, Economic Security, and Personal Development). The authors of this scale have labeled this the "Research Edition" to indicate that clinicians should be cautious in using it. There is a normative sample, but the authors recommend using an ipsative interpretation. *Ipsative interpretation* means the variables are compared to each other without reference to whether the client's values in that area are high or low compared to other people. Slaney and Suddarth (1994) wondered if even this cautious approach is warranted based on their review. They recommended that until there is more research, this instrument should only be used with adults in

conjunction with other measures. Hackett and Watkins (1995) agreed that
there were drawbacks with the instrument, but suggested it had cross-cultural
implications and did not appear to be gender biased. The Value Scale is used
in Super's C-DAC approach (Osborne et al., 1997), which stands for Career
Development, Assessment, and Counseling.

Salience Inventory. The focus of the *Salience Inventory* (Nevill & Super, 1986)
scale is on which *roles* the individual values. This scale is based on Super's concept that the saliency of different roles will vary during an individual's life
cycle. Super (1980) identified five major roles that are measured in the
Salience Inventory: student, worker, homemaker (including spouse and parent), leisurite, and citizen. On the Salience Inventory, each of these five roles is
assessed three ways: the Commitment Scale, the Participation Scale, and the
Value Expectation Scale. This instrument can assist adolescents in examining
their current roles and ones they are interested in committing to in the future.
It can also be helpful for women with issues of multiple roles and possible role
overload. This instrument is also an integral part of Super's C-DAC model (Osborne et al., 1997).

Minnesota Importance Questionnaire. The *Minnesota Importance Questionnaire*
(MIS, Weiss, Dawis, & Lofquist, 1981) is related to the *theory of work adjustment* and is often used in research related to this theory. The authors contended that it can be used in practice to assess needs and values. The instrument is appropriate for clients 16 and older. The MIS assesses 21 needs (e.g.,
Ability Utilization, Compensation, Co-workers, and Recognition) and six underlying work values (i.e., Achievement, Altruism, Autonomy, Comfort, Safety,
and Status). Brooke and Ciechalski (1994) rated its psychometric qualities
positively but questioned whether it actually assessed values.

Integrative Career Assessment Programs

As noted earlier, a number of interest and aptitude assessment are now offered
in conjunction with each other. In this section, a few of the programs that combine interests, abilities, and values assessments will be discussed.

COPSystem. The *COPSystem* is published by EdITS/Educational and Industrial Testing Services and combines separate interests, abilities, and values inventories. These instruments can be used alone or in tandem with each
other. Using the Comprehensive Career Guide, the results from the interests,
abilities, and values assessment can be interpreted with the results from all
three assessments using the same occupational classification system. Depending on the needs of the client, the practitioner can select from several
versions of the COPSystem Interest Inventory (COPS). In assessing interests,
there is a general form (COPS-Revised), a professional-focused instrument
(COPS-P), one appropriate for elementary through high school (COPS-II),

and a pictorial instrument (COPS-PIC). The values instrument, the Career Orientation Placement and Evaluation Survey (COPES), was revised in 1995. The instrument measures eight values using a continuum (e.g., Investigative vs. Accepting, Practical vs. Carefree, Independence vs. Conformity). Thus, the counselor can use the results to interpret which area is valued over the other on the continuum and identify from the eight areas the ones that are most valued. The ability measure is the Career Ability Placement Survey (CAPS), which consists of eight subtests. Each of the subtests only lasts five minutes and, therefore, it is not a comprehensive test of those eight abilities. The COPSystem continues to be revised and improved. It can provide an integrative program for career exploration, but sometimes clients will benefit from more thorough assessments. Furthermore, as Knapp-Lee, Knapp, and Knapp (1990) suggested, there is a need for longitudinal validation studies on this assessment system.

Integrative assessment does not have to involve only one system such as the COPSystem, for counselors can integrate a number of separate career assessments together. The Career Development Assessment and Counseling Approach (C-DAC, Osborne et al., 1997) involves integrating the results from at least five career assessments: the Adult Career Concerns Inventory, the Career Development Inventory, the Strong Interest Inventory, the Values Scale, and the Salience Inventory. In addition, career assessment does not always have to involve formal assessment instruments; some informal exercises have been shown to be valid tools (e.g., the Occupational Daydream exercise in the Self-Directed Search). Integrating information on interests, abilities, and values needs to be a part of the career counseling process. In terms of integrative career assessment, Spokane and Jacob (1996) found that there is a renewed interest in portfolio assessment. This approach could facilitate the integration of interests, abilities, and values assessment. This approach also makes sense in terms of career development, because students could keep in their portfolio career counseling exercises and results of assessments. The portfolio then could be used by school counselors to integrate career information gathered on students throughout their academic careers. Hence, an interest inventory taken in middle school could be compared to an interest inventory taken in high school. Portfolios are beginning to be used in many schools, with an example being the Get A Life program developed by the American School Counseling Association and the National Occupational Outlook Information Coordinating Committee.

Career Choice Process

The previous discussion addressed assessments of individual differences that are used to assist clients in making career decisions. These instruments assess various *contents* (e.g., interests, values) that have been shown to be related to sound career choices. The focus is now moving toward instruments that measure where clients are in the career decision-making *process*. Typical measures of career process variables are related to level of decidedness or certainty and level of career maturity (Oliver & Spokane, 1988; Whiston et al., 1998).

Career Decision Making

It is often helpful in career counseling to have an indication of where the client is in terms of career decisions or career indecision. The interventions a counselor selects would probably be very different with a client who has made a career decision as compared to clients who are undecided. A distinction should be made between clients who experience normal developmental undecidedness and indecisiveness. The term undecided means the client has not yet made a career decision, while the term indecisiveness indicates chronic indecision (Betz, 1992). There are a number of instruments that have been found to be useful in assessing clients' places in the decision-making process.

The most widely used instrument in this area is the *Career Decision Scale* (CDS, Osipow, 1987). The CDS has 19 items of which the first two measure the level of certainty the individual feels in making a career decision. The next 16 items measure the level of career indecision. The last item provides an opportunity for individuals to describe their career indecision if none of the other items seemed appropriate. The Career Decision Scale is generally regarded as a reliable instrument with evidence related to validity as a measure of overall career indecision (Harmon, 1994). An impressive amount of research was done in the development and subsequent evaluations of the CDS (Savickas, 1990; Herman, 1985). There is some debate, however, about how to score the instrument. Osipow (1991) argued for the use of one total score, while others have suggested using four subscale scores based on the results, reflecting that there are four stable factors (Vondracek, 1991). It is important to note that the CDS provides a measure of career indecision, but it does not provide an indication of the source or type of indecision.

Another measure often used in this area is Holland, Daiger, and Power's (1980) *My Vocational Situation* (MVS). There are three subscales on the MVS: the Vocational Identify scale, the Occupational Information Scale, and the Barriers scale. The Vocational Identify scale is often considered a measure of indecision and assesses the clarity and stability of one's career-related attributes. Both the CDS and the MVS are not only used to gather information about clients, but they are also used extensively to evaluate the effectiveness of career counseling. Another indecision instrument is the *Assessment of Career Decision Making* (Harren, Buck, & Daniels, 1985), which is a 94-item instrument that measures major, career, and academic decision-making styles. Rather than focusing on whether the client is undecided, this instrument focuses on what decision-making style the client uses (e.g., Rational, Intuitive, or Dependent). There are, however, some psychometric limitations with this instrument and it should be used cautiously.

Career Maturity

Betz (1988) defined career maturity as the "extent to which the individual has mastered the vocational tasks, including both knowledge and attitudinal components, appropriate to his or her stage of career development" (p. 80). Career maturity is examined developmentally and compares the individual to others in terms of career development. Essentially, career maturity measures the client's level of readiness for mastering career development tasks. Career maturity measures are used to identify limitations or deficiencies in terms of an individual's career maturity and as an evaluation tool to determine if career counseling increased the client's career maturity. There are two instruments that are frequently used in this area: the Career Development Inventory and the Career Maturity Inventory.

The *Career Development Inventory* (CDI, Super, Thompson, Lindeman, Jordaan, & Myers, 1988b) measures career maturity using Super's theory. The scales of Career Planning, Career Exploration, Decision Making, and the World of Work correspond to Super's theory with the exception of Reality Orientation. An overall career maturity measure, called the Career Orientation Total, is also available. The CDI is produced in two forms that vary based on the age of the client: the High School Form and the College Form. The results can also be scored into two broad areas to determine if interventions should focus on attitudes or knowledge. Some reviewers (Hackett & Watkins, 1995; Pinkey & Bozik, 1994) have criticized the variation in the reliability of the scales. The greatest strength of the CDI is its ability to measure a cogent model of career development (Savickas, 1990). Although there is compelling validation evidence in terms of Super's concept of career maturity, there are questions about some of the individual scales. A somewhat related instrument is the *Adult Career Concerns Inventory* (ACCI, Super, Thompson, Lindeman, Jordaan, & Myers, 1988a), which evolved from the Career Development Scale (Adult Form). Super suggested that the term *career adaptability* is more appropriate for adults than the term career maturity. The ACCI does not follow the same format as the CDI, and it focuses just on the planfulness dimension of Super's model. Whiston (1990) suggested that the ACCI is a useful instrument, particularly since there are few instruments for adults in this area. She, however, further argued for cautious use of the ACCI because of limited validation information.

The other common measure of career maturity is Crites' (1978) *Career Maturity Inventory* (CMI). The CMI is composed of an attitudinal scale and five competency tests. Assessment of both attitudes and competencies is geared toward students in grades 6 through 12. The Attitude Scale assesses decisiveness, involvement, independence, orientation, and compromise in career decision making. The Competency Test measures more cognitive variables such as Self-Appraisal, Occupational Information, Goal Selection, Planning, and Problem Solving. There is substantially more support for the Attitude Scale as compared to the Competency Test. Nevertheless, others have criticized the content of the

Attitudinal Scale (Savickas, 1990). A major limitation of the CMI is that it has not evolved in recent years and has not been updated since the middle 1970s.

Computer Assessment in Career Counseling

As will be discussed in Chapter 16, computers are having a significant influence on the field of assessment in counseling. In the career area, computers have been used for a number of years to both assess and provide occupational information. In fact, these programs are so widely used for career counseling that they will be discussed briefly in this chapter. Computer-assisted career assessment and information systems should not be considered as a replacement for career counseling; research has clearly shown that a counselor is needed in the process (Sexton et al., 1997).

Computerized Career Assessment Systems

There are two dominant computerized career assessment and information systems: the DISCOVER Program and the SIGI-Plus (Garis & Niles, 1990). These programs are widely used, and studies have indicated that students and counselors react positively to both of these systems (Kapes, Borman, & Frazier, 1989).

DISCOVER. *DISCOVER* is one of the predominate computer-assisted career guidance systems and was developed by the American College Testing Program. The high school version and the college and adult version of DISCOVER include the Unisex Addition of the ACT Interest Inventory (UNIACT), a self-assessment of skills, and a values inventory. This system also uses the World-of-Work Map. Results from other assessment instruments (e.g., ASVAB, ACT, and Strong Interest Inventory) can be entered, with the computer taking those results into consideration when providing occupational and training information. DISCOVER provides many interactive activities, where clients can gather extensive career information.

SIGI-Plus. The System of Interactive Guidance and Information Plus (SIGI-Plus) is a product sold by Educational Testing Services. The philosophical foundation of SIGI-Plus is values identification and clarification. Originally SIGI focused on the assessment of values, but it has been expanded to include an interest assessment and an analysis of skills. Individuals can use SIGI-Plus to move through nine separate modules, with the second module being Self-Assessment. Other modules are designed so that individuals interact with the computer to gain more knowledge about themselves and possible occupations. SIGI-Plus focuses on occupations that require two or more years of college and, therefore, may not be appropriate for all clients. SIGI-Plus is quite comprehensive and the average client spends more than three hours using it.

Strengths and Limitations of Computer-Assisted Career Systems

One of the major advantages of computer-assisted career assessment and information systems is the interactive nature of these systems. Clients can take multiple career assessment tools and then, based on the results of these assessments, retrieve relevant occupational information. Computers are very adept at storing large amounts of information that can assist clients in the career decision-making process. These computer-assisted programs often have an image of being fault-less and accurate (Sampson, 1986). There are, however, some limitations to these useful resources that need to be considered when counseling clients. One of the limitations according to Gati (1994) is that the occupational databases in these programs often consist of "soft" information. These databases are considered soft because the sorting of occupations often is based on expert judgment rather than empirical inquiry. As an example, experts would judge which occupations have a high degree of independence or lack of variety. Gati also argued that some occupations might be eliminated from a client's list without sufficient justification. There are no well-defined minimal or maximal cutoffs for entering a particular occupation or for success or "satisfactoriness" in them.

Another problem concerns the perception that these computer-assisted programs can provide the answer rather than encouraging the client to make informed career decisions. Because of the technological nature of computers, some clients are likely to see these programs as providing a definitive evaluation of their abilities. The career decision-making process is complex and these computer-assisted programs have addressed this with sophisticated approaches. These sophisticated approaches, however, reinforce the perception that the computer is accurate and unerring. Finally, no matter how sophisticated a computer-assisted career assessment and information system becomes, it can never take into account the uniqueness of all the different clients using these systems. The research clearly indicates that these systems are more effective when they are used in conjunction with a counselor rather than alone (Garis & Niles, 1990; Niles & Garis, 1990).

Issues in Career Assessment

In recent years, one of the major issues in this area has been related to gender difference on many career-assessment instruments. Research related to women's career development abounded in the 1980s and 1990s, and as a result, problems with career assessment with women were identified. As Betz (1992) argued, interest inventories have historically yielded different result patterns for men and women, which may result in continued stereotyping of occupations. Interest inventories typically use questions that are reflective of differential experiences. For example, the answers to questions like "I like to fix car engines" and "I like to take care of children" may be connected to the opportunities to participate in these activities. Therefore, it is not surprising that there are gender differences in interest inventory results. Using results from inventories utilizing Holland's theory, females are more likely to have higher scores on the Social, Artistic, and Conventional themes, while males tend to have higher scores on the Realistic, Investigative, and Enterprising themes. Females' lower scores on the Realistic, Investigative, and Enterprising themes decrease the likelihood that they will explore occupations in the skilled trades, medicine, science, engineering, law, and business (Betz, 1992).

Gender-role stereotyping has been found to influence gender differences in career assessments (Betz & Fitzgerald, 1987). In interpreting these instruments with women, Forrest and Brooks (1993) suggested that counselors explore the client's level of gender role socialization and perceived sociopolitical barriers. Women's answers may be reflective more of their socialization than their career interests. Forrest and Brooks recommended using sentence-completion exercises to assess gender-role socialization and perceived sociopolitical barriers. Examples of their sentence-completion exercises are "Since I am a woman, I am required to _____ ; I am allowed to be _____ ."

Some steps taken to address gender differences are the elimination of sexist language and the inclusion of gender-balanced items. Betz (1992) and Hackett and Lonborg (1993) suggested that interest inventories use same-sex normative scores rather than combined norms. With same-sex norms, females' interests would be compared to those of other females, which would increase the likelihood that nontraditional interests would be identified. For example, a female who is interested in a number of Realistic activities may receive a score of moderately high interest in this area when compared to other females, but her score may only appear as average or even as having below average interest if half of the norming group is male. Separate norming groups, however, can have a subtle influence on the manner in which clients view the results, and counselors also need to address sexual stereotyping in their interpretations of interest inventories.

There are also issues related to ethnic and cultural differences in career assessment. Subich (1996) suggested that fully integrating an appreciation of diversity into the practice of career assessment requires revealing and rejecting models and methods of assessment that assume cultural uniformity of clients. The research related to general ability and aptitude assessment with different cultural groups is particularly relevant when those measures are used in career counseling. A culturally biased instrument could affect clients' perceptions of opportunities that are available to them and unfairly influence clients' career decision making. In addition, work values inventories cannot incorporate all the values of the dominant ethnic groups, and their use with clients other than European-Americans has been questioned (Betz & Fitzgerald, 1995).

Career researchers have also examined the appropriate use of interest inventories with racial and ethnic minorities. Although early research cast some doubt about the use of Holland's hexagonal model with ethnic minority samples in the United States (Rounds & Tracy, 1996), more recent research has supported a common vocational interest structure among racial and ethnic minorities (Day & Rounds, 1998; Fouad, Harmon, & Borgen, 1997). The Day and Rounds results are particularly noteworthy since their sample was over 49,000 and involved large groups of minority students. Their multidimensional scaling analysis provided support for traditional methods of assessing career interests by indicating that individuals from diverse ethnic groups use the same cognitive map or structure of preference when examining career interests.

Related to other issues in career assessment, Chartrand and Walsh (in press) suggested that career assessment must keep pace with our changing work environments. They argued that the focus on occupational titles on many interest inventories may be less relevant because occupational information is moving toward a job-tasks and skills focus. For example, O-NET (the Occupational Information Network), which is being developed to replace the Dictionary of Occupational Titles, is skill-based rather than based on occupational titles. Chartrand and Walsh also asserted that personality and cognitive assessments need to be considered part of the career assessment domain. Research has indicated that characteristics such as flexibility, adaptability, and self-control are related to job success. With this broader definition of career assessment, the focus needs to be on learning and clients' cognitive processing. The focus on cognitive processing is certainly consistent with the abundance of research reflecting the importance of self-efficacy and cognitive processing.

Summary

Assessment tools have often been considered an integral part of career counseling. There are a number of well-developed measures of clients' individual attributes. Clients' interests are a good indicator of career direction or choice. In terms of interest inventories, John Holland's theory has had a significant influence. One of the instruments influenced by Holland is the Strong Interest Inventory, which is one of the most widely used instruments in counseling. The purpose of the Strong is to identify interest patterns. The Strong Interest Inventory provides results related to 6 General Occupational Themes, 25 Basic Interest Scales, and 211 Occupational Scales. Counselors can have the most confidence in interpreting the General Occupational Themes and the Basic Interest Scales, and less confidence in the results from the Occupational Scales and the Personal Style Scales. Other interest inventories that are often used by counselors are the Career Assessment Inventory, the Kuder Occupational Interest Survey, the Kuder General Interest Survey, and the Self-Directed Search.

Aptitude tests are often used in career counseling because they are significant predictors of occupational success. There is also research that supports the use of self-estimates of abilities. The exploration of clients' aptitudes and abilities should include an analysis of their self-efficacy beliefs. Self-efficacy beliefs directly influence the tasks attempted by clients and, thus, should be considered when clinicians are engaged in any therapeutic relationship.

The assessment of values is sometimes neglected even though it is an important part of the career assessment process. Work values have been found to be highly correlated with work satisfaction. Any values instrument is not inclusive of all values; hence, these assessments need to be supplemented with other exercises when working with clients. Gender and racial issues need to be considered by the clinician when using an interest inventory, an abilities or aptitude assessment, or a values scale.

Rather than focusing on individual differences, some career assessment tools focus on where clients are in the career decision-making process. Typical measures of career process variables are related to the level of decidedness or certainty and amount or stage of career maturity. These instruments can be helpful in selecting career interventions that are appropriate for the client. In addition, these instruments are used to evaluate career counseling to see if clients became more vocationally mature or decided about their occupational choice as a result of the counseling.

Computers are very adept at storing large amounts of information. Some individuals saw that this capacity made computers an excellent tool for combining career assessment with the delivery of career information. A number of computerized systems have been developed that integrate career assessment and career information. Thus, clients can use the computer to take a career assessment, get the results, and then immediately access career information. Computerized assessments, however, also need to be evaluated in terms of the reliability, validity, norms, and suitability for the client.

There are a number of relevant issues related to career assessment. One issue concerns gender differences on many career assessments and the need for counselors to be sensitive to gender stereotypes. A similar issue concerns ethnic and racial differences on career instruments and the need to take cultural differences into account. There is also concern about whether career assessments are keeping pace with the dramatic changes in the world of work. These issues are being addressed in the field and many existing instruments are being revised in response to these issues. In addition, there continues to be development of new methods and instruments in the career area that are appropriate for clients with diverse needs.

CHAPTER 10

Appraisal of Personality

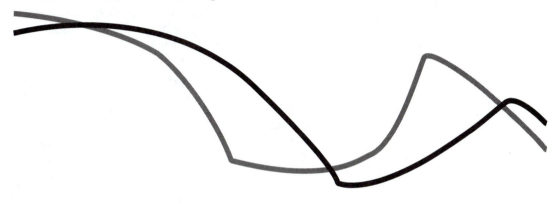

*T*he term *personality* is used in everyday conversation and has certain connotations in the mental health professions. It is not uncommon to hear someone say, "She has a good personality." If, however, we attempt to define personality, we find that it is a somewhat illusive construct. The term *personality* comes from the Greek term *persona,* which was a role-play by an actor in a play. Like other psychological constructs, there are different theoretical views about the facets of personality. Recent research, however, has contributed to a greater understanding of the structure of personality. Although we know more about personality than we did 20 years ago, there is still debate about what it is and how it can best be measured.

The assessment of personality has been around for thousands of years. The early hunters and gatherers probably assessed each other's personalities to determine who would be a better hunter or gatherer. Nonetheless, the field of formal psychological assessment of personality is less than a century old. During this century, both public sentiments and professional views toward personality assessment have varied. Although there have been times when personality assessment was somewhat unpopular, Butcher (1995) argued that personality assessment has increased in the last 20 years. Butcher cited three reasons for this expansion: (1) the increased research on the use of personality assessment; (2) the fact that personality assessment is more attractive to professionals than it was in the past; and (3) the increased use of personality assessment in forensic and industrial settings.

There are times when it can be beneficial to incorporate personality assessment into the counseling process. Personality assessment can, at times, provide a shortcut in identifying client problems (Butcher, 1990). In selecting interventions and making decisions about treatment, counselors can frequently benefit from having information about the client's personality. Personality probably influences coping styles, needs and desires, responses to environmental stressors, interpersonal patterns, and intrapersonal sensitivity. Counselors can use client personality information to assist them in structuring the counseling relationship and selecting specific interventions to use with that client.

This chapter provides an overview of the topic of personality assessment. The information contained in this chapter is not sufficient for anyone to use these assessments without considerable additional training and supervision. Many of the instruments discussed in this chapter can be administered, scored, or interpreted by master's level practitioners; however, some formal instruments (e.g., Rorschach) cannot. Nonetheless, counselors often work in multidisciplinary teams and need to have a basic understanding of these instruments

Within the area of personality assessment, there are numerous informal and formal assessment tools. Within formal personality assessment, there are two major categories: **structured personality instruments** and **projective techniques**. Structured instruments (e.g., the Minnesota Multiphasic Personality Inventory-2) are formalized assessments in which clients respond to a fixed set of questions or items. Projective techniques vary from standardized instruments in that the client is asked to describe, tell a story, or respond in some other way to relatively unstructured stimuli. The intent of the personality assessment is less obvious with projective techniques than with a structured inventory. The unstructured format presumably guards against faking because the examinee is not sure what the examiner is evaluating. With projective techniques, clients are believed to "project" their personality characteristics in their responses. Thus, projective techniques are considered by their proponents to be an effective method for uncovering latent, hidden, or unconscious aspects of personality.

This chapter examines both informal and formal personality assessment techniques. Informal assessment techniques are frequently used and clinicians need to consider methods for improving the reliability and validity of these measures. Informal techniques, just like formal instruments, need to be analyzed for their soundness. After the discussion of the informal techniques of observation and interviewing, there is a discussion of formal personality instruments. This includes an overview of the most commonly used structured personality inventories and projective techniques.

Informal Assessment Techniques

Observation

When you think of personality assessment, you may only consider formal assessment instruments such as the Minnesota Multiphasic Personality Inventory 2 (MMPI-2). If you believe personality assessment only includes standardized instruments, then you would ignore the most common method counselors use to assess personality: observation. When you meet someone, you may begin to make judgments about his or her personality based on such factors as attire, stance, choice of words, and facial expressions. The counselor observes the client from the first meeting and begins to make clinical judgments based on those observations. Counselor training is often designed to produce individuals with refined observational skills. Social psychology research, however, has found that mental health practitioners tend to be biased in the interpretations of their observations. When clinical decisions are based on observation, there are problems with selective recall, selective interpretation, and the power of preexisting assumptions (Dawes, 1994). Clinicians often selectively remember certain aspects of what clients say and how clients behave. Practitioners also have "themes" concerning what they remember, and clinicians have been found to recall similar information about a number of different clients. In addition, clinicians tend to be selective in their interpretations. Clinicians tend to focus on certain behaviors and draw conclusions on those behaviors. Social psychology research has also shown that people tend to see things with which they are familiar. Hence, a counselor who works primarily with clients who have eating disorders is more likely to see a new client as having an eating disorder (Dawes, 1994). Subjectivity is a persistent problem in observation. In fact, you may have had experience with subjectivity in observation, where a friend or family member has a very different view of an event.

Practitioners cannot afford to be subjective in their observations when assessing personality. Observation is an assessment tool and, therefore, we should evaluate it in the same manner that we evaluate other assessment tools (e.g., the reliability and validity of our observations). Let's consider reliability in terms of observation. *Unsystematic error* has a way of slithering into counselors' observations of their clients. Counselors, like other humans, tend to get an occasional cold, get stuck in traffic, or have a disagreement with a family member. All of these may lead to unsystematic error in their observations. Furthermore, the client may contribute to the unsystematic error. A counselor may perceive a client as being disinterested, when the sluggish speech and yawning are more related to staying up late the night before. Counselors need to examine the reliability of their observational methods, for there may be a high degree of error in these methods. Counselors can adapt some of the traditional methods of determining reliability to examine the consistency of their observations. For example, counselors could systematically conduct a test-retest situation by noting observations in one session and then comparing these to recorded observations of a second session. A counselor could split a session into halves or systematically attend to observations at specific time intervals in a session and examine the consistency of these observations. Sattler (1993) found that reliability can be increased in observation when there are clear and precise definitions of the behaviors and a systematic method of observing. Trained observers also tend to be more reliable in the observations than nontrained observers. Attending to the concept of reliability in observation has the potential to increase the validity of the counselor's observations.

There also can be problems with the validity of counselor observations (Hoge, 1985). When counselors are observing, they need to consider the *representativeness* and the *generalizability* of their observation (Sattler, 1993). In terms of representativeness, the time the client spends with the counselor is not long and the client may not be completely natural with the counselor. Therefore, the validity of the observations may be restricted because only a small sample of behaviors was observed, which might not represent typical client behavior. If the counselor's observations are inadequate, then it limits the counselor's ability to generalize to how the client behaves outside of counseling. For example, a client in the counseling sessions may act reserved, when outside of counseling the client's behavior may be very domineering and aggressive. One method for enhancing the representativeness of the observations is to increase the amount of time when the individual is observed. For school counselors this can be accomplished by observing students in the classroom, during lunch, during physical education, or on the playground. In other settings, counselors may want to have clients keep a log, which is essentially a self-observation technique. Another technique to increase the sample of observation is to have another person (e.g., a family member) record certain behaviors.

In conclusion, counselors often use observation to assess personality, but in doing so, they need to consider certain factors. Clinicians need to consider how they organize the observations and the conceptual framework for their conclusions. Furthermore, clinicians should evaluate their working models of personality that may influence this process. Counselors also need to consider whether their observations are filtered through their biases and beliefs.

Interviewing

Interviewing is another widely used method of personality assessment. In this context, an interview is defined as a face-to-face verbal exchange in which the counselor is requesting information or expression from the client. Vacc and Juhnke (1997) found that structured clinical interviews fell into the categories of either *diagnostic assessments* or *descriptive assessments*. The intent of diagnostic interviews is to identify issues and possible disorders consistent with a diagnostic taxonomy (e.g., the *Diagnostic and Statistical Manual of Mental Disorder—Fourth Edition*). Chapter 13 will address interviews with the specific purpose of diagnosis. Descriptive interviews are used when the purpose is to describe aspects of the client. The focus here is on descriptive interviews for the specific purpose of describing personality.

The same characteristics of a good intake interview discussed in Chapter 6, such as being warm and encouraging, also apply here. The quality of the questions that counselors use in assessing personality has a substantial influence on the value of the assessment. Poorly developed questions that are not conceptually related to personality assessment will probably add little to the counselor's understanding of the client's personality. Sometimes, counselors will use questions related to the client's problems and situation as the primary mechanisms for personality assessment. Questions only peripherally related to personality may not provide clients with the opportunity to explain their personality. Therefore, when the major focus is on understanding the client's personality, counselors should ask clients questions that directly assess personality. The discussion of reliability and validity of observation also applies to interviews. Counselors need to focus on the reliability and validity of their interviewing techniques.

Structured Personality Inventories

In order to understand the most commonly used personality instruments in counseling, it is important to have a foundation in the methods of constructing personality inventories. Anatasi and Urbina (1997) suggested that there are four basic methods of constructing self-report personality inventories. The first type of personality instrument is the *content-related procedure*. Here the focus is on the content relevance of the items. Developers use a rational approach to item development, where the items are directly related to the personality attributes being measured. The content scales of the MMPI-2 are examples of this type of procedure. There are some difficulties with content-related procedures because many times the instruments are easy to fake or to have a response set. A response set exists when an individual answers one question a certain way and then falls into the habit of answering other similar questions in the same way.

The second method of constructing personality inventories concerns using *personality theory* as the base for development. The items are developed based on the theory. Once the instrument is developed, then construct validation procedures are implemented to determine if the instrument does measure the tenets of the theory. Thus, the validation information is interpreted concomitantly with the theory. An example of a theory-related instrument is the Myers–Briggs Type Indicator (MBTI) that is based on Jungian theory.

The *empirical criterion keying* method is the third method of constructing personality inventories. Rather than content, items are selected based on their relationship to some external criterion. The MMPI is an example of the empirical criterion keying method, for items were selected that separated people who were considered to be normal from those people who were diagnosed with some form of psychopathology. The occupational scales of the Strong Interest Inventory were developed using this same method, with only items that differentiate between people working in that occupation from people not working in that occupation being used in scoring each occupation scale.

The last method involves the statistical technique of *factor analysis.* This strategy involves examining the interrelationships of items and determining the similarities of the items that group together. Researchers have used factor analysis to investigate personality and some current researchers have found five factors (nicknamed the "Big Five"). The NEO Personality Inventory—Revised is designed to measure these five factors of personality.

The precise number of self-report personality inventories is difficult to determine but there are at least several hundred. Rather than discuss all of these instruments (which would mean reading this book for a very long time), this section will summarize the instruments most used by counselors. The Minnesota Multiphasic Personality Inventory-2 is the most widely used structured personality inventory. The NEO-PI-R has a rich research base and is being increasingly used by practitioners. Finally, the Myers–Briggs Type Indicator is another popular instrument that is used in diverse settings.

Minnesota Multiphasic Personality Inventory-2

The *Minnesota Multiphasic Personality Inventory-2* (MMPI-2) (Butcher, Dahlstrom, Graham, Tellegen, & Kraemmer, 1989) replaced the original MMPI in order to improve on this widely researched and used instrument. The MMPI-2 also replaced the MMPI as the most widely used personality instrument. Soon after the publication of the MMPI-2, another form was introduced, the *Minnesota Multiphasic Personality Inventory-Adolescent Version* (MMPI-A, Butcher et al., 1992) for children ages 14 to 18. The MMPI and the MMPI-2 are empirical criterion keyed instruments, which means the items were not selected for their content but rather for their relationship to a criterion. The criterion in the original MMPI was the identification of psychopathology. The MMPI was designed to differentiate between those with a psychopathology as compared to normal individuals. The manual of the MMPI-2 reflected that it is a "broad-based test to assess a number of the major patterns of personality and emotional disorders" (Butcher et al., 1989, p. 2). Therefore, the MMPI-2 is used to diagnose emotional disorders, but it is also intended to be used in nondiagnostic activities.

One of the major reasons for revising the MMPI was the original norming group was tested in the 1930s and was primarily white, middle-class individuals from Minnesota. The norming group for the MMPI-2 was selected to match the 1980 census data. This norming group of 2,600 matches the portion of ethnic groups, geographic representation, and age distribution of the United States population. The MMPI-2 norming group has been criticized, however, for including a high proportion of individuals with advanced educational backgrounds and in higher-status occupations. Although there is greater representation of minority individuals in the MMPI-2 than in the MMPI, there continues to be debate about the racial bias (Newmark & McCord, 1996). Graham (1990) and Timbrook and Graham (1994) found that the differences among ethnic groups on the MMPI-2 were not statistically significant. Anyone using the MMPI-2 or the MMPI-A with minority clients, however, should be knowledgeable about ethnic differences on both the validity and clinical scales in order to ensure proper interpretation. Furthermore, others have argued that with minority clients, clinicians need to take into account acculturation (Anderson, 1995), socioeconomic status, and education (Long, Graham, & Timbrook, 1994).

The MMPI-2 booklet contains 567 items and the MMPI-A has 478 items. The items are statements (e.g., I am sure I get a raw deal from life, I cry easily) in which the client responds by indicating whether the statement is true or false. The MMPI-2 has an eighth-grade reading level, although clinicians can purchase an audiocassette version for clients who cannot read. The basic scoring of the MMPI-2 and the MMPI-A involves three validity scales and ten clinical scales. There are numerous other scales that have been developed that indicate a variety of personality characteristics or personal issues.

The interpretation of the MMPI-2 is complex and specific training is needed in order to use the results appropriately. A proper interpretation involves examining the entire profile together and not just each clinical scale in isolation. Newmark and McCord (1996) argued the MMPI-2 could be dangerous in the hands of the casual user who has not mastered its intricacies. Even though a T-score of 65 is usually considered the cutoff, a clinician does not consider one elevated score to indicate the disorder with which that scale is labeled. This is one of the reasons the clinical scales are usually referred to by number rather than by name (*see Figure 10.1*).

Validity scales. In interpreting a personality inventory, it is often quite helpful to understand individuals' attitudes while they were taking the inventory. For example, it might be helpful to know if the client is trying to put his or her "best foot forward," or if someone on trial for murder is attempting to appear as if he or she is psychologically disturbed. The validity scales of the MMPI-2 are designed to provide that type of information; in other words, these scales reflect the validity of the profile. Three Validity Scales, **L**, **F**, and **K**, are plotted on the MMPI-2 (*see Figure 10.1*). Not only do these scales provide information on the attitudes of the test taker, the results can also be used in treatment planning (Butcher, 1990). The **?** scale is not plotted on the MMPI-2 as it was on the original MMPI. For most clients, the typical number omitted is between 0 and 6, and Duckworth and Anderson (1997) suggested further investigation if the number omitted is 7 or larger.

L Scale   The L scale, or the Lie Scale, provides an indication of the degree to which the individual is trying to look good. Higher scores indicate the individual wants to report socially correct behaviors, while lower scores suggest the

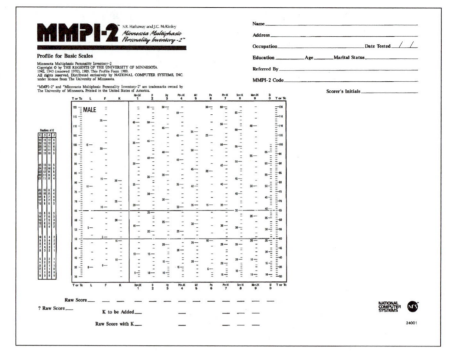

ability to acknowledge general human weaknesses. This scale should not be interpreted to represent overall honesty or the tendency to lie. A high L scale may indicate the counselor will need to work on being seen as trustworthy in order to encourage the client to be more self-disclosing.

F Scale   The second validity scale, the F scale, is the Infrequency Scale. Endorsing a large number of these items indicates the test taker is presenting an extreme symptomatic picture not found in the general population. There may be a tendency to exaggerate symptoms or attempt to "fake bad." However, Duckworth and Anderson (1997) found that in mental health clinics and college counseling centers, a high F scale represents the degree to which an individual's thoughts are different from the general population and only rarely an indication of purposefully faking bad.

K Scale   The K scale, or Correction Scale, measures defensiveness or guardedness. It is more subtle than the L scale but measures the same dimension of trying to present oneself in an overly positive manner. The context in which the person is taking the MMPI-2 must be considered when interpreting the K scale. For example, one might expect a higher K scale if the MMPI-2 is a part of a hiring process as compared to a client seeking counseling. In counseling situations, an elevated K scale (above 65) may indicate the individual will have difficulty recognizing his or her own contributions to problems.

Other Validity Scales   There are three other validity scales that can be scored to provide additional information: the F_B, VRIN, and TRIN. The F_B is an extension of the F scale and measures items that are infrequently endorsed by the general population. The validity scales are in the first part of the MMPI-2 in case practitioners use the shortened version. The F_B is on the back portion of the MMPI-2 and can verify the score on the F scale or indicate the person may be responding randomly on the second half of the test. The VRIN and TRIN scales look at consistency in responses and can be helpful in determining if the person is randomly marking answers or is having difficulty understanding the items. VRIN consists of paired items in which the content is very similar or opposite. Thus, if the responses are not in the expected manner, then the inconsistencies are reflected in the VRIN score. VRIN can be helpful in interpreting whether a higher F scale is related to responding randomly or attempting to fake. TRIN is designed to measure "yea-saying" or "nay-saying." These are paired items with consistency being indicated by answering true one time and false the other time. This scale will identify those individuals who mark all the items true or all the items false.

Clinical scales. The clinical scales of the MMPI-2 and the MMPI-A are drawn from the clinical scales of the MMPI (Butcher & Williams, 1992; Duckworth & Anderson, 1997). Table 10.1 lists the ten scales, each with a number, an abbreviation, and a formal name. As with the validity scales, the clinical scales are not interpreted in isolation since the entire profile is taken into account in interpreting the MMPI-2. In MMPI-2 interpretation, the term *elevated* is often used to indicate that the T-score on that scale is above 65. In addition, an interpretation may include the term moderately elevated, which generally indicates that the T-score is between 60 and 65. Sometimes a practitioner will

TABLE 10.1

The clinical scales of the MMPI-2

Number	Abbreviation	Formal Name
1	Hs	Hypochondriasis
2	D	Depression
3	Hy	Conversion Hysteria
4	Pd	Psychopathic Deviate
5	Mf	Masculinity-Femininity
6	Pa	Paranoia
7	Pt	Psychasthenia
8	Sc	Schizophrenia
9	Ma	Hypomania
0	Si	Social Introversion

focus only on the scales where the scores are elevated; however, other scales should also be examined in order to identify possible strengths and coping skills. The following overview of each of the clinical scales is designed to provide a basic understanding of the scales and an introduction to how the scales are combined in interpretation.

Scale 1: Hypochondriasis   Scale 1 is related to excessive concerns with health as indicated by reporting the presence of bodily complaints. This scale assumes that there is little or no organic basis for these complaints. If you have a client with a chronic illness or a client who was physically ill while taking the MMPI-2, then you need to be more cautious in your interpretation. It is believed, however, that scale 1 represents a characterological preoccupation with bodily concerns rather than a situational attentiveness to physical complaints. In addition to the physical complaints, elevated scores indicate a tendency to be self-centered, selfish, and pessimistic. The complaints center on health issues but spread to complaining or whining about other issues. Markedly elevated scores may indicate the tendency to manipulate others with their physical complaints and to use these complaints to avoid responsibility and meet dependency needs.

Scale 2: Depression   Elevated scores on scale 2 suggest feelings of discouragement, hopelessness, and isolation. Lower scores on the scale indicate the tendency to be optimistic, gregarious, and alert. Duckworth and Anderson (1997) indicated that scale 2 is frequently elevated for people voluntarily seeking counseling. As scores increase, the client's attitudes change from sadness or gloom to a pervasive pessimism about the world. This pessimism extends to the self, with high scale 2 scores often indicating self-deprecation and overriding feelings of hopelessness.

Scale 3: Hysteria   Scale 3 concerns conversion disorders that are a complex combination of denial and social flamboyancy. Moderate elevation may only reflect a tendency to think positively about people. Elevated scores reflect the tendency to deny issues, and these individuals often react to stress and anxiety with physical symptoms. Elevations on scale 3 are also indicative of individuals who are extroverted but somewhat superficial. They have a tendency to lack insight into both their own motivations and actions and insight into others' motivations. Rarely is a person with an elevated scale 3 diagnosed as being psychotic. These first three scales of the MMPI and MMPI-2 are often examined in combination. Sometimes these three scales are labeled the "neurotic triangle," which is a somewhat misleading title. The patterns within this triad of scales are examined and there is empirical support for certain interpretations based on certain patterns.

Scale 4: Psychopathic Deviate   An elevation on scale 4 suggests that the client is "fighting something" but does not identify the specific conflict. Higher scores reflect hostility toward social convention, authority figures, and possibly family members. Descriptors of individuals with elevated scale 4 scores are moody, irritable, resentful, and impulsive. These individuals tend to blame other people for their difficulties. In addition, these individuals often have difficulties with law enforcement and may be incarcerated. It is important for counselors to explore the context of an elevated 4 scale. If the scores are markedly elevated, the prognosis for change in therapy is poor.

Scale 5: Masculinity-Femininity   Scale 5 provides a measure of whether the individual's emotions, interests, attitudes, and perspectives on social relationships and work are consistent with men or women in general. This scale is scored separately, so that men's attitudes are compared to men and women's to women. High scores indicate their general perspective is nontraditional from others of their same gender. Hence for males, elevated scores are associated with having a wide range of interests, especially aesthetic interests. On the other side, low scores for males indicate more of a "he-man" attitude. Higher scores are also associated with nontraditional attitudes for women, with elevated scores indicating interest in masculine activities, being assertive, competitiveness, and self-confidence. Women with lower scores have endorsed more items indicative of stereotypically feminine interests. Low scores for women on scale 5 may indicate passivity and submissiveness. The interpretation of scale 5 needs to incorporate ethnicity, socioeconomic status, and educational level.

Scale 6: Paranoia   Scale 6 considers whether there is a pattern of suspiciousness, mistrust, delusional beliefs, and marked interpersonal sensitivities. Some of the items also address self-centeredness and insecurity. Moderately elevated scores are characteristic of a sensitive individual. An elevated scale 6 indicates the individual has the tendency to misinterpret the motives and intentions of others. They tend to be suspicious and believe that others' actions are somehow aimed at them. Research on the MMPI-2 indicated that scale 6 was associated with severe pathology. Markedly elevated scores are indicative of disturbed thinking and psychotic behaviors.

Scale 7: Psychasthenia   This scale is related to some of the symptoms associated with anxiety and obsessive-compulsive disorders. It measures generalized anxiety and distress, as well as a position of high moral standards. Moderate scores may reflect the ability to be methodical, organized, and punctual. Elevated scores indicate a tendency toward self-blame accompanied by anxiety, rumination, and feelings of insecurity. Extremely high scores are usually associated with some obsession and rigid efforts to control impulses.

Scale 8: Schizophrenia   The developers of the original MMPI constructed scale 8 with patients manifesting various forms of schizophrenia. Because various forms of schizophrenia are measured with this scale, there are a large number of items that may appear somewhat strange to some clients. Scale 8 includes a wide range of strange beliefs, unusual experiences, and emotional problems. Elevated scores reflect an unconventional lifestyle and feelings of alienation from others. It may be difficult to follow the individual's train of thought and mental processes. High scores are usually characterized by people who are isolated and alienated. These clients are unconventional, eccentric, and nonconforming. Extremely high scores are associated with individuals who show blatantly psychotic symptoms.

Scale 9: Hypomania   Scale 9 was constructed to measure manic or hypomanic behaviors. These behaviors include being energetic, hyperactive, and euphoric. Moderately elevated scores (not uncommon in graduate school) suggest highly energetic, involved, and gregarious people. As the scores increase, individuals are expending more energy but are less efficient (spinning their wheels). Elevated scores are indicative of overactivity, flight of ideas, and emotional excitement. Clients can be easily frustrated and fluctuate between euphoria and irritability.

Scale 0: Social Introversion   High scores on scale 0 are associated with a preference for being alone, while low scores indicate a preference for being with others. With many of the scales of the MMPI-2 and MMPI-A, clinicians have a tendency to assume that low scores are positive and high scores are negative. This conclusion on scale 0 is incorrect since introversion is not necessarily a deficit. Clients with moderately elevated scores on this scale prefer to be alone or with select friends. Increased scores usually indicate more social withdrawal and anxiety associated with being around people. Individuals with high scores have a tendency to worry and be guilt-prone. Examining other scales can provide an indication of the type and level of the social adjustment problems.

Additional scales. In the time since the original MMPI was published in the 1940s, many other scales have been developed to supplement the original validity scales and clinical scales. Some of the supplementary scales can be hand-scored, but because of the time investment, most practitioners use computer-generated supplementary scales. Clinicians use these additional scales to both augment and confirm their interpretation of the clinical scales' results. Most of the supplemental scales were developed with a specific purpose in mind (e.g., addiction problems, marital distress). One set of scales is the *Supplementary Scales*, which were selected by the revisers of the MMPI to supplement the MMPI-2. Examples of these scales are: A, Anxiety; R, Repression; Es, Ego Strength; and MAC-R, MacAndrew Alcoholism Scale. There are also *Content Scales* that address issues such as Anxiety, Fears, Obsessiveness, Depression, and Health Concerns. On the MMPI-A, 11 of the content scales are the same as the MMPI-2, but there are also content scales related to School Problems, Low Aspirations, Alienation, and Conduct Disorder. The Harris–Lingoes Subscales is another set of additional scales used by practitioners.

Psychometric qualities. There is some debate concerning whether the MMPI-2 is equivalent to the MMPI and, as such, can build from the vast amount of validation information already existing. In their reviews of the MMPI-2, both Archer (1992) and Nichols (1992) contended that, for better or worse, the instruments are closely related. Certainly, Butcher et al. (1989) provided a compelling case for the comparability of the two instruments. The test-retest reliability coefficients for the clinical scales range between .67 and .92 for men and .58 and .91 for women. Already there is substantial validity information concerning the MMPI-2 and to a lesser extent the MMPI-A. Archer and

Krishnamurthy's (1996) major concern about the MMPI-A is the instrument's ability to detect psychopathology and the possibilities of false-negatives (the instrument indicates they do not have a psychopathology when they do have a disorder). Austin (1994) criticized the MMPI-2 for not responding to recent developments concerning conceptual classification in psychopathology. Chapter 13 will address diagnosis and some instruments (e.g., Millon Clinical Multiaxial Inventory) that are directly tied to a prominent diagnostic system.

In conclusion, the MMPI-2 and the MMPI-A are widely used instruments and have clinical applications for counselors. The counselor must have in-depth knowledge about this complex instrument in order to use it appropriately. Computer-generated interpretative reports have almost eliminated hand-scored and interpreted reports. The use of a computer-generated report, however, does not exonerate a clinician from understanding the instrument.

Another instrument associated with the MMPI is the *California Psychological Inventory* (CPI). The current version of the CPI is the Third Edition (Gough & Bradley, 1996), which drew almost half of its 434 questions from the MMPI. The CPI scales stress more normal aspects of personality compared to the clinical scales of the MMPI. For example, the CPI provides measures of social expertise and interpersonal style; maturity, normative orientation and values; achievement orientation; and personal interest styles. The CPI can be used in many counseling settings with clients 13 years old and older. The CPI has a rich history and has been researched for over 40 years. It doesn't appear, however, to be as popular currently as some other instruments such as the Myers–Briggs Type Indicator.

Another instrument developed from the MMPI is the *Personality Inventory for Children—Revised Format* (PIC, Wirt, Lachar, Klinedinst, Seat, & Broen, 1982), which is completed by a parent or caregiver of the child. This inventory also has validity scales: Lie, Frequency, Defensiveness, and Adjustment. There are also 20 Clinical Scales (e.g., Social Skills, Delinquency, Family Relations, Achievement) that can be translated into 4 Broad-Band Factor Scales (Undisciplined/Poor Self-Control, Social Incompetence, Internalization/Somatic Symptoms, and Cognitive Development). Recently, Lachar and Gruber (1995) published the Personality Inventory for Youth (PIY), which is an extension of the PIC. The major difference is that the child or adolescent completes the PIY. The PIY is similar in terms of reliability to the PIC, but because of its recent development, it does not have the extensive validity information of the PIC.

NEO-PI-R

There are some exciting advancements in personality research that directly pertain to personality assessment. There is substantial research to indicate that personality can best be described by five factors (Digman, 1990; Goldberg, 1994; McCrae & John, 1992). Researchers have gathered multiple descriptors of personality, and using factor analysis, they found that all these different descriptors fall into one of the five factors (e.g., Digman & Takemoto-Chock, 1981; Goldberg, 1992; McCrae & Costa, 1987). The prominence of these five factors has lead some to label them as the "Big Five." These Big-Five factors have traditioally been numbered and labeled: Factor I, Surgency or Extra-version; Factor II, Agreeableness; Factor III, Conscientiousness; Factor IV, Emotional Stability or Neuroticism; and Factor V, Intellect or an Openness to Experience.

Not only is there substantial research that personality can be described by these five factors, but it also appears the factors may apply across diverse cultures. McCrae and Costa (1997) found, with a very large sample, that the American personality factors showed remarkable similarity to the factor structure in German, Portuguese, Hebrew, Chinese, Korean, and Japanese samples. They contended that their findings, along with other research, indicate that the structure of personality is universal. These results are encouraging and suggest that instruments based on the Big Five may be appropriate with clients from diverse backgrounds.

Two researchers have been instrumental in developing instruments that operationalize the five factors. Costa and McCrae (1992) developed the Revised NEO Personality Inventory (NEO-PI-R) and an abridged version, the NEO Five-Factory Inventory (NEO-FFI). The scales were developed by using a combination of rational and factor analytic methods with both normal adults and clinical samples. These instruments represent one of the few commercially available tests based on the five-factor model of personality (Botwin, 1995). The NEO-PI-R is a comparatively recent addition to the area of personality assessment; however, it is gaining in prominence. Caprara, Barbaranelli, and Comfrey (1995) found the NEO to be among the personality tests most heavily researched in the 1990s.

There is some debate about the appropriate names for the five factors. In the NEO-PI-R, Costa and McCrae (1992) have labeled their domains Neuroticism, Extroversion, Openness, Agreeableness, and Conscientiousness. In the NEO-PI-R, the *Neuroticism* (N) Scale provides a measure of adjustment or emotional stability. High scores are associated with a general tendency to experience negative feelings such as fear, sadness, embarrassment, anger, and guilt. Although clinicians make distinctions between types of emotional distress (e.g., anxiety, anger, depression), Costa and McCrae have found that if individuals are prone to one of these emotional states, they are more likely to experience the others. Thus, this domain measures a tendency toward coping poorly with stress, difficulty controlling impulses, and a proclivity toward irrational thoughts.

The *Extroversion* (E) Scale concerns the individual's tendency to be sociable, assertive, active, and talkative. High scores are associated with being upbeat, energetic, and optimistic. Costa and McCrae (1992) have found that introverts are not unhappy, hostile, and shy. Their studies indicated that introverts are reserved rather than unfriendly, independent as compared to followers, and even-paced as compared to sluggish.

The third dimension of personality according to Costa and McCrae (1992) is *Openness* (O). The openness scale measures the degree of openness to a variety of experiences. Elements associated with openness are an active imagination, aesthetic sensitivity, attentiveness to inner feelings, and intellectual curiosity. This is perhaps the most controversial of the domains on the NEO-PI-R,

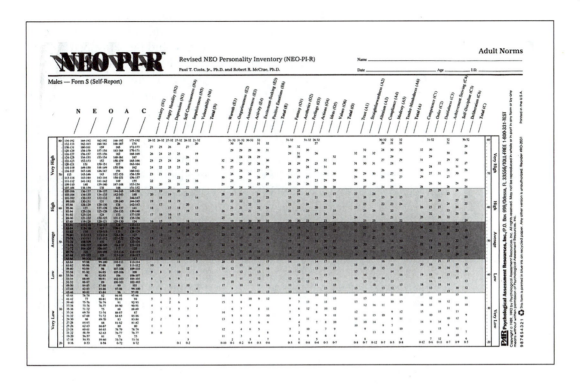

FIGURE 10.2

NEO-PI-R Profile

Reproduced by special permission of the publisher, Psychological Assessment Resources, Inc. From the NEO Personality Inventory—Revised, by Paul Costa and Robert Mc-Crae, ©1978, 1985, 1989, 1992 by PAR, Inc. Further reproduction is prohibited without permission of PAR, Inc.

for other researchers have labeled this factor Intellect and contend that the openness label does not adequately address the factor (Goldberg, 1994; Widiger, 1992). Costa and McCrae contended that this is the most researched scale of the NEO-PI-R and that a preference for the familiar as compared to a preference for novel experiences is one of the five factors.

The *Agreeableness* (A) Scale measures a tendency to be sympathetic, a desire to help others, and a belief that others will reciprocate and assist them. Low scores on this scale are associated with a tendency to be antagonistic, egocentric, and skeptical of others' intentions. Costa and McCrae (1992) argued that extremes at either end of this scale are problematic. Low scores are associated with narcissistic, antisocial, and paranoid behaviors, while high scores are associated with dependency problems.

The last domain is *Conscientiousness* (C), which is related to the individual's ability to control impulses. This domain measures self-control and the ability to plan, organize, and carry out tasks. Low scores are associated with being more lackadaisical in the pursuit of goals. Extremely high scores can indicate fastidious behaviors, compulsive neatness, and workaholic tendencies.

Each of the five domains (N, E, O, A, C) has six facets. As reflected in Figure 10.2, the facets for the Neuroticism Domain are Anxiety, Angry Hostility, Depression, Self-Consciousness, Impulsiveness, and Vulnerability. Form S is the self-report version of the NEO-PI-R and contains a total of 240 items with each of the facets containing only 8 items. There are three statements at the end of the instrument that address the validity of the profile. These, however, are simplistic statements (e.g., asking if they responded honestly and accurately). A check of the accuracy of the responses could be performed by having someone else (a family member, friend, or colleague) complete Form R, which is the observer-report form of the NEO-PI-R. There are two versions of Form R, one for women and one for men. These observer forms correspond to the self-report version except the items are in third person. Form S of the NEO-PI-R has both normal adult norms and college-age norms for men and women, while the norms for Form R are just for normal adults.

The NEO-PI-R has been the recipient of some criticisms. Part of the criticism focuses on the use of the NEO-PI-R in the identification of psychopathology, which Costa and McCrae (1992) advocated. Juni (1995) contended that this use is questionable since the instrument was developed with normal adults and that the model is based on common characteristics of personality, not on pathology. Hogan, Hogan, and Roberts (1996) found that when the five-factor model was measured with a well-developed instrument, such as the NEO-PI-R, it was a valid predictor of performance in virtually all occupations. Furthermore, they found that measuring personality in this way did not result in adverse impact for job applicants from minority groups. This research supports McCrae and Costa's (1997) research, which found that the NEO-PI-R could be used cross-culturally.

Myers–Briggs Type Indicator (MBTI)

The Myers–Briggs Type Indicator® (MBTI®, Myers, 1962; Myers & McCaully, 1985) inventory is a widely used instrument that is based on Jungian theory. In 1998, a new version of the Myers–Briggs Type Indicator (Form M) was published. The theory suggests that variations in behavior are related to basic differences in the ways individuals prefer to perceive and then make judgments about what they have perceived. Furthermore, Jung proposed that individuals have different attitudes in which they use their perceptions and judgments. The different forms of the Myers–Briggs Type Indicator inventory are designed to assist people in understanding their preferences as measured on four bipolar dimensions (see Figure 10.3). The MBTI is a typology instrument in which scores on the four dimensions result in individuals being categorized into 16 psychological types. The Murphy–Meisgeir Type Indicator for Children (Murphy & Meisgeir, 1987) is an instrument that measures MBTI types for children between ages 7 and 12.

The first dimension indicates preference in attitudes in terms of *extraversion-introversion*. Jung described extraversion and introversion as being complementary attitudes. He suggested that everyone feels a pull between extraversion and introversion and the MBTI is designed to measure the individual's preference along a continuum. The extraverted attitude (E) on the MBTI is not a simple indicator of being socially outgoing. The extraverted attitude reflects that attention

---

®Myers-Briggs Type Indicator and MBTI are registered trademarks of Consulting Psychologists Press, Inc.

FIGURE 10.3

Myers–Briggs Type Indicator Report Form

The test user, in selecting or interpreting a test, should know the purposes of the testing and the probable consequences. The user should know the procedures necessary to facilitate effectiveness and to reduce bias in test use. Although the test developer and publisher should provide information on the strengths and weaknesses of the test, the ultimate responsibility for appropriate test use lies with the test user. The user should become knowledgeable about the test and its appropriate use and also communicate this information, as appropriate, to others.

MYERS-BRIGGS T Y P E I N D I C A T O R® — STEP **I** / REPORT FORM **FORM M**

Name _____ Date _____

The MBTI® reports your preferences on four dichotomies. There are two opposite preferences on each dichotomy, as shown below.

E–I Dichotomy Where you like to focus your attention	**E Extraversion** You prefer to focus on the outer world of people and things	**I Introversion** You prefer to focus on the inner world of ideas and impressions
S–N Dichotomy The way you like to look at things	**S Sensing** You tend to focus on the present and on concrete information gained from your senses	**N Intuition** You tend to focus on the future, with a view toward patterns and possibilities
T–F Dichotomy The way you like to go about deciding things	**T Thinking** You tend to base your decisions primarily on logic and on objective analysis of cause and effect	**F Feeling** You tend to base your decisions primarily on values and on subjective evaluation of person-centered concerns
J–P Dichotomy How you deal with the outer world	**J Judging** You like a planned and organized approach to life and prefer to have things settled	**P Perceiving** You like a flexible and spontaneous approach to life and prefer to keep your options open

YOUR REPORTED TYPE AND PREFERENCE CLARITY CATEGORY

Your reported type comprises four letters representing the four preferences you chose. Your preference clarity category (pcc) shows how consistently you chose one preference over the other. High points indicate a clear preference; note, however, that the pcc does not measure abilities or development. To determine your pcc, follow these steps:

1. Refer to the "Points" chart on page two of the answer sheet. For each dichotomy, identify the preference with the greater number of points, and record that letter and number in the "Your Reported Type" column.
2. For each dichotomy, circle in the chart below the range that includes the number next to your preference.
3. Identify the preference clarity category ("slight," "moderate," etc.) shown above each circled range and record it below. If you did not answer all of the items, your points may be lower than the lowest range of numbers on the chart. If so, use "slight" as your pcc.

YOUR REPORTED TYPE	DICHOTOMY		PREFERENCE CLARITY CATEGORY				YOUR PREFERENCE CLARITY CATEGORY
			Raw Points Ranges				
			Slight	Moderate	Clear	Very Clear	
		E–I	11–13	14–16	17–19	20–21	_____
		S–N	13–15	16–20	21–24	25–26	_____
		T–F	12–14	15–18	19–22	23–24	_____
		J–P	11–13	14–16	17–20	21–22	_____

Each type, or combination of preferences, tends to be characterized by its own interests, values, and unique gifts. On the back of this page is a brief description of each of the sixteen types. Find your reported type and see whether the description fits you. If not, the person who administered the MBTI to you can help you identify a better-fitting type. Whatever your preferences, you may still use some behaviors that are characteristic of contrasting preferences. For a more complete discussion of the sixteen types and applications, see *Introduction to Type®*, Sixth Edition (Myers, I. B., 1998, CPP) or *Gifts Differing* (Myers, I. B., with Myers, P. B., 1995, Davies-Black).

 CONSULTING PSYCHOLOGISTS PRESS, INC.
3803 E. Bayshore Road • Palo Alto, California 94303 • www.mbti.com

6134

---

seems to flow out or be drawn out to people and objects in the environment. An introverted attitude (I) is a preference for drawing energy from the environment and consolidating it within one's own position. Extraverts prefer to focus their energy on the outer world, while introverts prefer to focus their energy on the inner world of ideas and concepts.

The preference in terms of perception is indicated on the second dimension, which is labeled the *sensing-intuitive* dimension. A higher sensing (S) score indicates a preference for perceiving using the five senses. These individuals use the senses to perceive what exists and they often develop skills in perceiving detail, observing the situation, and remembering specifics. Those with higher scores on the intuition (N) side of the continuum perceive more using "hunches" and perceptions of patterns. Those with an intuition preference perceive relationships, meanings, and possibilities. As an example, a sensing person will be able to describe the color of the carpet and the amount of wear on the furniture, while the intuitive person will contend the room had a depressed feel to it.

The third dimension concerns how the individual processes or makes judgments about the information brought in through the second dimension. This dimension measures where individuals prefer to make judgments on the *thinking-feeling* continuum. The thinking (T) function is a preference for processing perceptions using rational, cognitive abilities. A higher T score reflects a preference toward making judgments logically and impersonally. A preference toward feeling (F) indicates the individual primarily uses personal or social values in making judgments. These individuals are attuned to the values of others as well as their own in making decisions.

The last dimension describes the process an individual primarily uses in dealing with the outer world. The MBTI assessment focuses on how individuals perceive information and make judgments about that information, and this dimension reflects the *judgment-perception* preference in dealing with the external world. Those who prefer judgment (J) favor arriving at a decision or conclusion (using either thinking or feeling) more quickly than those that prefer perception. Those who prefer perception like to perceive situations and, thus, will favor putting judgments off in order to spend more time perceiving. This dimension was not explicitly addressed in Jung's discussions of psychological types and there are questions about whether it is truly independent from the other dimensions (Hood & Johnson, 1997).

The preference on the four dimensions of the MBTI assessment result in a four-letter code. The different methods of combining the letters produce 16 personality types. For example, an ESFP would reflect an extravert who uses his or her senses to perceive information and processes the information using feeling, while his or her orientation to the outer world is perception. An INTJ is an introvert who perceives using intuition and makes judgments by thinking, while his or her orientation to the outer world is judgment. Item Response Theory was used in the 1998 Revision of the Myers–Briggs Type Indicator inventory and there are some indications that this may alleviate some of the problems regarding estimates of types. Counselors, however, need to be careful and not "pigeon-hole" clients based on their personality types because there is wide variation within each of the 16 personality types. Often there can be an inherent link between types and stereotypes, and counselors using any kind of typology instrument need also to consider the uniqueness of the individual.

One of the reasons for the popularity of the MBTI inventory rests in its philosophical stance that all types are valuable and that the preferences are not correct or incorrect. The developers of the MBTI stress that the preferences are just differences rather than indicators of health or pathology. Myers (with Myers P. B., 1980) explained this concept in detail in *Gifts Differing*, which is suggested in the manual as a basic reference for anyone using the MBTI. There are also a wide variety of other resources available to aid in the interpretation of MBTI results.

There is detailed reliability information on the MBTI. The split-half reliability coefficients and the measures of internal consistency are mostly in the .70s and .80s. A problem with the MBTI is that, rather than viewing the results as continuous scores, the instrument uses types (i.e., the client is an E even if the score is just over the line). This leads to the question of stability of type, where the evidence is not as compelling. Hood and Johnson (1997) cited evidence that when retaking the MBTI inventory, there was only a 50-50 chance of having an identical four-letter code.

The Myers–Briggs Type Indicator assessment has been used in a wide variety of settings and for diverse reasons (e.g., family counseling, career counseling, team building, hiring decisions, determining promotions). The widespread use of the MBTI is one of its major problems. As you will remember from Chapter 4, an instrument is not either valid or invalid; validity concerns the support for specific interpretations and uses of an instrument's results. In my opinion, the MBTI inventory has been used for purposes where there is little validation evidence. Therefore, a counselor considering using the MBTI needs to be familiar with the validity evidence. A new manual was published along with the revision of the MBTI, which includes more recent validation studies. Jungian theory also has to be considered in using the MBTI, for unlike some personality instruments, this instrument is based on a theory.

There are a number of criticisms of the Myers–Briggs Type Indicator inventory. One of the consistent criticisms centers on the dimensions being dichotomies or bipolar discontinuous types (e.g., the client is either an E or an I). There is support for the dimensions being viewed as continuous variables that may even approximate a normal curve (Pittenger, 1993; Wiggins, 1989). A second line of criticisms is related to the constructs being measured and whether they are sufficient to describe personality. Dahlstrom (1995) argued that typologies, in general, cannot describe the complexities of personality.

Other Standardized Personality Instruments

The three personality instruments previously discussed are commonly used instruments in counseling and also are examples of the different methods of constructing instruments. The empirical criterion keying method was used to construct the MMPI-2; the NEO-PI-R was constructed using factor analysis; and the Myers–Briggs Type Indicator is an example of an instrument based on personality theory. Another commonly used personality instrument is the *Sixteen Personality Factor Questionnaire* (Cattell, Cattell, & Cattell, 1993), which is commonly called the *16PF.* This is also an instrument constructed using factor analysis, where Cattell started with compiling personality adjectives. Cattell identified 17,953 adjectives that were reduced to 4,504 "real" traits, which an examination of commonalties reduced to 171 traits. Through a series of factor analyses, he identified at first 12 pure factors and then 16 pure factors of personality. The 16PF is now in its fifth edition and includes measures of 16 factors and five Global Factors: Extroversion, Anxiety, Tough-Mindedness, In-dependence, and Self-Control. The 16PF is an instrument for adults, but there are extensions of it that are appropriate for younger clients. The High School Personality Questionnaire is appropriate for those ages 12 through 18, the Children's Personality Questionnaire is for ages 8 through 12, the Early School Personality Questionnaire is for ages 6 through 8, and the Preschool Personality Questionnaire is for ages 4 though 6.

Douglas Jackson has influenced the area of personality assessment by con-structing two instruments. Through the use of high-speed computer and de-tailed item selection procedures, Jackson (1996c) constructed the *Personality Research Form* (PRF). The PRF measures 20 traits (e.g., Abasement, Affiliation, Autonomy) that were for the most part drawn from Murray's theory. The PFR focuses on areas of normal functioning rather than on the identification of pathology. The PRF has been used primarily in research. Another Jackson (1996a) instrument, the *Jackson Personality Inventory—Revised* (JPI-R) has more of a practice oriented approach than the PRF. The JPI-R contains 15 subscales that are organized in terms of five higher-order clusters: Analytical, Emotional, Extroverted, Opportunistic, and Dependable. The item selection procedures for the instrument were also technically sophisticated. Both of these instru-ments are easy to score by hand and there is now software available to gener-ate computer reports. The Jackson instruments are psychometrically sound and well-researched instruments but are not used in counseling practice as much as some other instruments.

Limitations of Standardized Personality Inventories

One of the limitations of standardized personality inventories is that the ma-jority of them are self-report instruments. Research has shown that when indi-viduals are motivated to distort the results of a self-report personality inven-tory, they are quite adept at it (Strickler, 1969; Wiggins 1966). However, outright lying on a self-report personality measure is not that common in counseling and hiring situations (Schwab & Packard, 1973). Some individuals may be motivated to "fake bad" as a part of a trial defense. Some clients may attempt to "put the best foot forward" in order to present a more positive image to the counselor. Bornstein, Rossner, Hill, and Stephanian (1994) found that when a personality trait could be easily identified from the item (i.e., the item had high face validity), the item was more likely to receive a socially desirable response. Providing a socially desirable response is a common response set to personality instruments, but it is not the only one. Some individuals will have a tendency toward acquiescence, where they commonly select the "true" or "yes" response. On the other hand, some individuals may have a tendency to select the uncommon or less socially desirable responses. Other may have a tendency to select the extreme choices on almost all of the items.

As the previous discussion indicates, some instruments have validity scales that control for misrepresentation. Another method for controlling for faking and response set use is to inform the client of the purpose of taking the inventory and how the results will be used (e.g., for the counselor to understand them better or the couple to have a better understanding of their different personalities). In addition, it is often helpful to instruct the client to answer each question honestly. Having them focus on each of the questions will sometimes decrease the tendency to endorse items in a similar manner.

Projective Techniques

As indicated earlier, counselors often use a combination of informal and formal techniques in assessing personality. Within formal personality assessment, there are two major categories: standardized instruments and projective techniques. Projective techniques address some of the limitations of standardized instruments by providing the client with a relatively unstructured stimulus to respond to. The intent is that clients will have more difficulty faking their responses because they will be unsure what the unstructured stimuli are designed to measure. With projective techniques, there are no right or wrong answers since there are no specific questions. The client responds to the stimuli and the examiner takes those responses and interprets the meaning.

Many individuals trace the use of projective assessments to the early 1900s and the rise of psychoanalytic theory. The psychoanalytic concept of projection concerns individuals' tendency to project their own drives, defenses, desires, and conflicts onto external situations and stimuli. Thus, projective techniques encourage clients to project their personality in their responses to the unstructured stimuli. Projective techniques are thought to uncover more of the client's unconscious and, thus, provide an indication of the covert or latent traits.

Projective techniques originated in clinical settings such as psychiatric hospitals and many remain in these settings. Some projective techniques, such as drawings and sentence completions, are being used in counseling settings. There is significant subjectivity in the interpretation of projective techniques and extensive training is needed to use these instruments appropriately. In addition, there is no professional consensus on how any of these techniques should be specifically interpreted. Lindzey (1959) categorized projective techniques into five categories: *associations* (inkblots, word associations), *construction* (of stories or biographies), *completions* (of sentences or cartoons), *arrangement* or *selection* (toys or verbal options), and *expression* (drawing or dance).

Association Techniques

Rorschach Inkblot Test. The Rorschach Inkblot Test is a very well known association technique. There are ten inkblots, with five cards that are in shades of black and gray; two more are black and gray with additional touches of bright red; and the three others have several pastels. There are numerous methods or systems for using these ten cards. Typically the inkblots are presented in two phases. In the first phase, the association phase, the cards are presented and the examinee responds. The second phase is the inquiry phase where the examiner goes back through the cards and in a nondirective manner questions the examinee on what prompted their responses. This information is also used in the scoring and interpretation of the responses.

One of the more widely used systems is Exner's Comprehensive System, which is based on research with the Rorschach Inkblots as compared to clinical practice. In fact, this system is so detailed that some argue that the Rorschach is not a projective instrument. His system takes into account the location, determinants, and content in terms of scoring and interpreting the responses. *Location* refers to the section of the inkblot that the examinee's response focuses on. Some individuals will focus on the entire blot while others will focus on common details, and still others will describe unusual details, white space, or some combination of these areas. The *determinants* include the form and movement of the blot and the color and shading. For example, there is some evidence that the type of movement, whether it be human, animal, or inanimate, is associated with different psychological processes. The last scoring category is *content*, where there are common popular responses and other less common views concerning the content of the inkblot. Exner and his colleagues have gathered considerable psychometric data. When this method is used the reliability coefficients are significantly higher than with other systems. Also, there is better validity information than what previously existed. However, no matter what scoring and interpretive system is used, the Rorschach Inkblots should never be used without extensive training and supervision.

Early memories assessment. Munroe (1955) asserted that the analysis of a client's early memories was the first projective technique utilized. Anastasi and Urbina (1997) contended that the resurgence in use of autobiographical memories for personality assessment is one of most promising developments in recent projective assessment. The interest in early childhood experiences is not new to the field, for certainly Freud and Adler were interested in these memories. Adlerian counselors have incorporated assessment of early childhood recollection as a routine part of their counseling process. The work of Bruhn and his associates in the 1980s and 1990s has brought new interest and empirical support for the assessment of early memories. Bruhn (1995) approached early memories from a cognitive-perceptual model and suggested individuals do not remember useless, antiquated beliefs. He argued that if individuals remember certain situations then those memories hold some clinical significance.

Bruhn (1989) standardized the process of assessment of autobiographical memories with the *Early Memories Procedure* (EMP). He suggested that the 32-page booklet should usually be completed after the intake session and before the second session. The EMP contains a combination of spontaneous memories that deliberately avoid any specific schemes or situations. These spontaneous memories avoid the problems associated with directed memory probes. The EMP also includes direct memory probes such as first memory of school and first family memory. The EMP does include questions related to memories of an inappropriate sexual experience and memories of being physically and sexually abused; however, the form contains a place for individuals to indicate that they did not have those experiences. Bruhn (1995) argued that these questions are at minimal risk of encouraging false memories of sexual abuse if there have been no other suggestions by the therapist. The EMP can be scored using the Comprehensive Early Memories Scoring System—Revised (CEMSS-R, Last & Bruhn, 1991). This system is adapted from the Klopfer scoring system for the Rorschach. The CEMSS examines concepts such as setting, characters, content and process themes, relation to reality, object relations, and damage aspects. Bruhn and his associates are continuing to gather empirical evidence about the EMP and are analyzing results with specific samples (e.g., delinquents). It is difficult, at this point, to predict if this technique will become more common in counseling practice.

Construction Techniques

Thematic Apperception Test. The Thematic Apperception Test (TAT) is an example of a construction projective technique, where the examinee constructs a story based on a picture shown to him or her by the examiner. The TAT was developed by Murray and his colleagues in 1938 as a measure of Murray's theory of needs and presses. The current version (Murray, 1943) has a total of 31 cards, 30 of which are black and white pictures and one that is blank. Depending on the examinee's age and gender, there are 20 specific cards that can be shown to them (19 pictures and 1 blank). The pictures primarily depict people in ambiguous situations (e.g., a young boy is staring at a violin that is placed on a table in front of him). The examinee then constructs a story based on each picture presented. Rarely does someone construct a story for all 20 pictures. The story is recorded verbatim and then analyzed by the examiner.

Like the Rorschach Inkblot Test, numerous methods for scoring and interpreting the TAT have evolved over the years. There are some quantitative scoring systems that yield acceptable interrater reliability coefficients. These scoring systems, however, are somewhat time consuming and are not used very frequently. There are also normative data on the TAT, but clinicians often rely more on clinical experience when interpreting the TAT. This can be problematic since research has indicated that conditions such as lack of sleep and being hungry can influence performance. Another criticism of the TAT is that the pictures are somewhat out of date. Some clinicians do feel the TAT provides a good method of entering the client's "world," while also providing a way for the client to open up. Nevertheless, clinician's interpretations are often quite diverse and can even contradict one another. Therefore, like other projective techniques, one needs to be cautious in interpreting the responses and seek verification from other sources of information.

Completion Techniques

Rotter Incomplete Sentences Blank. Completion techniques involve providing a stimulus to the examinee and he or she then completes the task. A frequently used projective technique in this area is the sentence-completion exercises. Here examinees are provided with incomplete sentences and asked to complete the sentence in their own words. Examples of sentences are "I hope . . ." "People . . ." "At home . . ." "I get upset when . . ." Some counselors have developed their own incomplete sentence assessments to address various types of issues and problems. Incomplete sentence instruments can be constructed to address family conflict, transitional issues such as going to middle/junior high school, career satisfaction, and self-concept.

A carefully constructed and standardized sentence-completion test is the *Rotter Incomplete Sentences Blank, Second Edition* (Rotter & Rafferty, 1992). There are three levels of the Rotter Incomplete Sentences Blank: high school, college, and adult. The client completes 40 sentences that are scored for conflict, positive response, and neutral responses. An overall adjustment score can also be calculated from the responses. Aiken (1996) suggested that research findings indicate that the Rotter Incomplete Sentences Blank can be used as a screening tool for overall adjustment. Practitioners often do not score this instrument but analyze the responses clinically. The norms have recently been updated and the new manual provides new information on reliability and validity.

Rosenzweig Picture-Frustration Study. The *Rosenzweig Picture-Frustration Study* is derived from Rosenzweig's theory of frustration and aggression. The three forms of the instrument are based on age with one for adults, another for adolescents, and the third for children. The individual is presented with a series of cartoons that represent frustrating situations. In these cartoons, one of the character's speech bubbles is blank. The examinee then fills in the empty cartoon bubble with a response to the frustrating situation. For example, one cartoon contains two people sitting in a car saying to the person standing beside the car, "I'm very sorry we splashed your clothing just now though we tried hard to avoid the puddle." The examinee would then fill in the empty cartoon bubble with the response for the person who was splashed. There is considerable research related to the Rosenzweig, and clinicians need to be familiar with this research when using this instrument because there are cultural, developmental, and gender differences that must be taken into account when interpreting this instrument (Rosenzweig, 1977, 1978a, 1978b, 1988).

Arrangement or Selection Techniques

Assessment involving individuals selecting and arranging objects can avoid the difficulties associated with traditional assessment procedures, particularly with young children because they often have difficulty answering questions or completing a paper-and-pencil exercise. Sandplay or the use of sand trays has become of increasing interest to counselors in the last twenty years. There is some disagreement whether the sand tray should be used as a diagnostic or clinical assessment instrument or as a therapeutic tool. The International Society for Sandplay Therapy has supported the psychotherapeutic application of the sand tray as compared to diagnostic uses (Mitchell & Friedman, 1994). According to Mitchell and Friedman, the Sandplay literature indicated that five areas are predominantly considered when interpreting a sand tray: (1) how the sand tray is created; (2) the content of the tray; (3) developmental perspective of a series of trays; (4) the Sandplay story; and (5) the therapist's feeling response.

Most of the research on Sandplay or the use of sand trays has been individual case studies, with very few empirical investigations. This technique has not been investigated extensively and, therefore, does not have the empirical base of other projective techniques. Without more research its use as an assessment tool is questionable. A problem with the use of sand trays is the lack of standardization. There is not a universal standard on the size of the tray, the amount of water available, nor the number, size, or nature of the miniatures used. This lack of standardization severely hampers the research that can be performed or the ability to generalize from one sand tray to another. It may be easier to validate a projective technique such as the Scenotest (Straabs, 1991) where there is uniformity in the figurines and materials.

Children's selection, arrangement, and playing with toys in general have been used as a projective technique for many years. Because play allows for the natural expression of children's thoughts and affects, it lends itself to interpretation at multiple levels. The research on how to interpret play is not as extensive as other projective techniques such as children's drawings. Schaefer, Gitlin, and Sandgrund (1991) included three of the more promising projective play assessments. Interestingly, two of these projective techniques involve working with the entire family. One of these techniques involves having the family do a collaborative drawing exercise that encourages participation of both adults and children. Each member of the family contributes to the drawing, which is used to aid in the understanding of the family functioning. Another technique entails using puppets with the family and methods for having the family members reenact recent problematic situations. The third technique also involves the use of puppets in diagnostic interviews with children. This technique focuses particularly on analyzing the form and content of the child's play with the puppets.

Expression Techniques

Drawing techniques. It makes logical sense that the methods people use to express themselves may provide a window into their personality. The method of self-expression that has received the most study in terms of being a projective technique is art or drawing. One of the first formal techniques to incorporate drawing was Machover's (1949) *Draw-a-Person Test* (D-A-P). In the D-A-P, the client is first given a piece of paper and a pencil and told to draw a person. Once the first figure has been drawn, the examiner instructs the individual to draw a person of the opposite sex. After the drawing is completed, the examiner either asks the individual to tell a story about each figure or asks a series of questions concerning age, education, occupation, ambitions, and other pertinent details. Machover's interpretation of the D-A-P has been questioned and criticized (Swenson, 1968). Machover contended that individuals tended to project acceptable impulses on the same-sex figure and unacceptable impulses on the opposite-sex figure. In addition, certain characteristics of the drawing were thought to be indicative of certain personality traits. For example, hands behind the back were indicative of introversion; dark, heavy lines and shading suggested hostility and aggression; small drawings were related to low self-esteem; and disproportionately large heads indicated organic brain damage.

There are a number of different approaches to interpreting human figure drawings. Generally interpretations examine pencil pressure, stroke and line quality, lack of detail, placement, erasures, shading, and distortions (Handler, 1996). Experts in this field stress that no single sign has only one fixed and absolute meaning. Therefore, a child drawing a face with a frown does not always indicate the child is depressed. It is also important to take into consideration the child's educational background and developmental level. Koppitz (1968, 1984) compiled information on large numbers of children's drawings and identified "emotional indicators" of possible emotional problems.

One of the outgrowths of the human figure drawings is the popular *House-Tree-Person* (H-T-P), which was originally published by Buck (1948), with the latest revision being Buck (1992) (revised by Warren). In H-T-P, the individual draws three separate drawings of a house, a tree, and a person. The individual is then given the opportunity to describe, define, and interpret each of these drawings. In general, Buck suggested that the house reflects the home situation of the client, the tree represents the self in relationship to the environment, and the person represents the self.

Another influential name in projective drawing techniques is Burns. Burns (1987) adapted H-T-P into *Kinetic-House-Tree-Person* where the house, tree, and the person in action are drawn on one sheet of paper. This technique incorporates the interconnections among the three figures and the action of the person. Another technique that Burns (Burns, 1982; Burns & Kaufman, 1970 1972) is known for is the *Kinetic-Family Drawing* (K-F-D). A counselor using this technique would ask the child "to draw the family doing something." The incorporation of action into the drawing, according to Burns, allows for a clearer picture of family dynamics. The child can depict the family as an active, functioning unit, which can provide indications of family interactional patterns. Figure 10.4 is an example of a K-F-D of a 12-year-old boy. Burns (1982) suggested four major categories in interpreting a drawing: Actions; Distances, Barriers, and Positions; Physical Characteristics of the Figures; and Styles. *Actions* concern the overall content, theme, or activity of the picture. The *distances, barriers, and positions* analyze how the family is arranged and indications of relationships. *Physical characteristics* examine the formal aspects of the drawing (e.g., expressions, analysis of presentation of body parts, different size of the figures). *Style* variables are indicators of emotional problems or disturbance and interested readers are directed to Burns' publications. A resource for counselors working with children, both in school and nonschool settings, is Knoff and Prout's (1993) book *Kinetic Drawing Systems for Family and School: A handbook*. This book explores methods for examining children's difficulties both at home and in school.

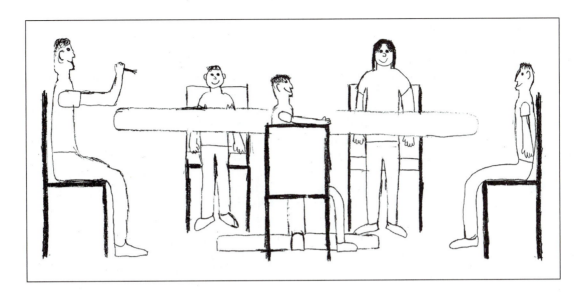

FIGURE 10.4

Example of Kinetic-Family-Drawing

Strengths and limitations of projective techniques. Projective techniques often address some of the limitations of standardized personality instruments, in that they are more difficult to fake and they can sometimes identify more complex themes and multidimensional aspects of personality. With some clients, projective techniques can serve as an effective method of establishing rapport. In addition, with young children and nonverbal clients some of the expressive techniques can provide an opening into the client's world that is difficult with other methods. On the other hand, projective techniques have some significant limitations. The reliability evidence for most of these techniques is quite low. As you have learned earlier, this means that there are higher proportions of error in these measures as compared to other measures. With these higher proportions of error, a counselor needs to regard the findings more cautiously. Certainly the examiner and the situation need to be taken into consideration when interpreting the results of a projective technique because both of these can have a significant influence on the process. The lack of normative data further compounds the problem. The central concern, however, with the use of any instrument is the validity of that instrument. The validation information on most of these techniques is often meager. In the wrong hands, a projective technique can be dangerous, for some clinicians could see every triangle any client draws as an indication that they were sexually abused. Anastasi and Urbina (1997) suggested that projective techniques be viewed not as tests but rather as clinical tools. As clinical tools, these techniques inform practice by identifying possible hypotheses to be further investigated in the counseling process. Thus, these tools would not serve to confirm a clinical judgment, but rather to generate hypotheses that would be further explored and investigated.

Self-Concept Measures

Some counselors would view self-concept as a construct closely related to personality, while others would define self-concept as a unique aspect of the individual. Self-concept is another area where there is debate and differing opinions on definition and characteristics. When the topic of self-esteem is added to the discussion, the matter becomes more tumultuous, for self-esteem in the last ten years has become a social/political issue. Leaving the debate over self-concept and self-esteem to other venues, this discussion will address some of the prominent measures in this area. In some form, these measures are related to individuals evaluating their performance or feelings about themselves. Counselors use self-concept or self-esteem measures in primarily two ways. First, counselors may want information on client attributes and may use these measures in the beginning of the counseling process to assess the level of self-esteem of the client. Second, counselors may want to use these instruments to examine the effect of counseling interventions. As an example, counselors might examine whether a group counseling experience raised the self-esteem level of the participants. It should be noted that research has shown that counseling interventions have *not* been found to have a consistent effect on self-esteem (Kahne, 1996; Whiston & Sexton, 1998). This may be related to difficulties associated with measuring self-concept and self-esteem.

Coopersmith Self-Esteem Inventories. The *Coopersmith Self-Esteem Inventories* (CSEI) consists of three forms: the School Form (for ages 8 through 15); the School Short Form (same ages); and the Adult Form (for ages 16 and above). The school forms both have 50 items, but the shorter form does not include the 8 Lie Scale items of the original School Form. The Adult Form is only 25 items and only provides a general measure of self-esteem. The School Forms provide measures of General Self, Social Self-Peers, Home-Parents, School Academic, Total Self, and Lie Scale. In reviewing these instruments, Adair (1984) found the standardization and normative data, reliability, and validity to be inadequate. In addition, the scoring provides percentile information but does not go any further in interpreting what the scores mean in terms of low to high self-esteem.

Piers-Harris Children Self-Concept Scale. *Piers-Harris Children Self-Concept Scale* (The Way I Feel About Myself) (Piers, 1984) is for students in grades 4 through 12 and consists of 80 items. Raw scores can be converted to both T-scores and percentiles on a total self-esteem measure and six cluster areas. The six cluster scores provide an indication of the child's self-esteem in the areas of Behavior, Intellectual and School Status, Physical Appearance and Attributes, Anxiety, Popularity, and Happiness and Satisfaction. Epstein (1985) evaluated the Piers-Harris as being highly reliable and favorably reviewed the validation evidence. Jeske (1985) contended that the Piers-Harris Children Self-Concept Scale was the best children's self-concept measure currently available. One limitation of the Piers-Harris is the normative sample, which is only from one school district in Pennsylvania and has not been updated from the original studies performed in the 1960s.

Tennessee Self-Concept Scale. Another of the frequently used self-concept scales, the *Tennessee Self-Concept Scale: Second Edition* (TSCS:2) was recently revised (Fitts & Warren, 1997). This instrument can now be used with children, adolescents, and adults. The results provide two summary scores, with one being a measure of total self-concept and the other a general measure of conflict. There are six specific self-concept scores: Physical, Moral, Personal, Family, Social, and Academic/Work. Furthermore, there are three supplementary scores and validity scores that take into consideration inconsistent responding and faking. This recent revision appears to be psychometrically sound, but additional research on the revised instrument is needed.

Summary

Assessing client personality is often incorporated into the counseling process. A client's personality is frequently intertwined with the problem and issues that motivated the client to seek counseling. In addition, the client's personality should be considered when making treatment decisions. Counselors often use both formal and informal personality assessment techniques. Observation is the most common technique in personality assessment. Counselors need to attend to the reliability and validity of their observations because personal biases and attitudes can influence their abilities to be skilled observers. Interviewing is another personality assessment technique that counselors often use. The quality of the interviewing questions will greatly influence the usefulness of the information gathered in an interview. Interviewing suffers from many of the same problems as observation, and counselors need to evaluate the psychometric qualities of their interviews.

Within formal personality assessment, there are two major categories: standardized instruments and projective techniques. In terms of standardized personality instruments, the most widely used is the MMPI-2. The interpretation of MMPI-2 results should be performed by individuals who are knowledgeable and well trained in the intricacies of this instrument. Other commonly used personality inventories are the Myers–Briggs Type Indicator, the NEO-PI-R, the 16PF, and the California Psychological Inventory. There are some limitations with these self-report instruments, particularly concerning clients' abilities to manipulate the results and the tendency to use a response set. Projective techniques are more difficult to fake or use a response set. Projective techniques, however, usually have lower reliability coefficients than standardized instruments and many are lacking in sufficient validation information. Self-esteem or self-concept measures are sometimes considered part of personality assessment. The area of self-esteem or self-concept assessment has problems in that there is a lack of consensus on what constitutes self-esteem and how to measure it.

CHAPTER 11

Assessment in Marriage and Family Counseling

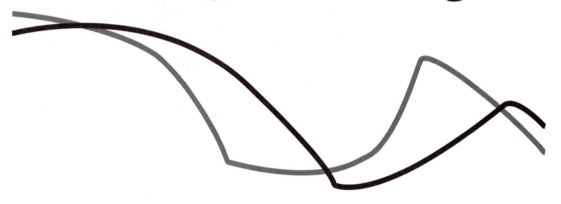

Thus far in this section, the focus has been on methods for assessing individuals; however, many counselors work with couples and families. Many marriage and family therapists or counselors use a systemic approach when working with couples or families. A systemic approach is holistic, where the focus is on the interactions that occur and the belief that all members of the family interact and influence each other. With this philosophical view, assessment would not be of individuals, but would focus on the dynamics or patterns that occur within the couple or family. Thus, testing each member within the family individually would not really be consistent with this systemic view. Sometimes instruments designed for individuals have been used in marriage and family assessment. The use of personality instruments is common in both couples and family counseling. For example, practitioners have used the Myers–Briggs Type Indicator to examine the differences in preferences for different members of the family. There are some difficulties, however, with using these tools because the assessment of individuals is essentially linear in concept, while many clinicians in marriage and family are frequently grounded in systemic theories.

Sporakowski (1995) argued that marriage and family counselors need to include assessment to gather information about the couple or family during counseling, as well as to evaluate the process and effectiveness of the counseling. There are numerous instruments for assessing couples and families. Straus and Brown (1978) found 813 instruments, and Touliatos, Perlmutter, and Straus (1990) had information on nearly 1,000. It does not appear, however, that these instruments are being used in practice. In a recent survey of marriage and family therapists, only 39% reported using standardized assessment instruments on a regular basis (Boughner, Hayes, Bubenzer, & West, 1994). This study also indicated that these clinicians do not use a specific battery of instruments, for no single assessment instrument was used by more than 8% of the sample. An inspection of the instruments used by marriage and family therapists reflects that the majority of these instruments were designed for individual counseling as compared to couples and family counseling. One reason for the dearth of instruments designed for assessing couples and families is that the field of family therapy or counseling is a comparatively recent development. Many of the theories or approaches for working with families were developed in the 1950s. Before that time, the dominant paradigm was individual therapeutic approaches. As therapeutic approaches designed for working with couples and families evolved, so did the beginnings of formal assessment instruments in this area. Hence, formal instruments designed specifically for couples and families do not have the long history that, for example, personality measures have. Another reason for the dearth of instruments designed for assessing couples and families concerns the difficulties associated with developing sound instruments in this area.

Difficulties with Assessment of Couples and Families

There are numerous difficulties associated with developing methods for assessing couples and families. One of the problems is determining what should be assessed within families. Assuming a clinician adheres to a systemic approach, what then is meant by a family's or couple's dynamics? Even if we use more specific terms such as interaction patterns, there continue to be multiple views on what constitutes interaction patterns. Some may argue that it is impossible to assess family interaction patterns because every family is so unique that these illusive dynamics cannot be quantified. Assuming that we do identify some dynamic or characteristic of a family, how do we then determine what constitutes a well-functioning family as compared to a dysfunctional family? Let's take for example family cohesion and determining the amount that is considered appropriate. Not all family theorists maintain that low cohesion is detrimental and high cohesion is positive in families. The Olson Circumplex Model (Olson,

Portner, & Lavee, 1985) suggested that cohesion should be viewed from a curvilinear perspective, where both too little and too much is problematic. In addition, what may be considered low cohesion for one family may function very well for another family. The difficulty in defining what constitutes functional as compared to dysfunctional becomes even more problematic when cultural differences are considered. Many differences exist between cultures in what are considered acceptable and unacceptable family behaviors. As an example, polygamy is accepted in some cultures and discouraged in other cultures.

Family assessment is a broad term, for in counseling we might want very diverse information depending on the problems or issues of the family. For example, a screening tool to determine if family counseling would be a suitable modality would be very different from an instrument to identify relational problems in a couple. Therefore, there is not just one area of focus in family assessment. In family assessment, the focus could be on couple's satisfactions, identification of communication patterns, perceptions of the family environment, self-reports of behaviors, analysis of relationships, identification of problems, or many other aspects of families. A family assessment device or technique could be extremely helpful in identifying the issues in one family but not appropriate for another family

Another problem with family assessment is that many of the variables assessed are fluid and fluctuate as compared to the more stable traits or characteristics of individuals. As an example of how family dynamics may vacillate, consider the variation in level of satisfaction a couple might report depending on whether they spent the night before at a wonderful French restaurant or completing their income tax forms. Not only are there situational fluctuations, there are also developmental changes. As Carter and McGoldrick (1988) have documented, families go through development stages within a life cycle. A family is at a different stage four months after the couple was married than it is when the couple has been married for 21 years and has two adolescent children. Individuals are also at different developmental levels. For example, some newlyweds may be 17 years old while others may be in their late 30s. Therefore, the assessment process needs to consider the developmental stage or level of both the family and the individual members within the family.

Another issue concerns getting multiple views rather than a single client's perspective. Often members within a family have divergent views on the problems and issues. This leads to a problem in the scoring of family assessments. Olson, Portner, and Lavee (1985) found low correlations between husbands' and wives' perceptions of family adaptability and cohesion. Thus, if the husband's perceptions are highly positive and the wife's very negative, do we add the scores together and take an average? Interpreting the results from the different family members' perspectives is more difficult than interpreting a single client's results. Another problem with gathering multiple perspectives concerns the confidentiality of the results of a family assessment. Sometimes there are problems with family members having access to each other's results. As an example, a child might be reluctant to disclose some information if the parents are going to be able to see the results. Thus, the counselor needs to consider how the assessment information is going to be used and who will have access to the results.

The final problem concerns the difficulties associated with developing adequate norming samples. It is time consuming and arduous to build adequate norms for instruments designed for individuals; however, with instruments for couples and families the norms need to be made up of couples and families. Therefore, an instrument developer must assess entire families rather than single individuals. Arranging to gather assessment information from each member of the family is complex and problematic. The instrument developer should also consider the ethnic makeup of the norming group. As Morris (1990) pointed out, many of the participants in family assessment norming groups are primarily Anglo-Americans. This overrepresentation of Anglo-Americans is problematic because not all ethnic groups share these same perspectives of family. The values of the culture have a notable influence on what is considered functional and dysfunctional in families. Therefore, it may not be appropriate to evaluate a family who recently immigrated to the United States from Iraq with an instrument that has a norming group from one midwestern state that is 90% Caucasian. Although problems with norming groups can be overcome, developing an instrument with a large and representative sample is difficult.

Even though there are numerous difficulties associated with the development of marriage and family assessment tools, a number of assessment devices have evolved that are departures from traditional paper-and-pencil instruments. Many of these assessment techniques involve completing a task with the family or observing the family in an activity. The most widely known of these assessment tools is the genogram (Coupland, Serovic, & Glenn, 1995), which will be discussed for those unfamiliar with this technique. These techniques are in many ways analogous to projective techniques, where there is a high degree of subjectivity in interpreting the results. The second area of assessment in marriage and family counseling involves instruments designed for use in individual counseling. Many counselors use instruments designed for individuals and administer these instruments to members of the family. A majority of these individually oriented instruments measure personality, although there are examples in the literature of counselors using the Block Design subscale of the WAIS-R to examine differences in couples' task approach skills. The third area of assessment encompasses instruments designed specifically for assessment of couples and families. These instruments strive to assess the dynamics that occur among family members. The next three sections of this chapter will address the multiple methods of assessing couples and families within context of tasks and observation techniques, instruments designed for individual counseling, and instruments specifically for couples and family assessment.

Tasks and Observational Activities

In assessment with couples and families, therapists are typically interested in the interactional qualities among the members of the couple or family. There are some limitations in paper-and-pencil instruments that typically ask clients to report on their behavior toward other members of the family. You might consider individuals in your family and how they might complete an instrument concerning family dynamics as compared to what a skilled observer may see when examining family interactions. With a paper-and-pencil instrument, it is nearly impossible to measure changes in tone, facial expressions, and nonverbal messages that often accompany verbal communications in families. On the other hand, there are problems with observational approaches because counselors can misinterpret nonverbal expressions and not accurately assess the family dynamics. To illustrate this point, let's examine the research related to differences in the amount of eye contact between distressed and nondistressed couples. Some clinicians might hypothesize that nondistressed couples are more likely to look into each other eyes, but Haynes, Follingstad, and Sullivan (1979) found that distressed couples had a higher rate of eye contact than nondistressed couples. Problems with observation are magnified as more clients are added to the process. A counselor cannot focus just on one client in a couple or family. With this additional level of complexity, the reliability of the observations decreases. Furthermore, both counselors' biases and past experiences influence the inferences they draw from the family's behaviors. These inferences may be sound or they may be distorted depending on the counselor's ability to be objective.

Some researchers in the area of marriage and family assessment have attempted to address the limitations in observation by developing coding systems. One coding system that is used by some is the *Marital Interaction Coding System—III;* it takes around two to three months of weekly instruction to learn how to use its 32 codes (Fredman & Sherman, 1987). Anothing coding system is the *Marital and Family Interaction Coding System,* which was developed by Olson and Ryder (1978) and is used in the Inventories of Premarital, Marital, Parent-Child, and Parent-Adolescent Conflict (Olson, 1983). These instruments all have the same format, in which the two individuals read the vignettes and then respond to questions about each vignette individually. The dyad then discusses the vignette, and the discussion is videotaped and coded using the Marital and Family Interaction Coding System. According to Olson, once the counselor is proficient with the coding, the exercise only takes about 30 minutes of her or his time.

Individuals trained in coding systems tend to be more reliable observers and are less likely to be biased in their interpretation of the behavior. Counselors who have the opportunity to receive training should certainly participate in that training. Many counselors, however, are in settings where training may not be easily obtained. These practitioners need to be cautious when adapting these observational techniques in their work with clients. An example of an observational technique is the *Family Task Interview* (Kinston, Loader,

& Sullivan, 1985). In this assessment, the family is given seven tasks; the therapist observes the family completing the tasks and evaluates them using a scale designed to measure family health. Examples of tasks are planning something together that must take at least an hour, building a tower out of blocks, and discussing the likes and dislikes of each member of the family. Counselors could adapt this activity by identifying relevant tasks for the family to complete in counseling, and while the family is completing these tasks the counselor could then concentrate on observing the interactions. The reliability of the observing could be improved if the counselor used a predetermined system for recording the observations. Another technique that can be adapted is the *Kvebaek's Family Sculpting Technique* (Cromwell, Fournier, & Kvebaek, 1980). The Kvebaek is one of the more structured sculpting techniques. It uses a board similar to a chess board, except there are 100 squares. The family members are instructed first individually and then as a family to place figurines on the board depicting the relationships among the family. The family first represents the relationships as they currently exist and then sculpts the family again from an ideal perspective. The sculptures are assessed by measuring the distances between the various placements of the figurines. Marriage and family therapists use sculpting techniques with a variety of objects, including having the family members arrange themselves in the room to depict the relationships. It is important to remember that sculpting techniques tend not to be very reliable. Relationships within a family are fluid, and these techniques only reflect the clients' current perspectives. Therefore, counselors need to be cautious in interpreting this information and not consider it as a stable representation of the family.

Genograms

Genograms are an assessment technique often incorporated into counseling with couples and families (Watts-Jones, 1997). Genograms are tasks counselors do with clients in which they draw a family tree that records information about family members and their relationships over at least three generations (McGoldrick & Gerson, 1985). Genograms are most closely associated with Bowen's family system theory (Bowen, 1978), but counselors with other theoretical orientations use them as well. Bowen contended that there are multigenerational transmissions of family patterns. The genograms can help identify which family patterns are being repeated by the family completing the genogram. With genograms, the clinician examines the previous generations and looks for patterns of functioning, relationships, and structure.

According to McGoldrick and Gerson (1985), creating a genogram involves three stages: (1) mapping the family structure, (2) recording family information, and (3) delineating family relationships. The first step involves the mapping of the family structure, which serves as the skeletal structure of the genogram. Typically the counselor asks questions about family structure and maps the genogram for the past three generations. Each family member is represented by either a circle if female or a square if male. Figure 11.1 provides examples of many of the symbols used in a genogram and Figure 11.2 is an example of a genogram. Married individuals are connected by lines, with separations being indicated by one slashed line and divorce by two slashed lines. All pregnancies, stillbirths, miscarriages, and abortions are mapped. If an individual has died then an X is drawn through either the circle or the square. In Figure 11.2, the genogram represents that the family of interest is made up of a father (Terance) and mother (Nan) who have two children (Samuel and Michael). Nan was married before and was divorced in 1979. The past generations are only of Nan's family and the genogram reflects that Nan's parents (Theodore and Marian) had four children (Nan, Katherine, Danielle, and Ann Elizabeth). There appears to be a close relationship between Nan's mother and her brother Daniel. Continuing the process and interpreting the symbols, one can see back three generations.

Once the skeleton of the genogram is assembled, the next step is to record family information. The recording of family information includes demographic information, functioning information, and critical family events (McGoldrick & Gerson, 1985). Demographic information includes marking the year of an individual's birth (e.g., b. 1953) and the year of death (e.g., d. 1999). Dates of marriages and divorces are also recorded on the genogram. Information on relatives' levels of functioning addresses the medical, emotional, and behavioral realms. This information is recorded next to the individual's symbol. Critical family events, such as losses, successes, or transitions, are also recorded. Although these critical events may have already been mapped, such as the death of a child, the events that the family deems critical are often noted again in the margins of the genogram.

FIGURE 11.1

Symbols used in a genogram

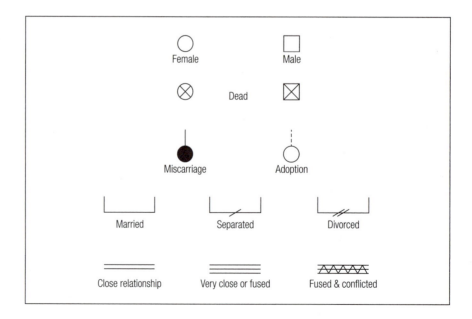

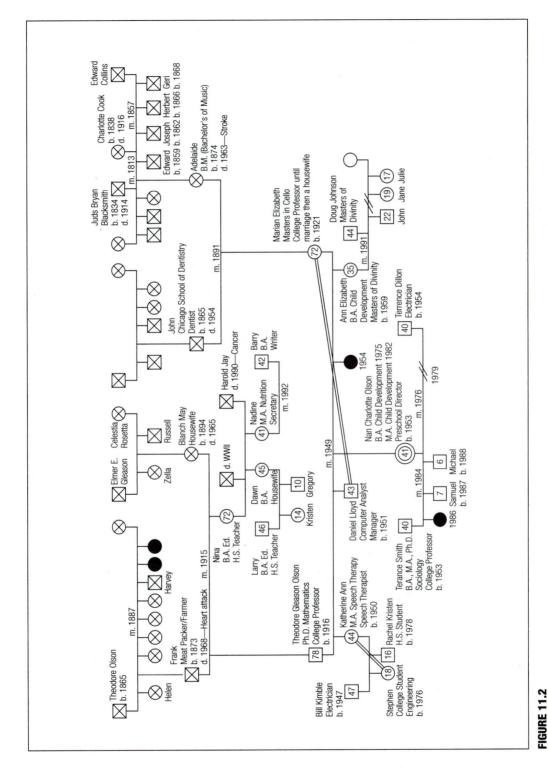

FIGURE 11.2
Example of a genogram

Watts-Jones (1997) advised clinicians to broaden the scope of the genogram when working with African American clients. She suggested that the practitioner not restrict the genogram to biological relatives but rather include "functional kinship." Functional kinship refers to nonbiologically related individuals who play a significant role in the individual's life. She argued that the African proverb "It takes a village to raise a child" has relevance to the administration of genograms with African American clients. Not restricting the genogram to biological relatives may provide pertinent information to clinicians in working with clients from other cultures. There are a number of cultures where large extended families are the norm, and restricting genograms to only biological relatives may skew the information gathered. Readers who are interested in how to draw this sort of genogram are directed to Watts-Jones's article.

The interpretation of the genogram involves the constructing of hypotheses that are later examined with the family. The counselor examines the relational structure and variables, such as whether the composition of the household is a nuclear family, involvement of extended family, the order of the siblings, and unusual family configurations. The family life cycle and stage should also be considered in interpreting a genogram. Furthermore, the theoretical base of genograms calls for the analysis of repetitive patterns across generations. Genograms are based on the premise that family patterns can be transmitted from one generation to the next and that by recognizing these patterns, the counselor can assist the family in avoiding ineffectual patterns. The genogram can also be used to analyze systemic connections among critical events that at first may not appear interrelated. In addition, the genogram may also provide insight into the relational patterns of the family. Relational patterns may appear through the recording of closed, fused, distant, and cut-off relationships (see Figures 11.1 and 11.2). Family therapists often focus on triangular relationships or triangles (see McGoldrick & Gerson, 1985 for an explanation). In a general sense, the genogram is designed to provide information on the family structure, roles, level of functioning, and resources. Genograms, however, are tasks that a counselor does with the family and the counselor observes the family as the information is recorded. Both the observation and the recorded information are used in the interpretation of the genogram.

There are some psychometric limitations that need to be considered if a practitioner is using a genogram. There have been very few studies on the reliability of the genogram (Coupland et al., 1995). Rohrbaugh, Rogers, and McGoldrick (1992) found poor interjudge reliability among practitioners in a medical setting. Coupland et al. (1995) found that doctoral students varied greatly in their accuracy in recording family information on genograms. This finding is even more disturbing because these advanced students had been trained in how to construct genograms. It also should be stressed that there is very little validation evidence for genograms. The lack of validation evidence is surprising, given the popularity of genograms. Clinicians should be extremely cautious in the conclusions they reach based on genogram information. Like other observational techniques, genograms are particularly susceptible to counselor bias. Counselors need to view their interpretations of genograms as only hypotheses that need to be confirmed or invalidated by gathering additional information about the family.

Structural Mapping

Structural mapping is another commonly used mapping technique, but it is based on another family systems' paradigm. Structural mapping is based primarily on the works of Minuchin (1974) and his model of Structural Family Therapy. The term structure in this model refers to the relatively enduring interactional patterns that serve to influence the comparatively constant relationships within a family. The family structure, thus, impacts the ways in which the family members interact. The purpose of structural mapping is to assist the clinician in identifying the family structures and transactional patterns.

The counselor performs structural mapping and, unlike the genogram, the family is not directly involved in the activity. The clinician meets with the family and during the discussion begins to "map" the family structure. As the sessions go on and more assessment information is gathered, the counselor then adds to or revises the map based on the additional information. The structural family therapist begins with mapping the *subsystems* of the family. Some practitioners will use circles for females and squares for males, while others will just use names. The second step is to map the *boundaries* between the subsystems. The symbols used to denote the boundaries are included in Figure 11.3. Boundaries concern the amount of information that is passed between subsystems within the family, and the continuum varies from rigid to diffuse. Rigid boundaries exist when very little information is shared, while diffuse boundaries exist when there are no limits. The third step in the structural mapping processes is to map the *transactions*. In examining transactions, the clinician examines the alliances, coalitions, and degree of involvement. An alliance reflects which two people are joined together for a shared purpose or interest. The mapping of the alliances also reflects the degree of involvement (i.e., clear and friendly, enmeshed or overinvolved, weak or unknown, and conflicted). A coalition forms when two people join together against a third person.

Figure 11.4 is an example of a structural map for a family, where one daughter is feeling very isolated from the family. The other daughter and the mother report being very close, but they are quite upset with the father. In this family, the map would reflect that there are two subsystems. One subsystem is made up of the mother, father, and one of the daughters, while the other subsystem is the second daughter. The boundary between these two subsystems is quite rigid and little information is passed to the second daughter, nor is information received from her. The transactions are characterized by an enmeshed alliance between the mother and one daughter. The other daughter has weak alliances with the other members of the family. The mother and one

FIGURE 11.3
*Structural map-
ping symbols*

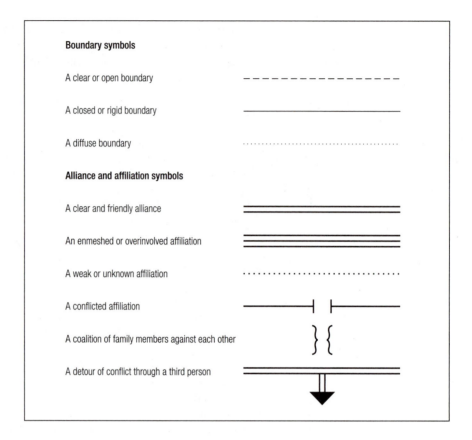

daughter are joined against the father, which is symbolized by the coalition
symbol.

Other Mapping Techniques

L'Abate (1994) suggested that the evaluation of a family involve a battery of
techniques, which might include a genogram and other mapping techniques.
One of the mapping techniques described by L'Abate is the *ecomap*. The
ecomap gathers information about the larger context of the family and the

FIGURE 11.4
*Example of a
structural map*

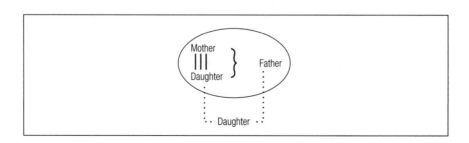

home. The information drawn is a collaborative process involving the counselor and all members of the family. The process is started by positioning the home in the center of a piece of paper, and then having each member of the family draw how far and where other resources are that are necessary for his or her "survival." The family members typically map schools, grocery stores, shopping, church, and recreational activities. The counselor can ask questions as the family creates the ecomap. The process the family uses to complete the ecomap may provide some indications of the dynamics in the family (e.g., Does one member dominate? Does one member not participate?). The ecomap needs to be interpreted very cautiously because there is little psychometric information. This technique, however, can provide insight into how the family spends their time and their priorities. The ecomap also helps in identifying relational patterns and areas of social support.

Another mapping technique suggested by L'Abate (1994) is the *house floor plan*. Like the ecomap, the family rather than the counselor draws this map. The process is begun by asking who wants to draw a plan of their house. The process requires the family to draw the floor plan of their home, indicating where each member sleeps and spends time. With this technique, the counselor needs to be skilled in facilitating the involvement of every member of the family. Different colored pencils can be used to add information on each family member. As the family draws the floor plan, the clinician asks questions about who does what, who spends time together, what activities are typically performed where, and other questions relevant to the family. This technique can provide some indication of isolation or conflict among family members.

In conclusion, observation activities should not be used as the sole means of family assessment because of the problems with reliability and the limited validation information. When using a more subjective assessment tool, such as observation, the counselor will need to balance the process with other more objective techniques. As is often repeated in this book, multiple forms of assessment are preferred because using multiple pieces of information provides a more thorough picture of the client or, in the case of family assessment, the clients.

Use of Instruments Designed for Individuals

A number of instruments initially constructed for use in individual counseling have been adapted for use in couples and family assessment. The prevalence of using an assessment instrument for individuals in marriage and family therapy is documented in Boughner, Hayes, Bubenzer, and West's (1994) findings. They found that the most frequently used assessment instruments in marriage and family therapy were either the Myers–Briggs Type Indicator, the Minnesota Multiphasic Personality Inventory-2, or the Taylor–Johnson Temperament Analysis. Other individually oriented instruments that marriage and family therapists reported using were the 16PF, the Millon Multiaxial Inventory, and the Beck Depression Inventory. In using these individually oriented instruments, the counselor working with a family will often use the information to identify how differences in personality or preferences may contribute to the family issues. For example, a counselor may use the Myer–Briggs Type Indicator to discuss how the couple's differences in perceiving information and then processing that information may affect the way the couple communicate with each other.

All of the instruments just listed are discussed in other sections of this book with the exception of the *Taylor–Johnson Temperament Analysis* (T-JTA, Taylor & Morrison, 1996). The Taylor–Johnson Temperament Analysis was originally designed as a measure of an individual client's personality. The authors later developed a feature called "criss-cross" testing, which can be very useful in couples counseling. With the criss-cross technique, each individual takes the instrument for herself or himself and then takes it a second time answering as he or she believes the other person would answer. The profile contains both the individual's self-appraisal and the other person's view of her or him. In marital and premarital counseling, the counselor then can use the criss-cross testing results to look at congruence in the couple's personalities and, also, congruence between how individuals view themselves and how their spouses view them. Boughner et al. (1994) found the Taylor–Johnson Temperament Analysis to be the second most widely used instrument in premarital therapy and the third most popular in marital counseling.

Some clinicians, in the past, have objected to the profile sheets of the T-JTA, because the sheets contained four shaded areas that corresponded to certain percentile scores. These shaded areas were labeled with the clinical designations of Excellent, Acceptable, Improvement Desirable, and Improvement Needed. Due to the complaints about the labels, it is now possible to purchase profile sheets with or without these clinical designations. Another previous problem with the T-TJA was an inadequate norming sample. The Taylor–Johnson Temperament Analysis was recently renormed and the new sample is 2,600 individuals who are 13 and older. The sample is also broken down into four age groups: adolescents, young adults, general adults, and senior adults.

Fredman and Sherman (1987) asserted that some of these well-known individually oriented instruments can provide therapists with insights into the family. These instruments, however, do not provide insight into level of satisfaction, qualities of the relationship, areas of conflict, or measures of parenting skill. During the last fifty years, researchers have studied marriages and families (Touliatos et al., 1990). This rich body of knowledge, however, is not reflected in instruments designed for individuals. Practitioners also want instruments designed for assessing couples and families from a theoretical perspective. Many clinicians working with couples and families use a systemic approach (Sporakowski, 1995). Individually oriented instruments may describe the individuals within the system, but they do not describe the family system. Therefore, there has been significant interest in instruments designed specifically for assessing systemic family factors (Sporakowski, 1995).

Formalized Assessment Instruments
Specific to Marriage and Family

Assessment in Premarital Counseling

This section focuses on assessment instruments designed specifically for use with couples and families. The first area addressed is measures designed expressly for premarital counseling, followed by a couple's assessment, and, finally, family techniques and instruments. When considering instruments specifically for premarital counseling, Boughner et al. (1994) found that practitioners reported using the *PREmarital Personal and Relationship Evaluation* (PREPARE, Olson, Fournier, & Druckman, 1996). PREPARE is intended to assist those who are planning to marry in examining their relationships realistically. The instrument is designed, with the assistance of a trained counselor, to have the couple: (1) take stock of strengths and growth areas in their relationship, (2) evaluate their level of idealism, (3) explore important topics that they might otherwise avoid, and (4) begin to develop communication and conflict resolution skills.

There is another version, PREPARE-MC, which is for couples planning to marry who already have children. Other instruments closely associated to PREPARE are ENriching Relationship Issues, Communication and Happiness (ENRICH) for couples already married, and Mature Age Transitional Evaluation (MATE) for married couples over 50.

PREPARE is a 125-item inventory in which individual scores are computed as well as a combined couple's score. Although it was not designed to predict successful marriages, Fower (1983) found that PREPARE was 86% accurate in predicting those who would divorce and 78% accurate in predicting those who would report being happily married. Druckman, Fournier, Robinson, and Olson (1980) found that PREPARE was rated as being more useful if the results were combined with counseling rather than just receiving feedback. PREPARE and related instruments cannot be purchased by counselors until they have attended training provided by the publishers of the instruments.

Couples or Marital Assessment

The use of specific formal instruments in the area of marriage and family counseling is a comparatively recent addition to the field of assessment. One of the first widely used assessment instruments for couples was the Marital Adjustment Test (Locke & Wallace, 1959). This instrument was often referred to as the Locke–Wallace and has been used for validating many of the later marital scales. As an indicator of where the field was at this point, the *Marital Adjustment Test* contained only 15 items and the norming group was 118 husbands and 118 wives who were *not* necessarily married to each other.

Dyadic Adjustment Scale. The *Dyadic Adjustment Scale* (DAS, Spanier, 1976) is an instrument that is often used in marital counseling. It is intended to measure the adjustment quality of married couples or similar dyads. This 32-item instrument produces a total adjustment score and scores on four subscales: dyadic consensus, dyadic satisfaction, dyadic cohesion, and affectional expression. The overall reliability of this instrument is quite high (.96), but the norming group consists only of 218 white married individuals from Pennsylvania.

Marital Satisfaction Inventory. Recently, an instrument often used in couples counseling was revised, the *Marital Satisfaction Inventory—Revised* (MSI-R, Synder, 1997). The MSI-R is designed to assist couples in communicating about a broad range of relationship issues. In order to be appropriate for both traditional and nontraditional couples, some of the items were changed to use terms such as partner and relationship rather than spouse and marriage. The items are scored on 11 scales (see Figure 11.5). The first scale in Figure 11.5 is the Conventionalization (CNV), which is the validity scale. CNV reflects the tendency of the individual to distort the appraisal of the marriage in a socially desirable manner. The Global Distress Scale (GDS) is an overall measure of dissatisfaction. High scores on the MSI-R indicate dissatisfaction. The other ten scales measure specific sources of conflict: Affective Communication (AFC), Problem-Solving Communication (PSC), Time Together (TTO), Disagreement About Finances (FIN), Sexual Dissatisfaction (SEX), Role Orientation (ROR), Family History of Distress (FAM), Dissatisfaction with Children (DSC), and Conflict Over Childrearing (CCR). The items for the last two scales are only answered if the couple has children. The instrument was restandardized on 2,040 people (1,020 intact couples). The ages of the couples were from the late teens through the early 90s, and attempts were made to stratify the sample to approximate the U.S. population in regard to geographic region, education, and ethnicity. The reliability coefficients for the scales range between .80 and .97. The manual contains validity information, which is meager compared to personality instruments but substantial when compared to other marital assessments. Reviews of the previous edition of the MSI were positive (Burnett, 1987) and it appears that the revision has addressed some of the criticism concerning the small and underrepresented norming group.

Couple's Pre-Counseling Inventory. Counselors who want to focus on marital counseling, may want to explore Stuart and Jacobsen's (1987) *Couple's Pre-Counseling Inventory, Revised Edition.* This is a 16-page form that each member of the couple completes before counseling. In many of the sections in this detailed form, participants are asked to provide information about themselves and how they would expect their partners to answer. This inventory goes beyond evaluation of satisfaction and adjustment into desired caring behaviors, violence, substance abuse, evaluation of sexual relationship, decision-making structure, and division of responsibilities. Computer scoring is available and results are provided in 13 areas (e.g., Goals of Counseling, Communication Assessment, Conflict Management, Sexual Interaction, and Child Management).

FIGURE 11.5

Marital Satisfaction Inventory Profile Form

© 1997, 1998 by Western Psychological Services. Sample reprinted by permission of the publisher. Not to be reprinted in whole or in part for any additional purpose without the expressed, written permission of the publisher. All rights reserved.

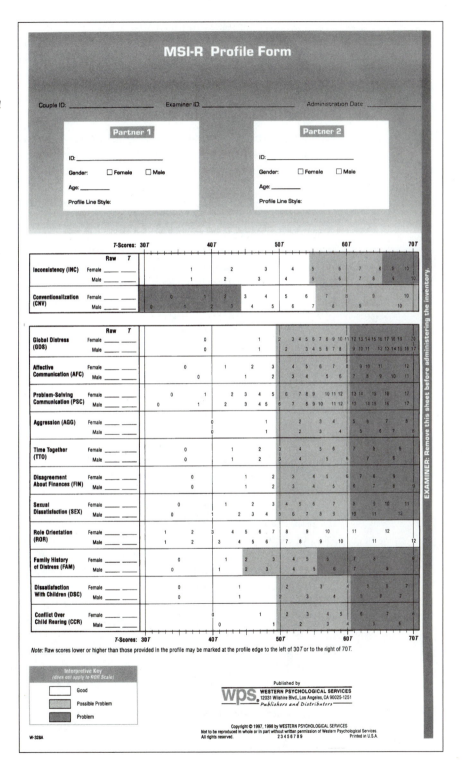

The normative sample with this instrument was 60 couples, including nonmarried heterosexual couples and homosexual couples. Because the Couple's Pre-Counseling Inventory is 16 pages long, it takes time for clients to complete it. The results, however, are quite detailed and can be useful to clinicians.

Family Assessment Instruments

Family Adaptability and Cohesion Evaluation Scale—III. A very widely used measure of family dynamics is Olson, Portner, and Lavee's (1986) *Family Adaptability and Cohesion Evaluation Scale* (FACES-III). FACES-III is a 20-item instrument that is based on the Circumplex Model of family functioning. In the model, there are three central dimensions of family behavior: cohesion, adaptability, and communication. FACES-III measures the dimensions of cohesion and adaptability. There are, however, some discrepancies between the model and the FACES-III instrument. The model describes a curvilinear relationship between the dimensions of cohesion and adaptability in family functioning. In this curvilinear relationship, too little or too much of either cohesion or adaptability results in difficulties for the family. For example, with cohesion, too little cohesion often results in feelings of alienation, while too much cohesion can result in feeling of enmeshment. FACES-III, however, measures both cohesion and adaptability in a linear (low to high) manner rather than in a curvilinear manner. FACES-IV is expected to be published in the near future.

Family Assessment Measure. In the comprehensive assessment battery of problem adolescents, the National Institute on Drug Abuse (NIDA) is using the *Family Assessment Measure* (FAM-III) by Skinner, Steinhauer, and Santa-Barbara (1995). The FAM-III consists of three interrelated instruments. The first is the General Scale (50 items) that focuses on the general functioning of the family. The second instrument, the Dyadic Relationship Scale (42 items), measures the quality of the relationship between two specific family members (e.g., mother and father). The third scale is the Self-Rating Scale (42 items), where the individual evaluates his or her own level of functioning in the family unit. Each of these three scales provides information on seven dimensions: Task Accomplishment, Role Performance, Communication, Affective Expression, Involvement, Control, and Values and Norms. The FAM-III is available in both paper-and-pencil and computer formats. The reported Cronbach's alpha for each of these scales is comparatively high for both adults and children, with the range for adults being between .89 and .95 and that for children being from .86 to .94. The validity information is relatively limited but is growing rapidly. There is also a computer version, in which clients can take either the FAM-III or the Brief FAM at the computer. The software will then score and write an interpretative report.

Family Environment Scale. The *Family Environment Scale* (FES, Moos & Moos, 1994) has evolved out of Rudolf Moos's work on assessing social climates. Assessment of social climates is closely related to environmental assessment, which examines how environmental factors influence the behavior of the individual. Moos (1973) contended that three dimensions provide insight into a social climate or environment: (1) a relationship dimension, (2) a personal development or personal growth dimension, and (3) a system maintenance and system change dimension. According to Moos, these dimensions provide insight into family environments as well as other social climates or environments. Table 11.1 describes the subscales related to each of the three dimensions in the Family Environment Scale.

There are three forms of the FES: (1) the Real Form (Form R) measures individuals' perception of their current family; (2) the Ideal Form (Form I) measures preferences for an ideal family environment; and (3) the Expectation Form (Form E) measures expectations about a family environment (e.g., prospective foster parents' expectations). Each form of the FES contains 90 items. These three forms can be used either alone or in combination in a variety of counseling interventions. Often, each family member's results are compared to examine differences in perceptions. For example, the counselor might want to explore discrepancies among the family members' perceptions of the environment. I once worked with a family where the mother and the children rated the conflict high while the father rated the conflict below average. Analysis of this discrepancy led to a useful discussion of the father's attempt to dismiss any opinion that varied from his stance on an issue. Another example of using the FES to examine differences in family perceptions is to examine the

TABLE 11.1

Dimensions and subscales of the Family Environment Scale

Relationship Dimension

Cohesion—the amount of commitment, help, and support family members provide for each other.

Expressive—the degree to which members of the family are encouraged to express feelings and act in an open manner.

Conflict—the amount of openly expressed conflict and anger in the family.

Personal Growth Dimension

Independence—the extent to which members are assertive, self-sufficient, and make their own decisions.

Achievement Orientation—the degree to which activities are framed in an achievement-oriented or competitive framework.

Intellectual-Cultural Orientation—the extent to which the family is interested and participates in political, intellectual, and cultural activities.

Active-Recreational Orientation—the level of participation in social and recreational activities.

Moral-Religious Emphasis—the amount of emphasis on values and religious and ethical issues.

System Maintenance Dimension

Organization—the extent to which organization and structure are clear in responsibilities and planning family activities.

Control—the degree to which set rules and procedures run family life.

difference in results between the Real Form and the Ideal Form. Sometimes, a family will have amazing similarities in their results on the Ideal Form, which can be a very effective intervention in unifying the direction of the counseling.

The normative sample is 1,432 normal families and 788 distressed families. The manual does not provide very specific information on the manner in which many of the normal families were selected. The internal consistency coefficients range from .61 to .78 on the nine subscales of the Family Environment Scale. There is also considerable validity information on this instrument, much of which concerns differences between normal and distressed families.

Other instruments. There are hundreds of other family instruments that measure various familial aspects such as family beliefs, extent to which families celebrate, coping behaviors, and family empowerment. Useful resources for identifying instruments were mentioned in Chapter 5, and practitioners might also want to examine Appendix B concerning Internet information that may be helpful. A word of caution, however, is warranted. Many of the instruments in the marriage and family area have very limited psychometric information. Counselors need to carefully evaluate these instruments before using them with a couple or family and understand their limitations. These instruments should be viewed more as a springboard for further discussion rather than as diagnostic tools.

Summary

In recent years, hundreds of instruments have been developed for assessing couples and families. These instruments are not as well established as some of the instruments developed for use with individuals (e.g., the MMPI-2, WISC-III). Developing instruments for use with couples and families is more difficult than developing instruments for individuals. This chapter addressed three areas of marriage and family assessment: tasks and observation techniques, instruments designed for individual counseling, and instruments specific to couples and family assessment.

Tasks and observation techniques can be very helpful because they afford the counselor the opportunity to observe family interactions. There are many different tasks that a counselor can initiate with a family to facilitate the gathering of relevant information. One of the most commonly used techniques is the genogram. Genograms are diagrams counselors construct with their clients in which they draw a family tree that records information about family members and their relationships over at least three generations. Genograms are based on the premise that family patterns can be transmitted from one generation to the next and that by recognizing these patterns the counselor can assist the family in avoiding these destructive patterns.

Clinicians counseling couples and families also use instruments designed for individuals. The instruments most commonly used by marriage and family therapists are the Myers–Briggs Type Indicator, the Minnesota Multiphasic Personality Inventory-2, or the Taylor–Johnson Temperament Analysis. The Taylor–Johnson has developed a system that allows the practitioner to examine congruence in the couple's personality and, also, congruence between how each client views himself or herself and how this person is viewed by the spouse.

Finally, there are instruments designed specifically for use with either couples or families. The most frequently used premarital instrument is PREPARE. In addition, there are a number of instruments that address marital satisfaction or issues after the couple is married. These instruments are typically used to identify issues and areas where the couple's perceptions may differ. Assessment of families is probably one of the most difficult areas in counseling due to the complexities of family interactions. Some of the family assessment instruments are based on theory, and the clinician must have an understanding of the theoretical implications when using the instruments. Assessment in the area of marriage and family counseling does not have the extensive history of intelligence and personality assessments. Therefore, the instruments in this area are not as well researched, nor has the field had time to address many of the limitations in current assessment devices.

Issues and Applications

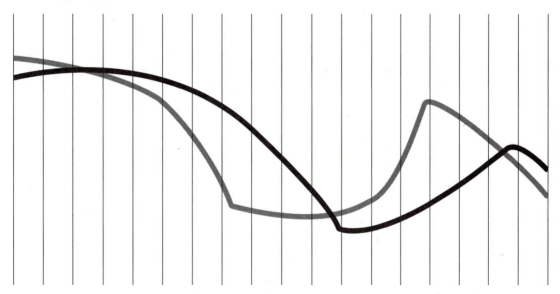

CHAPTER 12

Using Assessment in Counseling

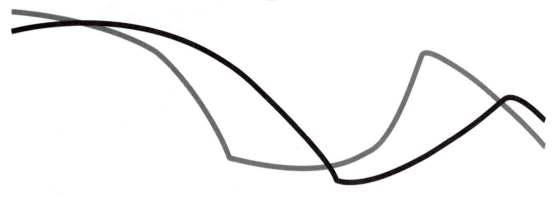

The subject matter of the last six chapters has been specific assessment areas with a description of the most commonly used instruments. The focus now shifts, with the theme of the remaining chapters centering on issues related to the uses of assessment tools in counseling. This chapter concerns using assessment information and how appraisal information can be integrated into counseling. The intent is to explore methods in which assessment practices can benefit the counseling process. Assessment appears to serve three major purposes in counseling. First, assessment is often used to inform the clinician and produce data that can be used in treatment planning. Counselors need information about their clients in order to make appropriate clinical decisions. Second, counselors may also use assessment instruments or techniques during the treatment phase of counseling. This second area concerns using assessment as a therapeutic intervention rather than a technique. As an example, clients often enter counseling for assistance in making a major decision (e.g., what career to pursue, whether to get a divorce, whether to quit drinking). Assessment results could be an integral part of the information-gathering phase necessary for effective decision making. The third area where assessment results play a crucial role in counseling is in evaluating the services provided to clients. There are increasing demands for counselors to provide accountability information, and many practitioners use assessment instruments to produce those data and information.

Treatment Planning

Counseling is not a process in which every client gets the exact same service. In counseling, the practitioner varies the therapeutic interventions depending on the needs of the individual client. According to Goodyear and Lichtenberg (1999), while working with clients, any mental health professional will make *some* assessment of a client's level and type of functioning. Therefore, counselors need to have sound information about the client or clients in order to select treatment approaches that have the best probability of succeeding. Beutler and Harwood (1995) argued that it was professionally irresponsible to counsel a client without considering client characteristics. Understanding clients' pretreatment characteristics does not just apply to individual counseling, as these factors also apply to group counseling and classroom guidance interventions. It is more likely that a school counselor will present a classroom guidance activity more effectively if she or he can gear the presentation to the students. Clinicians may often be able to use existing information (e.g., student achievement scores), or they may need to use additional assessment strategies to gather the necessary client information.

In discussing the uses of assessment results for treatment planning, a discussion of the role of diagnosis is warranted. Although in the past there was some disagreement about whether diagnosis was a part of the counseling process, there are some indications that many counselors are making diagnostic decisions (Hohenshil, 1996). The connection between appraisal and diagnosis is demonstrated in the Council for the Accreditation of Counseling and Related Educational Programs' (CACREP) Proposed Standards for 2001. In this document, the section addressing curriculum requirements related to appraisal (Section II) states that a counseling program must provide "an understanding of general principles and methods of case conceptualization, assessment, and/or diagnoses of mental and emotional status" (CACREP, 1997, p. 10). Diagnostic topics from the American Psychiatric Association's (1994) *Diagnostic and Statistical Manual of Mental Disorders*—Fourth Edition (DSM-IV) and other topics related to diagnosis will be covered in the next chapter. I would, however, argue that treatment planning involves more than just determining a diagnosis.

In planning treatment, counselors should use assessment techniques that answer questions related to: What are the issues and problems? To what degree are the problems affecting the client? Is there a disorder and is a diagnosis appropriate? What factors are contributing to the client's issues? What is the prognosis? Many of the techniques and instruments discussed in the previous section of this book could be used to answer some of these questions. Hummel (1998) presented compelling evidence of the usefulness of using tests in clinical decision making. He further documents that tests can lead to better understandings of clients, which has a direct influence on the effectiveness of the treatment.

Decisions related to the selection of specific strategies and techniques can be enhanced by the use of sound assessment information. For example, a client who scores very high on a measure of introversion would probably have a better outcome with individual rather than group counseling. Likewise, a high school student with low reading scores on an achievement test is probably not a good candidate for bibliotherapy. A client with a high score on the Realistic theme from an interest inventory may benefit from job shadowing, while a client high on the Investigative theme may benefit more from reading occupational information. Matching the treatment to the client is a common practice. Beutler and Clarkin (1990) supported matching and cited research indicating that client-counselor match was one of the strongest predictors of outcome. However, before appropriate matching can occur, the counselor must gather reliable client information.

Research has continually indicated that statistical or actuarial methods are much better predictors than clinician judgment (Ben-Porath, 1997; Dawes, Faust, & Meehl, 1989; Meehl, 1954). Some have responded to these findings that regression methods are better than clinical judgment by suggesting that clinical judgment needs to be more objective (Tracey & Rounds, 1999). The use of assessment instruments may contribute to more objectivity in clinical decision making. Gathering quality information and evaluating it with a scientific approach may assist clinicians in making better clinical judgments.

Using Psychological Reports

For some clients, the complexity of the case may result in the counselor deciding to refer the individual for a psychological evaluation. There are some settings in which counselors will perform these activities; in other settings, a psychologist conducts the evaluation. After completing the tests or assessments, the clinician will write a **psychological report**. A psychological report completed by a skillful clinician can provide an abundance of clinical information. For some clients, a psychological report may already exist that could be used in treatment planning. A detailed discussion on the writing of psychological reports is beyond the scope of this book. Counselors who need these types of skills are directed to Ownby (1997) and Sattler (1993). As many counselors will be the consumers of psychological reports, the following discussion is geared toward the evaluation of those reports.

Psychological reports are for disseminating assessment information to other *professionals*. The purpose of the report is to provide assessment information that can be helpful in making clinical decisions and in selecting treatment and educational services. Many psychological reports are not given to clients because the information is technical in nature and often focuses on diagnostic and clinical decisions. A well-written report will not merely report test results, but will also incorporate a wide array of relevant information. Thus, in evaluating psychological reports, counselors should expect a comprehensive overview of the client and an interpretation of the assessment results in a contextual manner. A psychological report should be carefully crafted, with attention to detail. The caliber of the report can be initially evaluated by examining typographical errors, use of vague jargon, careless mistakes, and lack of detail.

Common areas in a psychological report. In evaluating a psychological report, a counselor can expect it to contain certain information. A general outline for a psychological report is shown in Table 12.1. There are no established guidelines for writing a report, so not all reports will follow this outline. A quality report, however, will include all of these major areas. As Table 12.1 indicates, many reports will have a heading, such as PSYCHOLOGICAL REPORT: FOR PROFESSIONAL USE ONLY. This heading clearly identifies the document and stresses that the document is only for professional use.

Identifying Information   This section provides some demographic information on the client. The section is often done in outline format and includes the following information:

> Client's name
> Date of examination
> Date of birth
> Chronological age
> Date of report
> Grade (if applicable)
> Examiner's name
> Tests administered

Other information that may be included is the individual's sex, teacher's name, or parents' names. All of this is important information and is necessary introductory information to the reader of the report.

TABLE 12.1
Outline for psychological report

Psychological Report: For Professional Use Only
1. Identifying information
2. Reasoning for referral
3. Background information
4. Behavioral observation
5. Assessment results and interpretation
6. Recommendations
7. Summary
8. Signature

Reason for Referral   The second section of a psychological report typically addresses the reason for the referral for testing. Some practitioners will use the label of Reason for Counseling in order to broaden the focus. It should be noted that the term *psychological report* is typically associated with the reporting of assessment information. The information customarily included in this section is the name and position of the referral source (e.g., teacher); the reason for the referral; and a brief summary of symptoms, behaviors, or circumstances that led to the referral. The reason for the referral will often guide the practitioner in the selection of instruments or procedures. In evaluating a report, the practitioner should find a direct connection between the instruments or procedures used and the reasons for the referral.

Background Information   This section is critical for many readers because it provides a context in which to interpret the assessment results. The background information portion of the report should provide the reader with an overview of relevant information regarding the client. This section should provide sufficient information about the client's past in order for the reader to understand the current issues and concerns. The information in this section may come from interviews with the client, interviews with other family members (e.g., parents if client is a minor), or past educational, counseling, or health records. The focus of the background will vary depending on the reasons for the assessment, but it should include significant past events related to the assessment purpose. Often educational history is relevant, as well as the current family situation. Notable physical and mental health events in the client's life should be discussed. If other assessments have been performed there should be a summary of those assessment results and progress made since the prior evaluations. For adults, this section should include information on the current employment situation and any other past or present work-related information germane to the assessment.

Behavioral Observations   Practitioners unfamiliar with standard protocol may not include this important section of a psychological report. A well-written psychological report will describe what is observed during the assessment process. This information is critical to interpreting the results, for it addresses issues such as motivation, anxiety, concentration, and self-efficacy. The behavioral observations are reports of the client's behaviors while taking the instruments. The behavioral observation section will usually include a brief description of physical appearance, client comments and reactions to the process, responses to different assessment activities, unusual mannerisms or behaviors, variations in activities, and changes in voice tone and facial expressions. If inferences are made about the client's behavior, then they should be accompanied by descriptions of behaviors supporting the conclusions. For example, a report might include statements like "The client appeared somewhat tense and chewed her fingernails. She also reported that she was feeling anxious about the testing."

Assessment Results and Interpretations   This is the heart of the psychological report and will be the longest section. Topics included in this section are the assessment findings, the meaning of the results, and the clinical and diagnostic impressions. In the discussion of the assessment findings, the precise scores on every scale and subscale may not need to be presented. The focus should be on the pertinent findings and *interpreting* rather than just reporting these findings. The report should include sufficient detail so that a reader unfamiliar with the specifics of the instrument can understand the meaning of the results. Names of the instruments and descriptions of the scores and scales will help the reader understand the results. The interpretation of the results will often include an exploration of the client's strengths and limitations. Furthermore, there should be a discussion of both consistent and inconsistent scores and results. The reader will also expect to find an explanation or possible hypotheses about any notable results. The psychometric qualities of the instrument are not directly reported in the report, but the interpretation needs to incorporate any psychometric limitations. For example, limited validation evidence should be stressed. When a diagnosis is presented in a report, then there should be sufficient evidence to support that diagnosis. Consistent findings from different sources provide the sort of documentation expected for a diagnosis. The report should be organized in a manner that is easy to follow. Many practitioners organize their reports in a domain-by-domain framework. A summary is not needed at the end of the results and interpretation section because that will be provided later in the report.

Recommendations   The recommendations section extends the material presented in the report into future actions that will be beneficial to the client. The case for the recommendations should have been made in the previous sections of the psychological report. The recommendations should be realistic, with consideration of the client's resources and situation. There also needs to be sufficient detail in the recommendations so that they can be easily implemented. Many times this requires the clinician to have information about community resources.

Summary   The summary is a succinct summarization of the entire report, with a focus on the results and interpretation. The summary is usually only one or two paragraphs, but it contains the major aspects of the report. As one of my teachers once said, "Write the summary as if that will be the only thing anyone reads." The summary provides the opportunity to reiterate and emphasize important results. Sometimes the summary and recommendations will be combined into one ending section.

Signature   The report writer's name and professional title or capacity should be typed at the end of the report. The writer then signs her or his name above the typewritten name.

Evaluating the writing style. Besides examining the content of a psychological report, a counselor can evaluate the quality of a psychological report by examining the writing style. First, the writing needs to be specific and concrete as compared to vague and ambiguous. The writer should attempt to convey the *results* to a reader with little background in assessment. A vague statement is "Pat has low self-esteem." It is not clear what is meant by low, nor is it clear what is meant by self-esteem. Although the report should be clearly written, declarative statements about people can rarely be given. For example, a report should not say that "Michael is an extrovert." Michael may only be pretending to be extroverted. A report writer should report, "his answers on the Myers–Briggs Type Indicator *indicated* that Michael's preference is toward the extroverted function, which reflects a preference for . . . ." The focus should be on what the scores reflect or indicate, not on some specific label. A clinician cannot say Mary's IQ is 102 because the next time she takes an intelligence test her IQ may be 104! It would be more appropriate to present the results as "Mary's scores on the [insert test name] reflect that her IQ is around 102." A better strategy would be to use standard error of measurement and say "Mary's performance on the [insert test name] indicates that 68% of the time Mary's IQ could be expected to fall between 99 and 102."

Counselors should also evaluate a psychological report with the **Barnum Effect** in mind. The term *Barnum Effect* is related to the showman P. T. Barnum's statement, "There's a sucker born every minute." The Barnum Effect applies to *all* types of personality reports but is particularly relevant to computer-generated reports. Let's pretend that you have just taken a personality inventory and the following is your report:

> You are a person that some people are drawn to; yet, there are a few people who do not see your strengths. You tend to be warm and friendly at times but need to be by yourself at other times. People tend to see you as someone they can trust. You can be critical of yourself, particularly when you don't function to your full capacity. Presently, you are unsure of all of your skills and abilities. You are energetic when it comes to important matters. It is difficult for you to attain a balance in your life because you have a tendency to be drawn in different directions. You seek a certain amount of change and variation in your activities. While you are generally honest with others, you are most honest with those who know you very well. You can also be honest with yourself, which causes you to doubt some of your decisions.

For many people, the above description would probably fit because it is somewhat vague and general. The Barnum Effect is in effect when a report is written so vaguely that it applies to everyone. A number of research studies have used similar statements and found that many participants thought the description was a good or excellent description of their personality (Synder, Shenkel, & Lowery, 1977; Ulrich, Stachnik, & Stainton, 1963). Merrens and Richards (1970) found that individuals could not discriminate between bogus interpretations and bona fide interpretations. Computer-generated reports are more prone to Barnum Effect interpretation because there is no direct contact with the individual. Most generalized personality descriptions tend to include *double-headed* sentences (e.g., "You tend to be warm and friendly at times but need to be by yourself at other times."); *modal* statements, descriptive of virtually anyone (e.g., "You seek a certain amount of change and variation in your activities."); *vague* statements (e.g., "Presently, you are unsure of all of your skills and abilities."); and *favorable* statements (e.g., "People tend to see you as someone they can trust."). When counselors begin to see a number of these types of statements in a report, they should examine it more carefully and explore to see if a Barnum Effect may be present.

In conclusion, a thorough psychological report written by a well-trained clinician can provide a wealth of information that can be used in treatment planning. Practitioners using a report written by another professional will need to critique the report to determine the quality of the information. Most well-done reports will identify both strengths and limitations of the client. A quality report will not just provide the assessment results, but will also integrate other information to produce a thorough report. It should be stressed that practitioners do not need to have a psychological report to use assessment information in treatment planning.

Other Uses of Assessment Information in Treatment Planning

Counselors can use assessment information for more than the selection of specific strategies and techniques. For example, assessment information can be very helpful in determining how to structure the therapeutic relationship. There are no universal guidelines for developing a therapeutic relationship, and counselors need to adapt their style to the individual client (Sexton & Whiston, 1994). Both formal and informal assessment measures can provide information that can be useful in determining methods for enhancing the therapeutic relationship. Indications are that clinicians who monitor clients' progress with repeated assessments are able to adjust their approach and produce better results than those who do not use repeated measures. Treatment planning is not just done once and then forgotten; counselors need to continue to adjust and change as the counseling progresses. Hence, using assessment data may assist the practitioner in making more effective adjustments.

Sometimes counselors have a narrow view of assessment and believe that the term only applies when they have responsibility for selecting, administering, scoring, and interpreting the results. This narrow view may restrict their effectiveness because they may be eliminating a wealth of assessment information. Oftentimes, there is existing testing or assessment information that a counselor could use in effective treatment planning. For example, school counselors can easily access achievement test results, and many students' files will also contain general ability or group intelligence test results. This information can be used in making counseling decisions, such as whether a student might feel out of place with other students in a group because of his or her lower academic performance. Sometimes practitioners ignore existing assessment information and rely almost exclusively on information gained from the sessions. This seems like an unwise use of time and resources.

In conclusion, information gained from sound assessments can often assist the counselor in making effective treatment decisions. There is evidence that relying only on an interview may not be in the client's best interest. Clinicians can generate more comprehensive client information by supplementing subjective measures with more objective instruments. Using assessment information for treatment planning is by far the most common way that practitioners use assessment results. There are, however, other ways that assessment information can benefit the counseling process.

Achieving Counseling Goals Through the Integration of Assessment

The premise of this chapter is that assessment results can be used in counseling in three ways: (1) for treatment planning, (2) for achieving therapeutic goals, and (3) to evaluate counseling. Campbell (1990) suggested that assessment instruments are an alternate means of achieving certain counseling goals and can be a valuable addition to counseling practices. Assessment interventions can be geared toward providing client information and feedback that is related to the goals of the counseling.

Finn and Tonsager (1992; 1997) suggested a model in which the assessment itself is considered to be a therapeutic intervention. This *therapeutic assessment model* is compared to the traditional *information-gathering model*, in which assessment is viewed as a way to collect information that will guide subsequent treatment. The intent of therapeutic assessment is to promote positive changes in clients through the *use* of assessment instruments. The assessor's primary task is to be sensitive, attentive, and responsive to the client and to foster opportunities for the client to gain information about himself or herself. The process of therapeutic assessment involves establishing a working relationship with the client and then working collaboratively to define individualized assessment goals. The assessment results are then shared and explored with the client. Finn and Tonsager (1997) suggested that in feedback sessions, clinicians begin with the feedback that most closely matches clients' preconceived notions and then move on to more discrepant information.

There has been little attention in the past on the therapeutic effect of assessment, but recent research is encouraging. Two studies (Finn & Tonsager,1992; Newman & Greenway, 1997) found those who received therapeutic assessment with the MMPI-2 reported better outcomes than those who received supportive, nondirective counseling. There are also a number of case studies that support their model (Clair & Prendergast; Dorr, 1981; Waiswol, 1995). Hanson, Claiborn, and Kerr (1997) found some difference between career counseling clients who received an interactive interpretation as compared to a delivered interpretation. The clients who received the interactive interpretation considered their sessions to be deeper and rated the counselor as being more expert, trustworthy, and attractive.

Assessment results do not just have to identify deficits; these results can be used to help individuals identify strengths, assets, and coping strategies. At the onset of counseling in some settings, clients are given an instrument(s) that is used for treatment planning and decision making. That information may never be used after the initial stage of planning, nor is it often shared with the client. This information, however, can often be integrated into the counseling in a therapeutic manner.

Assessment results can also be used in a therapeutic manner in counseling by helping clients make effective decisions. Counselors can use information gained from assessment to help clients weigh the pros and cons of a decision and examine the probabilities of expected outcomes. Although this manner of using assessment information has been common in career counseling, counselors can also use assessment results related to other issues. Drummond (1996) suggested a decision making model that uses test information. His is a three-step decision making model:

Step 1: Preparation (which involves the following):
   1. Specifying the judgments and decisions to be made
   2. Describing the information needed
   3. Locating the information already available in files or records
   4. Deciding what information is needed and when and how this information can be obtained
   5. Selecting data-gathering instruments and tests to be used and reviewing the instruments for validity, reliability, usability, and interpretability

Step 2: Data Collection (which involves the following):
   1. Securing the information needed through test, observation, and other appropriate methods
   2. Recording, analyzing, and interpreting the information

Step 3: Evaluation (which involves the following):
   1. Forming hypotheses
   2. Making decisions or judgments
   3. Reporting decisions and judgments

In Drummond's (1996) decision-making model, he stressed that tests and appraisal instruments are only one source of information. He further argued that if the limitations of the assessment process are recognized, test information can be a valuable tool in decision making. In using assessment tools to assist clients in making decisions, the counselor needs to ensure that the information is disseminated in a nonbiased manner. Counselors often influence clients; therefore, counselors need to monitor their presentation of the assessment results so that their own preferences do not unduly influence the client. For example, if a counselor is not particularly interested in Realistic occupations, then the counselor should be careful in his or her interpretation of an interest inventory.

The view that assessment can be used in a therapeutic manner is sometimes contrary to how professionals often view testing and assessment. Counselors can, however, use assessment results to stimulate self-awareness and exploration. Furthermore, both formal and informal instruments can also be used to assist clients in making decisions.

Using Assessment for Evaluation and Accountability

The complexion of mental health services changed dramatically in the 1990s as a result of changes in our society. One of the major changes was the emergence of managed health care and the corresponding demands for accountability information from clinicians. Some managed health care organizations will not approve counseling services unless the clinician can show that that he or she is effective with clients. Therefore, many practitioners are examining methods that evaluate their own counseling effectiveness. In addition, accountability demands occur in counseling settings other than just mental health; school counselors, rehabilitation counselors, and career counselors also need to provide information to administrators, oversight boards, or governmental agencies indicating that the services they provide are worth the monetary investment.

Whiston (1996) advocated that practitioners can provide accountability information by easily adapting the methodologies and measures developed in counseling outcome research. Outcome research studies the overall effectiveness of counseling and what factors or approaches contribute to positive client change. Researchers have actively scrutinized the research methods for investigating the outcome of counseling for over 60 years. This scrutiny has resulted in a wealth of information that counselors can use in evaluating their own effectiveness.

In developing evaluation or accountability information, clinicians first need to consider what they are attempting to evaluate. Sometimes, a counseling organization will seek one method of developing accountability information on all of the different services they provide. Identifying one method of developing accountability information may be difficult because the services vary (e.g., individual counseling, group counseling, substance abuse services, parenting classes, brief crisis interventions). Thus, practitioners need to consider what services they want to evaluate. As an example, an elementary school counselor may decide to focus first on evaluating a series of classroom guidance activities performed with fifth graders to ease the transition into middle school, as compared to all the different services the counselor provides to the children in that school. Often better accountability information can be gathered by examining different types of counseling services separately because there needs to be a direct connection between the services provided and the outcome measures used.

Table 12.2 lists the most commonly used outcome measures that Sexton (1996) found in the outcome research. The selection of outcome measures is,

TABLE 12.2

Commonly used outcome measures

<u>**Individual Counseling**</u>

Beck Depression Inventory

Symptom Checklist 90

Hamilton Rating Scale for Depression

State Trait Anxiety Inventory

Social Adjustment Scale

<u>**Career Counseling**</u>

Career Decision Scale

Career Development Inventory

My Vocational Situation

Survey of Career Development

<u>**School Counseling**</u>

Elementary Guidance Behavior Rating Scale

Self-Esteem Index

however, more intricate than simply selecting one measure that appears to be appropriate. For example, research has consistently shown that the effectiveness of counseling varies depending on whether the client, the counselor, or an outside observer completes the outcome measure (Lambert, 1983, Orlinsky, Grawe, & Parks, 1994). Furthermore, counseling is complex and multidimensional and, therefore, simple outcome measures may fail to adequately evaluate the therapeutic services provided. Clinicians should consider incorporating current strategies in outcome research, which according to Lambert and Hill (1994) are to (1) measure change from multiple perspectives (client, counselor, and outside observer); (2) use symptom-based and atheoretical measures; and (3) examine, as much as possible, patterns of change over time.

Lambert, Ogles, and Masters (1992) developed a conceptual scheme to aid researchers in selecting multiple outcome measures that may also assist practitioners. Their system (see Table 12.3) is designed to assist researchers in selecting instruments that gather outcome data from a variety of viewpoints and domains. The first dimension is *content*, which includes the categories of intrapersonal, interpersonal, and social role. In relation to this dimension, a practitioner may want to select instruments where clients examine themselves (intrapersonal), their relationships with others (interpersonal), and how well they function in certain roles (social role). Within the category of intrapersonal there are subcategories of affect, behavior, and cognition. The second category in Lambert et al.'s classification scheme is *source*, which concerns who is reporting the information and includes self or client report and rating by coun-

TABLE 12.3

Classification scheme for outcome measures

Content	Source	Technology	Time Orientation
1. Intrapersonal Affect Behavior Cognition	1. Self-report	1. Evaluation	1. Trait
2. Interpersonal	2. Counselor rating	2. Description	2. State
3. Social role	3. Trained observer	3. Observation	
	4. Relevant other	4. Status	
	5. Institutional		

Journal of Counseling & Development Vol. 74, July/August 1996. ©1996 ACA. Reprinted with permission. No further reproduction authorized without written permission of the American Counseling Assn.

selor, trained observer, relevant other, and institution. An institutional source could be a grade point average or a supervisor's evaluation of job performance.

The third area is *technology* and concerns the methods used to collect outcome data. Examining the effectiveness of marital counseling can serve as an example of using the technology category to select outcome measures. The first area in technology is evaluation; this might involve having the couple complete a questionnaire evaluating the marital counseling they received. The second subcategory is description. Description involves having clients describe their current attributes, symptoms, or problems. An instrument such as the Marital Satisfaction Inventory would have couples describe their current levels of dissatisfaction in the marriage. This description measure could be used to see if the dissatisfaction decreased as a result of the marriage counseling. The third subcategory is observation and involves the client being observed by someone. In the marital counseling example, the counselor could observe the couple early in the counseling performing a communication exercise and then observe the same exercise at the end of the counseling. The status subcategory concerns physiological measures or other indicators of current status. In the marital counseling example, a status measure could be the couple's marital status at the end of the counseling (i.e., married, separated, or divorced). As reflected in Table 12.3, the last category in Lambert et al.'s (1992) classification scheme is *time orientation*. Time orientation in this system addresses whether the instrument is measuring a stable traitlike characteristic or an unstable statelike characteristic.

As an illustration of how a counselor might use this classification system, let's consider a facilitator of a group for mildly depressed clients. In order to gain more comprehensive information, the facilitator may begin by looking at the *content* subcategories and possibly using three instruments. The facilitator may search for an instrument that would measure changes in affect (intrapersonal), one that measures changes in the quality of relationships (interpersonal), and one that measures changes in the types and amount of activities (social role). Next, the facilitator would consider whom to get information from and use the *source* categories. For example, in terms of content, the clients could complete the Beck Depression Inventory—II (BDI-II) and the facilitator could complete the Hamilton Rating Scale for Depression (HRSD). Concerning the other source categories, it is often difficult to use trained observers, but the facilitator might also want to gather information from family members of the clients. The facilitator would move to the third category of technology, and since the facilitator has decided to use the BDI-II and the HRSC, the facilitator would not want to select another description type of measure. The facilitator would want to consider either an evaluation, observation, or status measure. An evaluation of the group counseling may provide indispensable information. The facilitator could then consider the last category, *time orientation*. As the BDI-II and the HRSD are more nearly state measures of depression, the facilitator might also want to consider using a personality instrument that may provide more of a trait measure. In assessing outcome, often multiple measures that draw relevant information from diverse sources provide the best measures. Therefore, clinicians need to consider a variety of factors when selecting measures to use in order to gather sound accountability information.

Some counseling practitioners shy away from gathering accountability information because they are unsure of how to analyze the data. New computerized statistical packages make data analysis simpler and more user friendly. Sometimes descriptive information rather than statistical analysis is sufficient, with practitioners describing the changes in the outcome measures. Thompson and Snyder (1998) advocated that researchers use effect size more because of practical applications. Effect size is traditionally calculated by subtracting the control group's mean from the experimental group's mean and dividing by the standard deviation of the experimental group (Glass, McGaw, & Smith, 1981). There are other methods of calculating effect size (see Hedges & Olkin, 1985; Rosenthal, 1991). Many times practitioners in the field do not have a control group, so instead they can calculate average effect size by subtracting the posttest score from the pretest score and dividing by the posttest standard deviation. Practitioners should also be aware that many researchers are often willing to consult with practitioners on methodological and statistical questions. Therefore, if clinicians are unsure of the correct methods for analyzing the data, they should consult with someone with expertise in that area.

In conclusion, there appears to be increased pressure for counselors to provide accountability information on their own effectiveness. Meeting the needs of third-party payers or administrators is not the only reason to gather accountability information. Providing outcome assessment results to clients can also have a therapeutic effect. Duckworth (1990) contended that graphically showing clients the progress they have made in counseling can often confirm their progress. Perhaps the most important reason for gathering accountability information is so that counselors can analyze factors that may contribute to their effectiveness and factors that may be lessening their own effectiveness. Therefore, professional development and better services to clients can be promoted through the process of gathering outcome information.

Summary   Assessment results can be used in counseling in primarily three ways: in treatment planning, in a therapeutic manner, and for evaluation purposes. Information gained from both formal and informal assessment strategies is often used in treatment planning. Counselors need information about their clients in order to structure the counseling to meet the client's needs. Research, however, indicates that clinicians are often biased in their clinical judgments. Incorporating quality assessment information into the clinical decision-making process may assist clinicians in making better treatment decisions. For many clients, there is assessment information that already exists (e.g., scholastic aptitude tests) that counselors can use. For some clients, a psychologist may have previously made an evaluation and a counselor can use the psychological report. Quality psychological reports can be very beneficial to the treatment planning process.

Second, counselors may also use assessment instruments or techniques during the treatment phase of counseling. This second area concerns using assessment as a therapeutic intervention rather than for informing the counselor. Finn and Tonsager (1997) proposed the therapeutic assessment model, where assessment results are used to encourage self-exploration and awareness among clients.

The third area in which assessment results play a crucial role in counseling is in evaluating the services provided to clients. There are increasing demands for counselors to provide accountability information, and many practitioners use assessment instruments to produce that information. Counselors need to use sound outcome measures and evaluate their services from multiple perspectives. There are also methods that practitioners can use to analyze the data and convey results to managed-care organizations, administrators, or other groups.

CHAPTER 13

Assessment and Diagnosis

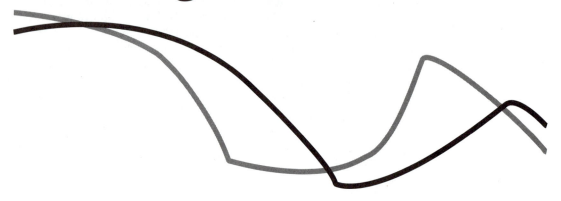

As we begin to explore the applications of assessment information, we need to consider that client assessment is performed for many different reasons and can have many different applications or uses. All clinical decisions are actually based on assessment, since counselors gather information and make treatment decisions based on the information they have gathered through formal or informal assessment techniques. In many ways, making a treatment decision is a form of diagnosis. Although some may argue that diagnosis contradicts the developmental philosophy of counseling, Hohenshil (1993, 1996) maintained that assessment and diagnosis of clients are now integral parts of the counseling process. He contended that thousands of counselors are in settings where they are expected by their employers, licensing agencies, and insurance companies to formally know how to diagnose mental disorders. Hohenshil further argued that all counselors diagnose, either formally or informally. When a developmentally oriented counselor determines that the problem is a normal developmental issue and not a psychopathology, this is essentially a form of diagnosis. Diagnosis does not just play a role in personal counseling, for career counseling also involves diagnosis. When a career counselor determines that a client is "vocationally immature," that also is a diagnosis. In fact, a number of researchers have called for a systematic diagnostic scheme for career clients (Oliver & Spokane, 1988; Rounds & Tinsley, 1984; Whiston et al., 1998). When a school counselor recommends to a mother to have her child evaluated by a psychologist, the counselor is initiating the diagnostic process.

Informal diagnosis, such as deciding if a client should be referred, has always been a part of counseling. In recent years, however, many counselors are required to be familiar with formal diagnostic systems and to have an understanding of diagnoses of mental and emotional status. There are numerous diagnostic systems that are used by mental health service providers. The American Psychiatric Association's (1994) *Diagnostic and Statistical Manual of Mental Disorders*—Fourth Edition (DSM-IV) is the most widely used resource for diagnosis in mental health settings. Another diagnostic system is the *International Classification of Diseases* (ICD-10). These diagnostic systems are designed to provide a common language for professionals, so that professional terms have a common meaning rather than individuals using their own unique definitions. For example, if I walked down the street and asked pedestrians their definitions of substance abuse, the definitions would probably differ dramatically. Some people may not consider a six-pack of beer every night as an indication of substance abuse, others may consider one drink substance abuse. Within a profession, there needs to be uniformity in definitions in order to communicate effectively. Diagnostic systems, such as the DSM-IV, attempt to provide a nosology or nomenclature for counselors, psychiatrists, psychologists, social workers, and other health and mental health professionals. Diagnosis should not be viewed as providing a punitive label but rather as providing a description of the client's symptoms that others can understand.

Diagnostic systems can also be helpful in conceptualizing cases. With certain client problems there is substantial empirical evidence on the most effective methods of providing counseling services (Sexton et al., 1997). A counselor, however, must first identify or diagnose the client problem and then match the appropriate treatment to the identified problem. In some settings (e.g., mental health clinics), formal diagnostic systems will be used as a framework for case conceptualization. In other settings (e.g., schools and career centers), counselors will not be required to use the DSM-IV or other formal diagnostic systems. Even for counselors who will not use these diagnostic systems, having knowledge of the disorders will help in the assessment and referral process. For example, when a school counselor begins to hear some symptoms indicative of a disorder, he or she can explore further to get a more complete picture. This more complete assessment can assist the counselor in making more appropriate referrals. The likelihood of counselors in various settings having clients suffering from mental disorders is quite high. Kessler et al. (1994) found that around 30% of their sample met the criteria for a mental disorder in the year previous to the study.

Diagnosis and assessment are intimately intertwined. Using one of the diagnostic systems requires a thorough appraisal of the client's problems, physical condition and symptoms, and environmental influences. A diagnosis is based on information about the client that is gathered through either informal assessment tools, formal assessment instruments, or a combination of both. Whether the diagnosis is formal or informal, assessment and appraisal skills are needed to make informed clinical decisions.

Using the DSM-IV

Increasingly, counselors are being requested by administrators and managed care organizations to determine if specific problems exist (e.g., substance abuse, depression, anxiety disorders). In many of those settings, counselors must diagnose client problems using the criteria from the *Diagnostic and Statistical Manual of Mental Disorders*—Fourth Edition (DSM-IV, APA, 1994). The DSM-IV is the most widely used diagnostic system in mental health settings. Substantive training in diagnosis is beyond the scope of this chapter. This chapter is intended to provide the reader with an introduction to diagnosis and an overview of disorders. For each diagnosis within the DSM-IV, there are specific criteria that must be met. This discussion of the disorders will provide counselors with a general understanding of the disorders in order to begin to know what should be looked for and how it is assessed.

In order to understand the *Diagnostic and Statistical Manual of Mental Disorders* (APA, 1994), counselors need to understand the term *mental disorder*. The definition of a mental disorder in the DSM-IV is

> a clinically significant behavior or psychological syndrome or pattern that occurs in an individual and that is associated with present distress (e.g., a painful symptom) or disability (i.e., impairment in one or more important areas of functioning) or with a significantly increased risk of suffering death, pain, disability, or an important loss of freedom (p. xxi).

Mental disorders are categorically classified in the DSM-IV based on the practitioner's evaluation of certain criteria. The DSM-IV covers a wide array of diagnostic categories, with applications for clinicians in educational, clinical, and research settings. Counselors are not trained to intervene with all of the disorders in the DSM-IV, but general knowledge of these disorders is now expected of all professionals in the mental health field.

The DSM-IV uses a multiaxial diagnostic system in which the practitioner uses five axes to ensure that information needed for treatment planning, prediction of outcome, and research is provided (Reid & Wise, 1995). Table 13.1 includes an overview of the five axes of the DSM-IV. For appropriate treatment planning, Fong (1993) recommended that counselors determine a full five-axial diagnosis for all clients. The practitioner uses *Axis I* and *Axis II* to describe the client's current mental conditions. Axis I includes all clinical syndromes except for Personality Disorders and Mental Retardation. For certain clients, a

TABLE 13.1
DSM-IV five-axial system

Axis	Description
Axis I	Clinical Disorders and Other Clinical Conditions That May Be a Focus of Attention
Axis II	Personality Disorders and Mental Retardation
Axis III	General Medical Conditions
Axis IV	Psychosocial and Environmental Problems
Axis V	Global Assessment of Functioning (GAF)

counselor will make multiple diagnoses on Axis I or diagnoses on both Axes I and II. The clinician provides information on the client's general medical conditions on *Axis III. Axis IV* is where information on psychosocial and environmental problems that influence treatment and prognosis of Axis I or II are listed. On *Axis V*, the counselor estimates the client's current level of functioning. The Global Assessment of Functioning (GAF) Scale contained in the DSM-IV is the specific scale used for this purpose.

The client's current conditions and mental disorders are described on Axis I and Axis II. Most clients will seek treatment for clinical disorders and other clinical conditions that are classified in Axis I. Whether diagnosing on either Axis I or Axis II, the clinician determines if the information about the client corresponds to a polythetic list of criteria (i.e., set of many types of symptoms, emotions, cognitions, and behaviors). The DSM-IV clearly stipulates the criteria that need to be present in order to meet the diagnostic conditions. For example the diagnostic criteria for Conduct Disorder (312.8) are as follows:

A. A repetitive and persistent pattern of behavior in which the basic rights of others or major age-appropriate societal norms or rules are violated, as manifested by the presence of three (or more) of the following criteria in the past 12 months, with at least one criterion present in the past 6 months:

Aggression toward people and animals
(1) often bullies, threatens, or intimidates others
(2) often initiates physical fights
(3) has used a weapon that can cause serious physical harm to others (e.g., a bat, brick, broken bottle, knife, gun)
(4) has been physically cruel to people
(5) has been physically cruel to animals
(6) has stolen while confronting a victim (e.g., mugging, purse snatching, extortion, armed robbery)
(7) has forced someone into sexual activity

Destruction of property
(8) has deliberately engaged in fire setting with the intention of causing serious damage
(9) has deliberately destroyed others' property (other than fire setting)

Deceitfulness or theft
>   (10) has broken into someone else's house, building, or car
>   (11) often lies to obtain goods or favors or to avoid obligations (i.e.,
>   "cons" others)
>   (12) has stolen items of nontrivial value without confronting a victim
>   (e.g., shoplifting, but without breaking and entering; forgery)

Serious violations of rules
>   (13) often stays out at night despite parental prohibitions, beginning
>   before age 13 years
>   (14) has run away from home overnight at least twice while living in
>   parental or parental surrogate home (or once without returning for
>   a lengthy period)
>   (15) is often truant from school, beginning before age 13 years

B. The disturbance in behavior causes clinically significant impairment in social, academic, or occupational functioning.

C. If the individual is age 18 years or older, criteria are not met for Antisocial
Personality Disorder (pp. 90–91).

These systematic descriptions of the disorders provide diagnostic criteria
that describe the frequency, duration, and severity of the symptoms. The
client must meet the specified criteria in order for a diagnosis to be given.
Clinicians need to ensure that the criteria are truly met, because an error in
diagnosis can be peculiarly harmful to clients. Diagnostic labels may not always be kept confidential by insurance companies and other organizations;
thus a client could be irreparably harmed by an incorrect diagnosis. An incorrect diagnosis could also prevent a client from receiving the correct treatment and prolong the suffering and expense of treatment. Training on the
uses of the DSM-IV and supervised experience are important to accurate
diagnosis.

Axis I

Axis I is for the reporting of clinical conditions, with the exception of the pervasive personality disorders and mental retardation. Table 13.2 lists the major
groups of disorders included on Axis I. Counselors can list multiple diagnoses
on Axis I. If they use more than one diagnosis, they need to indicate the primary diagnosis. In an outpatient setting, counselors need to list the *reason for
the visit* after the primary diagnosis, while in an inpatient setting they should
use the term *principal diagnosis* after the diagnosis on which treatment should
focus. The practitioner can also list specificers after the diagnoses (i.e., Mild,
Moderate, Severe, In Partial Remission, In Full Remission, and Prior History).
Because of the diversity of clinical disorders, it is impossible for any diagnostic
system to contain every possible situation. For this reason, each diagnosis on
Axis I has at least one Not Otherwise Specified (NOS) category.

TABLE 13.2

Axis I: Clinical Disorders and Other Conditions That May Be a Focus of Clinical Attention

- Disorders Usually First Diagnosed in Infancy, Childhood, or Adolescence (excluding Mental Retardation, which is diagnosed on Axis II)

- Delirium, Dementia, and Amnestic and Other Cognitive Disorders

- Mental Disorders Due to General Medical Condition

- Substance-Related Disorders

- Schizophrenia and Other Psychotic Disorders

- Mood Disorders

- Anxiety Disorders

- Somatoform Disorders

- Factitious Disorder

- Dissociative Disorders

- Sexual and Gender Identity Disorders

- Eating Disorders

- Sleep Disorders

- Impulse-Control Disorders Not Elsewhere Classified

- Adjustment Disorders

- Other Conditions That May Be a Focus of Clinical Attention

Disorders Usually First Diagnosed in Infancy, Childhood, or Adolescence

In most cases, clients who meet the criteria for the diagnoses in this category will be identified in childhood or adolescence; however, some individuals will not be diagnosed until adulthood. *Mental Retardation* is included in this section of the DSM-IV but the diagnosis is given on Axis II. Mental retardation is characterized by significantly subaverage intellectual functioning (typically an IQ of approximately 70 or below) with onset before the age of 18 years. The subaverage intelligence must be accompanied by concurrent deficits or impairments in adaptive functioning.

Learning Disorders are indicated when individuals' academic performance are substantially below what is expected for their age, schooling, and level of intelligence. The learning problems need to significantly interfere with academic achievement or daily activities in reading, mathematics, or writing skills. There is debate within the field on what constitutes a substantial discrepancy between achievement and intellectual level. According to the DSM-IV, "substantially below" is usually defined as a discrepancy of more than two standard deviations. The DSM-IV also addresses instances of where the discrepancy can also be smaller (e.g., considering individual's ethnic and cultural background).

Three other disorders that are usually first diagnosed in infancy, childhood, or adolescence concern developmental delays. *Motor Skills Disorders* includes the one diagnosis of Developmental Coordination Disorder, which is characterized by motor coordination substantially below what is expected. Difficulties in speech and language are included in the *Communication Disorders. Pervasive Developmental Disorders* are characterized by pervasive and severe impairments in multiple development areas. Examples of these pervasive disorders are Autistic Disorder, Rett's Disorder, and Childhood Disintegrative Disorder.

Attention-Deficit and *Disruptive Behavior Disorders* have received increased public attention in recent years. This category of disorders is characterized by socially disruptive behaviors that are often more distressing to others than to the client (Reid & Wise, 1995). The prominent symptoms for *Attention-Deficit/Hyperactivity Disorder* are inattention and/or hyperactivity-impulsivity. Subtypes are typically diagnosed in order to specify the predominant symptoms and include: Predominantly Inactive Type, Predominantly Hyperactive-Impulsive Type, and Combined. This section also includes disorders that are disruptive in nature, such as Conduct Disorder. The essential characteristic of *Conduct Disorder* is a repetitive and persistent pattern of behavior that violates the basic rights of others or major age-appropriate societal norms or rules. Similar to Conduct Disorder is *Oppositional Defiant Disorder,* where the essential feature is a pattern of negativistic, defiant, disobedient, and hostile behavior.

Feeding and Eating Disorders of Infancy or Early Childhood are included in this section but should not be confused with Anorexia Nervosa or Bulimia Nervosa that are included in Eating Disorders. Another diagnostic area is *Tic Disorders,* which are characterized by vocal and /or motor tics (e.g., Tourette's Disorder). *Elimination Disorders* includes *Encopresis,* the repeated passage of feces into inappropriate places, and *Enuresis,* the repeated voiding of urine into inappropriate places. The final category is *Other Disorders of Infancy, Childhood, or Adolescents,* which includes disorders not covered in the section such as Separation Anxiety Disorder.

Delirium, Dementia, and Other Cognitive Disorders

As reflected in Table 13.2, the second major category in Axis I is Delirium, Dementia, and Other Cognitive Disorders. Counselors are less likely to be involved with this diagnostic area as compared to others. This section is characterized by a clinically significant deficit in cognition or memory that is a significant change from previous functioning. The disorders in this section are further subdivided depending if the etiology is either a general medical condition, a substance (e.g., drug abuse), or a combination of these factors. A *delirium* is described as a disturbance of consciousness and a change in cognition that develops over a short period of time. *Dementia* involves multiple cognitive deficits that include impairment in memory. Dementia disorders are listed according to their presumed etiology (e.g., Alzheimer's Type, Vascular Dementia, Substance-Induced Persisting Dementia). An *Amnestic Disorder* also involves memory impairment but in the absence of other significant cognitive impairments.

Mental Disorders Due to a General Medical Condition

The third diagnostic section for Axis I involves mental disorders that are judged to be the direct consequence of a general medical condition. The term *general medical conditions* is consistent with what is coded on Axis III and these are conditions that are not considered "mental disorders." This section provides health care providers with a shorthand method of identifying when the disturbances are the direct physiological consequence of a general medical condition.

Substance-Related Disorders

In the DSM-IV, the term *substance* includes drugs of abuse (including alcohol), side effects of prescribed and over-the-counter medications, or a toxin. Therefore, these disorders are related to a wide range of substances. With these diagnoses, the substance class is identified and the substances are grouped into 11 classes (e.g., alcohol, amphetamine or similarly acting sympathomimetics, caffeine, cannabis, or cocaine). Furthermore, the substance-related problem could be Polysubstance Dependence and Other or Unknown Substance-Related Disorders (which include most disorders related to medications or toxins). Often clinicians do not consider the problems associated with prescribed or over-the-counter medications. Examples of prescribed and over-the-counter medications that can cause Substance-Related Disorders are: anesthetics and analgesics, anticonvulsants, antihistamines, corticosteriods, and muscle relaxants. Toxins could include heavy metals, rat poisons, pesticides, and carbon monoxide. The Substance-Related Disorders are separated into two major groups: *Substance Use Disorders* and the *Substance-Induced Disorders.*

When considering Substance Use Disorders, counselors need to consider the difference between *Substance Dependence* and *Substance Abuse.* With Substance Dependence, regular substance use leads to the development of impaired control of that substance use and the continued use of the substance despite adverse consequences. Typically there is a pattern of self-administration of the substance that results in tolerance, withdrawal, and compulsive drug-taking behaviors. Dependence is defined as a cluster of three of the following symptoms occurring in the same 12-month period.

- Tolerance is either (a) a need for markedly increased amounts of the substance to attain intoxication or desired effect or (b) markedly diminished effect with continued use of the substance at the same amount.
- Withdrawal is characterized by (a) the development of substance-specific syndrome due to the cessation or reduction of substance use, such as alcohol withdrawal that can involve hand tremors, nausea, or vomiting; psychomotor agitation; (b) the substance-specific syndrome causing significant distress or impairment with everyday functioning; and (c) the substance or something closely related being taken to relieve or avoid withdrawal symptoms.

- The substance is often taken in larger amounts or over a longer period than was intended.
- There is a persistent desire for the substance, or efforts to cut down or control use do not succeed.
- A great deal of time is devoted to activities necessary to obtain the substance, use the substance, or recover from its effect.
- Reduction or cessation of important social, occupational, or recreational activities are related to the use of the substance.
- Substance abuse continues despite the knowledge that it contributes to physical or psychological problems.

When a client meets the criteria for Substance Dependence, the actual diagnosis is for the substance he or she is dependent upon, using the categories listed earlier (e.g., 304.40 Amphetamine Dependence, 304.30 Cannabis Dependence).

The *Substance Abuse* diagnosis does not have the emphasis on dependency. Here the focus is on a maladaptive pattern of substance use leading to clinically significant impairments or distress. The substance use may result in repeated failure to fulfill major role obligations, repeated use in situations in which it is physically hazardous, multiple legal problems, and recurrent social and interpersonal problems. These problems need to have occurred repeatedly over a 12-month period. Once again, the actual diagnosis of Substance Abuse is related to the specific substance (e.g., 305.00 Alcohol Abuse, 305.60 Cocaine Abuse).

Substance-Induced Disorders are the second major group of disorders under the general category of Substance-Related Disorders. Related to Substance-Induced Disorders, the concerns are with *Substance Intoxication* and *Substance Withdrawal.* (As a note, there are other Substance-Induced Mental Disorders included in other sections of the manual such as Substance-Induced Delirium, Substance-Induced Psychotic Disorder, Substance-Induced Mood Disorder). Concerning Substance Intoxication, we need to consider that short-term or "acute" intoxication may have different signs and symptoms as compared to sustained or "chronic" intoxications. Intoxication requires recent use or exposure to a substance and the presence of maladaptive behaviors or psychological changes. Furthermore, these maladaptive behaviors or personality changes have to be related to the effect of the substance on the central nervous system. Substance Intoxication is often diagnosed in combination with Substance Abuse or Substance Dependency or with other diagnoses. The DSM-IV provides diagnostic criteria for each of the major substances in order to assist in differential diagnosis.

Substance Withdrawal diagnoses also frequently accompany other diagnoses. With Substance Withdrawal, the practitioner must be familiar with the substance-specific withdrawal syndrome (i.e., the behavioral, physiological, and cognitive symptoms for withdrawal from specific substances). Not all of the common substances have a withdrawal diagnosis. For example, withdrawal from caffeine is not included in the DSM-IV. With Substance Withdrawal diagnoses, the symptoms must develop as a result of the recent cessation or decreased intake of a substance after there has been prolonged and/or heavy use of the substance. Furthermore, significant impairment and distress are required.

Schizophrenia and Other Psychotic Disorders

All of the disorders in this section are characterized by having psychotic symptoms as the defining feature. Since counselors are primarily trained with a developmental approach, this area will only be briefly summarized. *Schizophrenia* is a disorder that lasts for at least six months and includes at least one month of active-phase symptoms (i.e., the client must exhibit two or more of the following: delusions, hallucinations, disorganized speech, grossly disorganized or catatonic behavior, or other negative symptoms). There are also subtypes of Schizophrenia that are Paranoid, Disorganized, Catatonic, Undifferentiated, and Residual. With *Schizophrenform Disorder,* the client must also exhibit two or more of the symptoms listed for Schizophrenia. The main difference between Schizophrenform and Schizophrenia is the duration of the disturbance; Schizophrenform can last from one to six months. There are also subtypes of Schizophrenform Disorder.

Mood Disorders

Before counselors can understand the criteria for diagnosing *Mood Disorders,* they need to first be familiar with the different Mood Episodes (Major Depressive Episode, Manic Episode, Mixed Episode, and Hypomanic Episode). Mood Episodes are *not* diagnosed as disorders, for they are the building blocks for the Mood Disorder diagnoses. A *Major Depressive Episode* is one in which the client is in a depressed mood or has lost interest or pleasure in nearly all activities for at least two weeks. In children and adolescents, the mood may be more irritability than sadness. In addition, the client must experience four or more of the following symptoms: (1) changes in appetite or weight; (2) changes in sleep (insomnia or, less frequently, prolonged sleeping); (3) psychomotor agitation or retardation; (4) fatigue or loss of energy; (5) feelings of worthlessness or guilt; (6) difficulty thinking, concentrating, or making decisions; or (7) recurrent thoughts of death or suicidal ideation, suicide plans, or attempts. These symptoms need to persist through most of the day and cannot be directly the result of a medical condition or bereavement. A *Manic Episode* is characterized by abnormally elevated, expansive, or irritable moods. In addition, other symptoms that are present are grandiosity, decreased need to sleep, flight of ideas, distractibility, increased activity, and involvement in risky activities. These symptoms need to be obvious and last for at least a week. This is not a normal feeling good about oneself, but rather becoming so driven that it causes marked impairments in occupational functioning, social activities, or relationships. A *Mixed Episode* is one in which on a daily basis the client has periods that meet the criteria for a Manic Episode and for a Major Depression

Episode. This rapid alternating of depressive and manic moods within a day has to continue for at least a week. These mood alternations need to be severe and cause marked impairment in activities. A *Hypomanic Episode* is similar to a Manic Episode in that there needs to be a persistently elevated, expansive or irritable mood. The Hypomanic Episode only has to last four days as compared to a week. Some of the same other symptoms need to be present (i.e., inflated self-esteem or grandiosity, decreased need to sleep, flight of ideas, distractibility, increased activity, and involvement in risky activities); however, these symptoms do not need to be so severe as to cause marked impairments.

The clinician then uses these four descriptions of episodes to diagnose Mood Disorders that can be categorized into three major areas: *Depressive Disorders, Bipolar Disorders,* and *Other Mood Disorders.* Within the Depressive Disorders, the first distinction is between the *Major Depressive Disorder* and *Dysthymic Disorder.* Major Depressive Disorders are characterized by one or more Major Depressive Episode without a history of Manic, Mixed, or Hypomanic Episodes. The Major Depressive Disorders are further delineated by whether it is a single episode or a recurrent problem and the current state of the disturbance. Dysthymic Disorders differ from other depressive disorders in that clients don't suffer from a Major Depressive Episode but rather experience a chronically depressed mood for a long period of time (at least two years for adults and one year for children). Individuals describe themselves as being "down in the dumps," although children may seem more irritable than sad. Symptoms that are present with Dysthymic Disorders are poor appetite or overeating, insomnia or hypersomnia, low energy or fatigue, low self-esteem, poor concentration or difficulty making decisions, and feelings of helplessness.

If a Manic, Mixed, or Hypomanic Episode develops in conjunction with a Major Depressive Episode, then the diagnosis should be a *Bipolar Disorder.* Bipolar I diagnoses indicate that the client has had at least one Manic Episode or Mixed Episode usually accompanied by a Major Depressive Episode. Bipolar II Disorders, on the other hand, are characterized by one or more Major Depressive Episodes in conjunction with at least one Hypomanic Episode. Somewhat different from Bipolar I and Bipolar II is the Cyclothymic Disorder. With Cyclothymic Disorder a client needs to have had numerous periods of hypomanic symptoms that do not meet the criteria for Manic Episode and numerous periods of depressive symptoms that do not meet the criteria for a Major Depressive Episode.

Within the general section of Mood Disorder in the DSM-IV there is a third major section besides Depressive Disorders and Bipolar Disorders titled *Other Mood Disorders.* This section includes mood disorders that are related to a specific medical condition and ones that are induced by substances.

Anxiety Disorders

One or more of the following conditions may be diagnosed in clients whose prominent symptoms are anxiety related. Morrison (1995) reported that most anxiety disorders begin when clients are relatively young. Similar to Mood Disorder, there are "building blocks" with Anxiety Disorder that are not codable diagnoses but are used to determine the precise Anxiety Disorder. The "building blocks" with Anxiety Disorders are *Panic Attacks* and *Agoraphobia.* A Panic Attack is a brief period during which the client feels intense apprehension, fearfulness, or terror. These feelings are often accompanied by a feeling of impending doom. During the attack, the client typically experiences physical symptoms such as shortness of breath, palpitations, chest discomfort, difficulty breathing, or a sense of losing control or "going crazy." With Agoraphobia, clients fear situations or places where they may have trouble coping or finding help if they become anxious or have a panic attack. Furthermore, the anxiety leads to avoidance of the places or situations in which the anxiety may occur.

In terms of Panic Disorders, there are two diagnoses: Panic Disorder with Agoraphobia and Panic Disorder without Agoraphobia. With both of these disorders there are recurrent and unexpected Panic Attacks. There is also a diagnosis of Agoraphobia Without History of Panic Disorder. Here the focus is on the Agoraphobia and the paniclike symptoms, but there is not a history of unexpected Panic Attacks.

The Anxiety Disorder section also includes diagnoses related to phobias. A *Specific Phobia,* such as a phobia of spiders, is characterized by clinically significant anxiety induced by exposure to that specific feared object or situation. With a phobia, the fear of a specific object or situation leads to avoidance behaviors that are problematic. Within the DSM-IV, there is a specific diagnosis for *Social Phobia,* which is associated with significant anxiety associated with certain types of social or performance situations.

Another Anxiety Disorder is *Obsessive-Compulsive Disorder.* The characteristics of Obsessive-Compulsive Disorder are recurrent obsessions or compulsions that are severe enough to be time consuming or cause marked distress or impairment. Obsessions are persistent ideas, thoughts, impulses, or images that interfere with normal activities. Compulsions are repetitive behaviors (e.g., checking the stove, hand-washing) or mental acts (e.g., counting, repeating certain words) with the goal being to reduce or prevent the anxiety. In order to meet the criteria for Obsessive-Compulsive Disorder, adults at some point must recognize that the obsessions or compulsions are excessive or unreasonable. This requirement of recognition does not apply with children because they may not have sufficient cognitive awareness to evaluate the situation. Simply checking the stove a couple of times will not meet the criteria for Obsessive-Compulsive Disorder since the obsessions or compulsions need to be problematic and/or time consuming (at least an hour a day).

Posttraumatic Stress Disorder is another diagnosis in the Anxiety Disorders section. Posttraumatic Stress Disorder is characterized by the reexperiencing of an extremely traumatic event. The reexperiencing can be in the form of distressing recollections, dreams, feeling as if the traumatic event were recurring, or other reactions to cues that might symbolize or resemble aspects of the traumatic event. Another criterion for Posttraumatic Stress Disorder is a persistent avoidance of stimuli associated with the trauma and a numbing of general responsiveness. Furthermore, the individual needs to have persistent symptoms of anxiety or increased arousal that were not present before the trauma (e.g., sleep problems related to nightmares, hypervigilance, exaggerated startle response, increased irritability or outburst of anger, difficulty concentrating). In addition, the posttraumatic symptoms are not just immediately following the traumatic event but continue for more than a month. A similar diagnosis is *Acute Stress Disorder,* which has many of the same symptoms as Posttraumatic Stress Disorder, except that additional symptoms are present in the first month after the traumatic event. In Acute Stress Disorder, the client experiences symptoms of dissociation during the event or just after the event.

Generalized Anxiety Disorder is somewhat different from the other Anxiety Disorders because it involves more generalized anxiety and worry that tends to persist for six months or more. The individual finds it difficult to control the worry. In addition, the anxiety and worry result in symptoms such as restlessness, feeling keyed up, being easily fatigued, difficulty concentrating, irritability, muscle tension, and sleep disturbance. Also in the Anxiety Disorder section of the DSM-IV are diagnoses of Anxiety Disorder Due to General Medical Condition and Substance-Induced Anxiety Disorders.

Somatoform Disorders

All of the *Somatoform Disorders* have the unifying feature of the presence of physical symptoms that suggest a medical condition, yet these physical symptoms cannot be fully explained by a general medical condition. In contrast to Factitious Disorders and Malingering, these physical symptoms are not intentional. If a counselor has a client for whom the somatic symptoms are the prominent reason for seeking counseling, then the counselor should examine the different types of Somatoform Disorders in this section of the DSM-IV.

Factitious Disorder

This is a section that includes only one disorder, *Factitious Disorder,* with subtypes. Factitious Disorder involves the intentional producing or feigning of physical or psychological symptoms. With Factitious Disorder the motivation is to assume the sick role; however, the reasons are not for economic gain or for other incentives. The client isn't trying to fool the insurance company or avoid responsibilities, but rather the individual is intentionally producing the symptoms to meet a psychological need.

Dissociative Disorders

Dissociation is the state in which one group of the normal mental processes become separated from other mental processes. In the DSM-IV, it is described as a disruption in the usually integrated functions of consciousness, memory, identity, or perceptions of the environment. The onset of the dissociation can be either sudden or gradual and the dissociation can disappear or remain chronic. The DSM-IV includes four Dissociative Disorders: Dissociative Amnesia, Dissociative Fugue, Dissociative Identity Disorder, Depersonalization Disorder, and also the common Not Otherwise Specified diagnosis. *Dissociative Amnesia* is characterized by the client's being unable to recall important personal information. The information is usually of a traumatic or stressful nature and is too extensive to be explained by ordinary forgetfulness. With a *Dissociative Fugue*, the client unexpectedly and suddenly travels away from home or his or her work environment. This unexpected travel is accompanied by the inability to remember the past and confusion about identity. In some cases, the client will assume a new identity. *Dissociative Identity Disorder* (formerly Multiple Personality Disorder) involves the presence of two or more distinct identities or personality states that recurrently take control of the client's behavior. These distinct identities or personalities are accompanied by the inability to recall important personal information that is too extensive to be explained by ordinary forgetfulness. Finally, in *Depersonalization Disorder* there is persistent depersonalization (i.e., a feeling of detachment or estrangement from oneself). Clients often have episodes during which they feel as if they were observing their actions from the outside. With Depersonalization Disorder, clients' abilities to test reality remain intact, they just view their reality from an outsider's viewpoint.

Sexual and Gender Identity Disorders

The Sexual and Gender Identity Disorders involve three major areas: Sexual Dysfunction, Paraphilias, and Gender Identity Disorders. With *Sexual Dysfunction* there is a disturbance in sexual desire and problems in the psychophysiological changes that characterize the sexual response cycle. The Sexual Dysfunction category is subdivided into disorders related to sexual desire, sexual arousal, orgasm, and sexual pain. The Sexual Dysfunction Disorders are often gender specific because sexual difficulties typically differ between men and women. The term *paraphilia* means abnormal or unnatural attraction. In *Paraphilia Disorders* the attraction or sexual-arousing fantasy generally involves: (1) objects or nonhuman animals; (2) humiliation or suffering of the individual or the partner; or (3) nonconsenting persons, including children. These diagnoses are made only if the urges have been acted upon or if there is marked impairment or distress. Furthermore, the paraphilia impulses and behaviors need to be the preferred methods of sexual excitement and expression, with the symptoms being present for at least six months or longer. The third major category of disorders in the section is Sexual and Gender Identity Disorders. Clients with *Gender Identity Disorders* feel intensely uncomfortable with their own biological gender. The diagnoses related to Gender Identity Disorder are not appropriate for clients questioning their own sexual orientation. These clients have a strong and persistent cross-gender identification. They either see themselves as being of the opposite sex or desire to become the opposite sex. This cross-gender identification is not because of perceived advantages of being the other sex, but rather they are intensely uncomfortable with their own assigned gender.

Eating Disorders

Eating Disorders involve severe disturbances in eating behavior and the DSM-IV includes two specific diagnoses: Anorexia Nervosa and Bulimia Nervosa. The central feature of *Anorexia Nervosa* is the inability to maintain a minimally normal body weight. The client, even though underweight, is intensely afraid of gaining weight and exhibits a significant disturbance in the perception of her or his body. Some individuals feel globally overweight, others are concerned with certain parts of their body being "too fat." Amenorrhea (the absence of at least three consecutive menstrual cycles) is a sign of Anorexia Nervosa since the severe dieting affects hormone levels. The mean age of onset is 17, although some studies indicate that there are peaks around the age of 14 and around the age of 18. There are two subtypes, one in which the food intake is severely restricted and the other of the binge-eating/purging type.

Bulimia Nervosa is an eating disorder characterized by binge eating and inappropriate compensatory behaviors to prevent weight gain. Clients with Bulimia have recurrent episodes of binge eating, during which within a two-hour time period they will eat large amounts of food. These binges are not slightly overeating, but the amount of food is large and often consists of starches and sweets. Clients report a sense of lack of control over eating during these binge episodes. To prevent gaining weight, the person uses compensatory behaviors (e.g., vomiting, use of laxatives or diuretics, or excessive exercise). The Bulimia Nervosa diagnosis is given when the binging and purging occur at least twice a week for a three-month period. Like clients with Anorexia Nervosa, clients with Bulimia have self-images that are unduly influenced by their body shape and weight. Clients with Bulimia, however, are much more realistic in their perceptions of their own body as compared to Anorexic clients. There are also two subtypes with Bulimia Nervosa: purging types (those who vomit or use laxatives, diuretics, or enemas) and nonpurging types (those who use fasting or excessive exercise as the compensatory behaviors).

Sleep Disorders

The Sleep Disorders are organized in the DSM-IV into four sections according to the presumed etiology (cause or origin of the disorder): Primary Sleep Disorders, Sleep Disorders Related to Another Mental Disorder, Sleep Disorder Due to a General Medical Condition, and Substance-Induced Sleep Disorder. In *Primary Sleep Disorders* the etiology is undetermined and not related to the other causes. These Primary Sleep Disorders are subdivided into Dyssomnias and Parasomnias. Dyssomnias involve abnormalities in the amount, quality, or timing of sleep. Parasomnias are characterized by abnormal behaviors while sleeping (e.g., sleep walking) or physiological events that occur in conjunction with sleep, in specific sleep stages, or in the sleep-wake cycle. The diagnosis of Sleep Disorders is not simple and involves systematic assessment of sleep complaints, physical condition of the client, and evaluation of substances and medicines. Furthermore, the clinician must be knowledgeable of the sleep stages and methods for measuring these. Practitioners also need to understand the typical variations in sleep across the life span.

Impulse-Control Disorders Not Elsewhere Classified

The central characteristic of the disorders in this section is the individual's failure to resist an impulse, drive, or temptation to perform a harmful act. For most of the disorders in this section, the client feels an increasing sense of tension or pressure before committing the act. After committing the act, the person then feels a sense of relief, pleasure, or gratification. Later this may be followed with regret, guilt, or remorse. *Intermittent Explosive Disorder* is related to discrete episodes of failure to resist aggressive impulses that result in serious assaults or destruction of property. These aggressive behaviors are markedly out of proportion to the situation or to any stressors. *Kleptomania* concerns the inability to resist impulses to steal objects that are not needed. The motivation for stealing is not anger or desiring the object, the motivation is to relieve the tension that mounts before the stealing behavior. With *Pyromania,* pleasure, gratification, or relief of tension is secured through a pattern of setting fires. *Pathological Gambling* is also classified as an Impulse Control Disorder and is characterized by persistent and frequent maladaptive gambling behaviors. The last disorder in this section is *Trichotillomania,* which involves the recurrent pulling out of one's hair for relief, pleasure, or gratification.

Adjustment Disorders

Adjustment Disorders involve the development of clinically significant symptoms in response to an identifiable psychosocial stressor(s). The significant symptoms must occur within three months of the beginning of the stress. Furthermore, the symptoms need to be beyond what is a typical reaction, or there is marked reaction that affects social or occupational functioning. The stressor can be a single effect (e.g., the ending of a significant relationship) or there can be multiple stressors (e.g., unemployment and marital discord). Stressors can be recurrent (e.g., seasonal business problems) or continuous. Stressors can also be a reaction to a developmental change (e.g., getting married, having a baby). A natural disaster could also be a stressor. In many ways, Adjustment Disorders are the focus of counselor training. The authors of the DSM-IV, however, suggested that this diagnosis not be used as a "catch-all."

Other Conditions That May Be a Focus of Clinical Attention

This category refers to conditions or problems that are *not* considered to be a disorder, but that may still be a focus of clinical attention. Many of the conditions in this section are coded with a V-code and sometimes these conditions are just called "V-Codes." All of these conditions are coded on Axis I, except for the one related to borderline intellectual functioning. Because of the developmental and preventive focus of counseling, counselors are particularly prepared to counsel clients with these conditions and problems. Table 13.3 lists some of the common codes that counselors might use from this section.

TABLE 13.3

Common V-Codes used in counseling

Relational Problems

V61.9	Relational Problems Related to a Mental Disorder or General Medical Condition
V61.20	Parent-Child Relational Problem
V61.10	Partner Relational Problem
V61.8	Sibling Relational Problem
V62.81	Relational Problem Not Otherwise Specified

Problems Related to Abuse or Neglect

V61.21	Physical Abuse of Child (995.54 for victim)
V61.21	Sexual Abuse of Child (995.53 for victim)
V61.21	Neglect of Child (995.52 for victim)
V61.12	Physical Abuse of Partner
V62.83	Physical Abuse of Someone Other Than Partner (995.81 for victim)
V61.12	Sexual Abuse of Partner
V62.83	Sexual Abuse of Someone Other Than Partner (995.83 for victim)

Additional Conditions That May Be a Focus of Clinical Attention

V71.01	Adult Antisocial Behavior
V71.02	Child or Adolescent Antisocial Behavior
V62.82	Bereavement
V62.3	Academic Problem
V62.2	Occupational Problem
313.82	Identity Problem
V62.89	Religious or Spiritual Problem
V62.4	Acculturation Problem
V62.89	Phase of Life Problem

Axis II

Axis II diagnoses are used to describe maladaptive personality disorders or forms of mental retardation. Diagnosis of the Axis II disorders uses the same approach as Axis I disorders, with a clinician examining a clustering of criteria around an essential feature. Personality Disorders are *enduring* patterns or personality traits that are inflexible and maladaptive and that cause significant functional impairment or distress. Thus, Axis II diagnoses differ from Axis I in that disorders are enduring and inflexible. Most clients seek treatment for an Axis I problem or a V-Code problem (not attributable to a mental disorder). An Axis II diagnosis can be present with an Axis I diagnosis or present without an Axis I diagnosis. The Axis II Personality Disorders are, in many ways, difficult to diagnose because the criteria are somewhat less precise and the client, as a function of the personality disorder, is less able to report symptoms accurately (Fong, 1995).

Because Personality Disorders are somewhat more difficult to diagnose, it is important for counselors to understand the general characteristics and early signs of these disorders. Clients with Personality Disorders will have long-term functioning difficulties since these disorders are categorized by traits. The onset of the pattern of inflexibility and maladaption is typically in adolescence or early adulthood. Although a client may seek counseling for difficulties in a reaction to a specific stressor or event, a counselor should determine if there is a chronicity of maladaption. Fong (1995) suggested that during the initial interview counselors ask clients questions about the duration of the problems and if the client can recall other such periods of distress or difficulties.

Clients' perceptions of personality disorders are described as *egosyntonic,* meaning that the disorder is an integral part of the self. Clients with an Axis I disorder will perceive the disorder as not part of themselves. Thus, a client with a Mood Disorder will not see the Mood Disorder as a part of him or herself. Clients with a personality disorder will see the maladaption as a part of themselves and see the situation as just being the way it is. Therefore, clients with personality disorders will view counseling as having low probability of changing their situations because the problems are immutable.

Another important feature of Personality Disorders is significant impairment in social and/or occupational functioning. Although clients occasionally experience anxiety or depression, the most dominant features of Personality Disorders are impairments in occupational and social functioning (Fong, 1995). Because Personality Disorders are related to enduring traits, difficulties will arise across situations. One way the inflexibility is evident is that the client continues to use the same maladaptive strategies over and over again.

A Personality Disorder may not be evident in the first counseling session where the focus may be on the immediate or acute difficulties. Fong (1995) proposed the following signs that may be indicative of a possible Personality Disorder: (1) the counseling seems to suddenly stall or stop after making initial progress; (2) the client does not seem to be aware of the effect of his or her behaviors on others; (3) the client seems to accept the problems; (4) the client is underresponsive or noncompliant with the counseling regimen; and (5) the client is often involved with intense conflictual relationships with institutional systems.

In the DSM-IV, there are 10 personality disorders that are organized under 3 clusters (see Table 13.4). The clusters are atheoretical and are grouped together because of shared features. *Cluster A* concerns the disorders with odd and eccentric dimensions, while *Cluster B* includes disorders that are characterized by dramatic-emotional features. *Cluster C* includes disorders with anxious-fearful characteristics.

Cluster A

Cluster A disorders are characterized by a lack of relationships, aloof behaviors, restricted affect, and peculiar ideas. There are three disorders within this cluster: Paranoid Personality Disorder, Schizoid Personality Disorder, and Schizotypal Personality Disorder. The essential feature of *Paranoid Personality Disorder* is a pattern of pervasive distrust and suspicion of others such that others' behavior is considered threatening or malevolent. Clients with this disorder will expect other people (including the counselor) to exploit, harm, or deceive them. They do not trust others and have great difficulty with interpersonal relationships. They feel they have been deeply and irreversibly injured and are preoccupied with doubts about the loyalty or trustworthiness of friends and associates. They are continually looking for confirmation of their paranoid beliefs. Because they are constantly wary of harmful intentions, they are often quick to identify some slight as an attack on their character or reputation. Furthermore, these individuals often react with intense anger to any perceived insults.

The central feature of *Schizoid Personality Disorder* is a pervasive pattern of detachment from social relationships and a restricted range of emotions. These individuals prefer to be alone and have little desire for personal relationships. They appear indifferent to the approval or criticism of others and are not par-

TABLE 13.4

DSM-IV clusters of personality disorders and diagnoses

Cluster	DSM-IV Diagnosis
Cluster A	Paranoid Personality Disorder Schizoid Personality Disorder Schizotypal Personality Disorder
Cluster B	Antisocial Personality Disorder Borderline Personality Disorder Histrionic Personality Disorder Narcissistic Personality Disorder
Cluster C	Avoidant Personality Disorder Dependent Personality Disorder Obsessive-Compulsive Personality Disorder

ticularly concerned about what others may think of them. These individuals do not have close friends or confidants, except possibly a first-degree relative.

The essential feature of the *Schizotypal Personality Disorder* is a pervasive pattern of peculiar ideation and behavior with deficits in social and interpersonal relationships. These individuals incorrectly interpret casual incidents as having particular and unusual meanings to the individual. They have odd beliefs or magical thinking that is inconsistent with the subcultural norms (e.g., superstitions, belief in clairvoyance). Paranoia, unusual perceptions, and odd beliefs are evident, but they do not reach the level of chronic delusional proportions.

Cluster B

Individuals with a Cluster B disorder will be very different from Cluster A clients, for these individuals will be quite emotional and try to impress the counselor. The behavior of individuals in this group tends to be erratic and unstable, with affect that is quite changeable and heightened. The first of the four disorders is the Antisocial Personality Disorder. The central characteristic of the *Antisocial Personality Disorder* is a pervasive pattern of disregard and violation of others' rights. This disregard begins in childhood or adolescence and continues into adulthood. This diagnosis, however, cannot be given until the person is at least 18 and has a history of some of the symptoms of Conduct Disorder before the age of 15. After the age of 15, the individual's disregard for others is a pattern reflected in the following: (1) repeated involvement in illegal behaviors; (2) deceitfulness, lying, or conning others; (3) being impulsive and not planning; (4) aggressiveness and repeated physical fights or assaults; (5) reckless disregard for the safety of self and others; (6) being consistently irresponsible; and (7) lack of remorse.

Borderline Personality Disorder is characterized by a pervasive pattern of instability in interpersonal relationships, self-image, and mood. This instability is also accompanied by impulsivity. Borderline clients may display frantic efforts to avoid real or imagined abandonment. Often their relationships are unstable and intense, fluctuating between idealizing to devaluing the other person. There is usually a marked and persistent disturbance of identity. There may be self-damaging behaviors and recurrent suicidal gestures or threats. The clients often have intense feelings and there is emotional instability. Others may perceive these individuals as overreacting, with brief but intense episodes of depression, irritability or anxiety. These individuals also have a tendency to feel chronically empty and have anger control problems.

The essential feature of the *Histrionic Personality Disorder* is an excessive and pervasive emotionality and attention-seeking behaviors. These individuals are dissatisfied unless they are the center of attention. Their interactions with others may be inappropriately sexual or provocative. Emotions change rapidly and their behavior is often considered inappropriately exaggerated, sometimes to the point of being theatrical. Their speech is dramatic and impressionistic but also tends to lack detail. They are often quite suggestible and perceive relationships to be more intimate than the relationships actually are.

With *Narcissistic Personality Disorder* there is a pattern of grandiosity, need for admiration, and lack of empathy. These individuals have a grandiose sense of self-importance and are preoccupied with their fantasies of success, brilliance, beauty, or ideal love. Narcissistic clients expect special regard from others but often devalue others' achievements and abilities. They require excessive admiration and expect to be catered to. They may exploit others and generally have a lack of empathy towards others. Often narcissistic clients are envious of others and expect that others are envious of them in return.

Cluster C

The disorders in this cluster are characterized by the client's being anxious and avoidant. Clients with these disorders rigidly respond to demands by passively enduring, changing self, or withdrawing. The three disorders are the Avoidant Personality Disorder, the Dependent Personality Disorder, and the Obsessive-Compulsive Personality Disorder. The essential feature of the *Avoidant Personality Disorder* is a pervasive pattern of social inhibition, feelings of inadequacy, and a fear of negative evaluation. These individuals avoid work, school, or even promotion opportunities because of these fears. They are unlikely to enter into relationships without strong guarantees of unrelenting acceptance. Because they are preoccupied with being criticized or rejected, they have a markedly low threshold for detecting such behaviors. These clients tend to see themselves as being socially inept, personally unappealing, or inferior.

Dependent Personality Disorder is characterized by a pervasive and excessive need to be taken care of. This need leads to submissive and clinging behaviors accompanied by fears of separation. These individuals have great difficulty making decisions. They want others to take the lead and are fearful of disagreeing with them. These individuals are fearful of being alone and will go to excessive lengths to obtain nurturance and support from others. If a relationship ends, they typically will urgently seek another relationship.

The central feature of *Obsessive-Compulsive Personality Disorder* is a preoccupation with orderliness, perfectionism, and interpersonal and mental control. The person's overly stringent standards continually interfere with her or his ability to complete tasks or projects. They strive to make every detail perfect and display excessive devotion to work and productivity. They rarely take time for leisure, and when they do, the focus is on performing the leisure activity perfectly. Harsh judgments of oneself and others are common. Some people will have difficulty discarding even unimportant objects and may be frugal in their spending in order to be prepared for a future disaster. These individuals tend to be rigid and stubborn and contend there is only a single "right" way to perform.

Axis III

Axis III is for the reporting of the client's current medical conditions that are possibly relevant to the individual's mental condition or disorder. Medical conditions that cause the disorder should not be coded here, but rather the appropriate code should be selected from the Axis I Disorders (e.g., 310.1 Personality Change Due to a General Medical Condition). Axis III is used to describe medical conditions that should be considered in treatment decisions but are not a direct cause of the disorder. Another reason for including Axis III information is that in some circumstances the reporting of Axis III conditions may affect the number of treatment sessions allowed by a managed care organization.

Axis IV

As indicated in Table 13.1, Axis IV is for the reporting of psychosocial and environmental problems that may influence the diagnosis, treatment, and prognosis of the disorder. This is where counselors report psychosocial or environmental issues that affect the Axis I or Axis II diagnosis. Examples of these problems are death of a family member, divorce, inadequate support, unemployment, or extreme poverty. Typical problems are grouped together in this section of the DSM-IV for convenient reference. If the psychosocial or environmental issues are the primary reason for seeking services, then the counselor should record these in Axis I, using the "Other Conditions That May Be a Focus of Clinical Attention."

Axis V

In Axis V, the clinician reports his or her professional judgment concerning the client's overall level of functioning. This information can be used in treatment planning and also to later assess the outcome of the counseling. The Global Assessment of Functioning (GAF) is typically used to report the client's level of functioning. With the GAF, the practitioner provides a single indicator from 0 to 100 reflecting the global functioning. The GAF Scale is reported on Axis V by "GAF= insert number." The GAF should only reflect psychological, social, or occupational functioning and should not include physical (or environmental) limitations. Furthermore, the GAF only reflects *current* level of functioning unless otherwise noted. For example, there may be times when a clinician will want to report the highest level of functioning over the past three months. On page 32 of the DSM-IV, practitioners will find an easy-to-use scale indicating the appropriate GAF codes.

Multiaxial Evaluation

The reporting of the multiaxial system of diagnosis will vary somewhat depending on the setting. Some agencies will require a full five-axial diagnosis for all clients, while other agencies or organizations will not. Fong (1995) suggested that counselors always provide a full five-axial diagnosis because of the relevance of the information to treatment. Table 13.5 provides some examples of how to record DSM-IV multiaxial evaluations.

TABLE 13.5

Examples of how to record DSM-IV diagnoses

Example 1

Axis I	309.81	Posttraumatic Stress Disorder, Acute
	305.00	Alcohol Abuse
Axis II	V71.09	No diagnosis
Axis III	446.0	Bronchitis, Acute
Axis IV		Lives Alone
Axis V	GAF = 45	(current)

Example 2

Axis I	315.00	Reading Disorder
Axis II	301.6	Avoidant Personality Disorder
Axis III		None
Axis IV		Unemployed
Axis V	GAF = 57	(current)

Example 3

Axis I	V61.10	Partner Relational Problem
Axis II	V71.09	No diagnosis
Axis III	250.00	Diabetes mellitus, type II/non-insulin-dependent
Axis IV		Discord with boss
Axis V	GAF = 62	(current)

Example 4

Axis I	312.81	Conduct Disorder, Childhood-Onset, Moderate
Axis II	V71.09	No diagnosis
Axis III		None
Axis IV		Death of brother
		Discord with teacher and principal
Axis V	GAF = 50	(current)
	GAF = 72	(highest level in past six months)

Considering the multitude of possibilities, diagnosis can be overwhelming to the novice clinician. This selection process becomes even more taxing when the consequences of the diagnostic decision are considered. Therefore, practitioners often need tools to guide them through the process of using the DSM-IV. The DSM-IV is a differential diagnostic system, in which the clinician uses a hierarchical system to differentiate among criteria to identify the appropriate diagnosis. Figure 13.1 provides an initial framework for using the DSM-IV for Axis I

FIGURE 13.1

Decision tree for DSM-IV

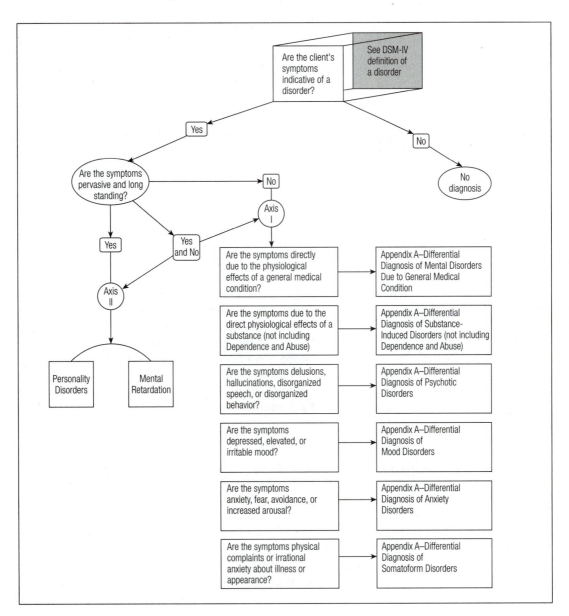

and Axis II diagnosis. In using the DSM-IV, the first question a counselor should consider is whether the client's symptoms and behaviors are indicative of a mental disorder according to the DSM-IV definition that was described earlier. If the answer is no, then the counselor should not go any further because the DSM-IV is only for diagnosing disorders. If the client's symptoms do correspond to the criteria of a disorder, the next question concerns whether the symptoms are pervasive and long standing. If the problems appear to be more pervasive, long standing, and trait-like, then the practitioners would examine Axis II Disorders (Personality Disorders or Mental Retardation). If the symptoms and behaviors appear more florid, then the clinician would be directed to Axis I Disorders. If on the other hand, there is a combination of pervasive personality problems and other more acute clinical symptoms, then the practitioner would examine both Axis I and Axis II Disorders because it is possible to diagnosis on both axes. When considering the symptoms for Axis I diagnoses, Figure 13.1 contains six pertinent questions (e.g., Are the symptoms directly due to the physiological effects of a general medical condition?). If the client's symptoms correspond to the question, then the clinician is referred to the appropriate section of Appendix A of the DSM-IV. Appendix A contains decision trees for the six areas, which can be very helpful to clinicians in determining the appropriate diagnosis.

The DSM-IV is designed to facilitate comprehensive and systematic evaluation. The determination of these diagnoses is important and needs to be performed carefully and with training. Cultural consideration should certainly be taken into account. Within the discussions of the disorders in the DSM-IV, there are some descriptions of the ways culture may affect the symptoms. In addition, the DSM-IV contains an appendix (Appendix I) related to cultural considerations in using the manual. There is an outline for cultural formulation that assists practitioners in considering cultural factors. There is also a glossary of "culture-bound syndromes" contained in Appendix I. These culture-bound syndromes include the name for the condition from the culture in which it was first described and a brief description of the psychopathology. The developers of the DSM-IV were sensitive to cultural issues in diagnosis, but the clinician has the ultimate responsibility to consider the client's cultural context in determining if a diagnosis is warranted.

Instruments Designed to Provide Diagnosis

This chapter is related to the application of assessment results in determining a diagnosis. Many assessment tools and instruments can assist the clinician in making this determination. Certainly, talking with and interviewing the client is one of the major methods for gathering information to determine a diagnosis. There are structured clinical interviews that are designed specifically for diagnostic assessment. At the conclusion of these structured or semi-structured interviews, clinicians should have sufficient information to determine a diagnosis using the DSM-IV. For adults, Vacc and Juhnke (1997) found that two published structured interviews and two published semi-structured interviews were noteworthy. The structured interviews that Vacc and Juhnke recommended were the Composite International Diagnostic Interview: Authorized Core Version 1.0 (CIDI-Core) and the Diagnostic Interview Schedule (DIS). Both of these instruments had good interrater reliability and had undergone extensive review. The CIDI-Core assesses Axis I disorders and is appropriate for those 18 and older. It takes between a half hour and one and a half hours. It can also be administered by clinicians or trained lay interviewers with clinical knowledge or experience. The DIS is designed for diagnosis on all axes of the DSM-IV. This interview does not require clinical judgments; however, the DIS must be administered exactly as given and the trainer must have participated in a training program. The DIS takes an hour to administer.

In terms of semi-structured interviews, Vacc and Juhnke (1997) found the Psychiatric Research Interview for Substance and Mental Disorders (PRISM) and the Structured Clinical Interview for Axis I DSM-IV Disorders (SCID-I) to be psychometrically sound. Once again the interrater reliability coefficients were good to excellent and these instruments were well researched. The PRISM assesses Axis I disorders and antisocial and borderline personality disorders. Trained clinicians usually are the ones to conduct this semi-structured interview, and the amount of time varies depending on the psychopathology. The SCID-I can only be administered by clinicians. It also assesses Axis I disorders and takes about one hour and a half to administer.

There are fewer clinical interviews published for children, yet, it appears that clinicians are increasingly using these tools. Vacc and Juhnke (1997) recommended two structured interviews for children: the Diagnostic Interview for Children and Adolescents (DICA) and the Diagnostic Interview Schedule for Children (DISC-IV). Both of these are structured interviews and can be performed by a clinician or a trained lay person. The DICA assesses a wide range of child and adolescent psychopathology and the DISC-IV assesses Axis I disorders.

There also are standardized instruments that were developed for the specific purpose of assisting in the diagnostic process. One instrument, the Millon Clinical Multiaxial Inventory (MCMI-III), is an interesting combination of a measure based on theory that is also designed to correspond with the DSM-IV. *The Millon Clinical Multiaxial Inventory* (Millon, Millon, & Davis, 1994) is based on Millon's theory of personality, in which he suggested that psychopathology could be described by using two dimensions. The first dimension pertains to the primary source from which individuals gain positive reinforcement or avoid negative reinforcement, which includes the types of Detached, Discordant, Dependent, Independent, and Ambivalent. The second dimension concerns the coping behaviors the client uses, which can be either active or passive. These two dimensions (5 × 2) produce 10 personality disorders that are listed under Clinical Personality Patterns in Figure 13.2. The Severe Personality Patterns are a combination of types within the theory. These two categories are consistent with the diagnoses in Axis II of the DSM-IV. The Clinical

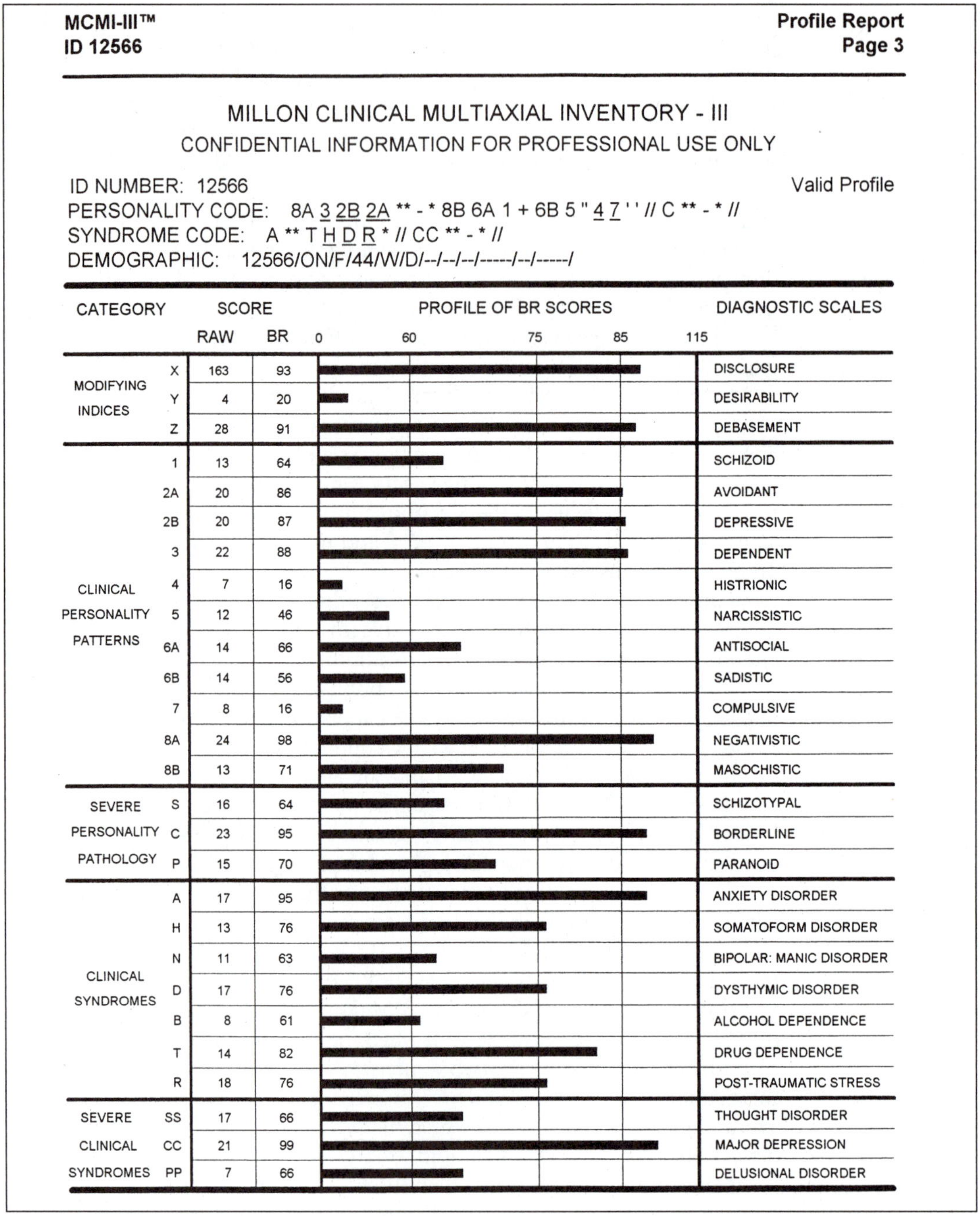

FIGURE 13.2

Profile of the Millon Clinical Multiaxial Inventory

©1994 DICANDRIEN, INC. Published and distributed exclusively by National Computer Systems, Inc., Minneapolis, MN 55440. Reprinted by permission of NCS.

Syndromes and the Severe Syndromes, on the other hand, include many of the disorders coded on Axis I (see Table 13.1). The MCMI-III also includes indices of the examinee's attitudes in the Modifying Indices, which are similar to the Validity Scales of the MMPI-2.

The primary use of the MCMI-III is to differentiate psychiatric disorders, and this focus on differentiation is reflected in the scoring process. The scoring system uses what is called *Base Rates,* which calculate the probability that the client is or is not a member of a particular diagnostic group. The scoring of the MCMI-III is quite complex and can only be done by computer. Rather than using measures such as two standard deviations above the mean to indicate psychopathology, the MCMI-III considers the actual prevalence of disorders in the clinical population. Prevalence rates do vary among settings and there can be some adjustments made in the scoring depending on the setting. It is important to note, however, that an individual's responses on the MCMI-III are compared to psychiatric clients.

For counselors, there are some important factors to consider with the MCMI-III. This instrument is *not* designed for normal functioning adults and should not be used as a general personality inventory. The MCMI-III should be used for diagnostic screening or clinical assessment. In addition, the computer-generated reports are written toward clients with moderate levels of pathology. Hence, for clients with lower ranges of psychological disturbance, the reports will probably overestimate the degree of difficulty. On the other hand, Fong (1995) recommended the use of the MCMI-III over other instruments with clients who may have symptoms of a personality disorder. There is empirical support for using the MCMI-III for diagnosing personality disorders (Craig, 1993). Millon's (1969) theory of personality functioning and psychopathology had an influence in the original formulation of Axis II personality disorders on earlier versions of the DSM. Most master's-level practitioners will not be able to use the MCMI-III unless they are supervised by someone with the appropriate qualifications.

Two other instruments have emerged from Millon's work. One of these is the Millon Adolescent Clinical Inventory (MACI, Millon, Millon, & Davis, 1993), which also is aligned with the DSM-IV diagnostic system. This instrument is appropriate for adolescents, ages 13 through 19. The second instrument, the Millon Index of Personality Styles (MIPS, Millon, 1994), is not for diagnosis or clinical assessment, but is intended for use with normal adults. This instrument incorporates Millon's theory with Jungian theory in an assessment of personality styles.

Summary

When counselors assess clients, the primary purpose is to gather information in order to effectively counsel clients. In determining the issues and problems that exist, the counselor will often either formally or informally diagnose the client. Hence, assessment and diagnosis are often closely connected. Sound assessment information is the precursor to sound diagnostic decision making.

This chapter has focused on the most widely used diagnostic system in mental health settings, the *Diagnostic and Statistical Manual of Mental Disorders— Fourth Edition (DSM-IV)*. The DSM-IV is a multiaxial system, where the practitioner provides information about the client on five axes. Axis I and Axis II are for recording the disorders, with Axis I being for clinical disorders and Axis II for personality disorders or mental retardation. Axis III is where the counselor reports any medical conditions that need to be considered in treatment. Psychosocial and environmental problems are also important to consider in counseling and those are listed on Axis IV. The last axis, Axis V, concerns the overall level of functioning of the client. A diagnosis for a client may not always remain within the confines of a counselor's office (e.g., reporting it on an insurance form). Therefore, clinicians need to be extremely cautious and careful in the diagnostic process. Social and cultural factors need to be examined and considered in this process. Counselors need to thoughtfully examine both the information about clients' behaviors and symptoms and the diagnostic criteria in order to determine appropriate diagnoses.

Issues Related to Assessment with Special Populations

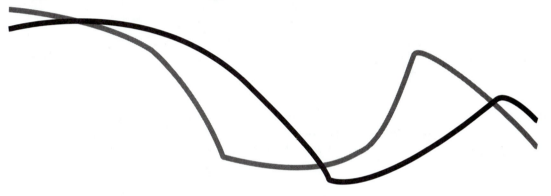

*I*n appraisal, there is the assumption that everyone has an equal opportunity to perform. The assumption may not always be correct, for there may be a variety of reasons why an assessment may be fair to some individuals but not fair to others. Individuals' backgrounds may vary and they may have different experiences and knowledge to draw from while being assessed. For example, let's say that that only people who could sing the Natrona County High School fight song could be hired as counselors in a counseling agency. Many counselors would be able to learn this song but were probably not exposed to it during their counseling classes. When it comes to assessment, questions related to equal opportunity to learn or to be exposed to material can often be an issue. In the case of the Natrona County High School fight song as an employment test, it is clear that those who attended Natrona County High School would have a clear advantage, but in many testing situations the influences of background and culture are not as blatant. Culture has a significant influence on all aspects of the individual, and problems can occur with instruments that do not consider cultural differences. In considering this ludicrous example of the fight song, we might also question its fairness for individuals who for some reason are physically unable to sing. Once again this example is somewhat obvious, but it is designed to make the point that assessments can be used that do not consider individuals from diverse backgrounds or with disabilities.

Knowledge about appraisal techniques with special populations is crucial. Many of the instruments discussed in this book were developed for European-American individuals and the norming groups are primarily made up of European-Americans. There is concern about the misuses of assessment instruments with women, ethnic and racial minorities, limited-standard-English speakers, and the physically challenged (Betz, 1990; Gregory & Lee, 1986). Many counseling-related ethical standards (e.g., the American Counseling Association, the American Psychological Association, and the American Association of Marriage and Family Therapists) contain specific information about assessment with special populations.

Multicultural Assessment

In the field of counseling and psychotherapy, many have proposed that there have been four major influences or four major forces (Ivey, Ivey, & Simek-Morgan, 1993). The first three of the forces have been related to theoretical approaches, which were Psychodynamic foundations, Cognitive-behavioral foundations, and Existential/humanistic foundations. The fourth force is multicultural counseling and therapy. Attending to multicultural issues is important, but there is probably no area within counseling where it is more important than the area of assessment. One of the most controversial issues in assessment concerns whether tests or assessment instruments are fair to individuals from different racial or ethnic groups (Padilla & Medina, 1996). There is, within the field of counseling, some debate on whether the term multicultural is related to only ethnic or cultural variations in groups, or if the term multicultural is broader and incorporates variations from the dominant culture in terms of sexual preference, physical and mental disabilities, and other group differences (Pedersen, 1991). In the first section of this chapter, the term *multicultural* refers to differences in ethnicity, race, and culture. The second section of the chapter, however, addresses some of the issues related to assessment with individuals who may be suffering from some physical disability.

The issues related to multicultural assessment become particularly pertinent because there is variation among different racial or ethnic groups on their average performance on some assessment instruments. For example, there are racial differences in how groups perform on instruments commonly used for employee selection (Gottfredson, 1994). In general, African-Americans tend to do less well than European-Americans and have a higher rate of failing these exams. This same trend is also found in intelligence or cognitive ability testing, with African-Americans scoring almost a standard deviation below European-Americans. The average scores for Hispanics or Latinos on intelligence tests tend to be between the average scores for African-Americans and European-Americans. There is some controversy concerning the average intelligence test scores for Asian-American individuals; however, there is consensus that their achievement scores far exceed the projection based on intelligence assessment (Neisser et al., 1996).

Although there are differences in average performance among ethnic groups, those findings should not be interpreted as indicating that any group is more culturally advantaged and other groups are culturally disadvantaged. As Sattler (1993) argued, "No one has the right to degrade a subculture because it does not conform to the patterns of the majority group. Different cultural mores and traditions expressed by minority groups may be both healthy and adaptive, for the lifestyles of these groups differ markedly from those of the majority culture" (p. 565). Furthermore, the reasons for ethnic differences on aptitude and intelligence tests are difficult to ascertain and are not due to one simplistic explanation. Research in this area indicates that both nature and nurture are intertwined in a complex relationship where biological, cultural, sociological, and environmental factors have an interactional effect on individuals' performances on these instruments (Neisser et al., 1996).

Individuals from different cultures vary in many ways, including their ways of viewing the world. According to Dana (1993), *worldview* involves group identity, individual identity, beliefs, values, and language. Worldview influences all perceptions and, thus, influences not only what is learned but also how people learn. Therefore, clients' culture and worldview can affect their performance on traditional achievement, aptitude, and ability tests. Assessment in the affective domain may also be influenced, because clients' worldviews influence responses to questions, nonverbal behaviors, and communication styles. Counselors need to understand differences in worldview in order to work effectively with diverse clients.

One of the factors to consider in multicultural assessment is the influence of culture and language. A postmodern perspective would suggest that language has a pervasive influence that affects perceptions of reality. The influence of language needs to be considered in the assessment techniques most commonly used by counselors, which are primarily verbal techniques such as questioning, clarifying, and reflecting. Cultures differ, for example, in terms of the degree to which self-disclosure, particularly to a nonfamily member, is encouraged. An insensitive counselor may perceive the client's reticence as resistant rather than due to cultural differences, which could encourage misunderstandings and problems in the relationship. The counseling process is predominantly a verbal process and the subtle influences on language need to be considered by a multiculturally competent practitioner.

Today, counselors need to be prepared to work with clients from diverse backgrounds. There are some projections that Anglo or European-Americans will constitute 50% or less of the population by the year 2050 (U.S. Bureau of Census, 1990). Assessment of clients from different ethnic and cultural backgrounds is complex and needs to be performed with professional care and consideration. Counselors need to be able to evaluate instruments that may be biased against certain groups and identify other methods for assessing these clients. In addition, counselors need to be competent in using assessment results with clients from diverse cultures appropriately. Using an instrument that is not culturally appropriate for clients can be problematic, for there are instances in which a lack of cultural sensitivity in the assessment process has resulted in clients being harmed. Counselors can expect to work with clients from cultures other than their own and they need to be skilled with cross-cultural assessment.

Types of Instrument Bias

In appraisal, it is assumed that all individuals are given an equal opportunity to demonstrate their capabilities or level of functioning during the assessment process. Even an instrument that is designed to be culturally sensitive and fair may be unfair depending on the circumstances of how it is used or with certain groups of individuals. The term **bias testing** refers to the degree that construct-irrelevant factors systematically affect a group's performance. Thus, there are factors not related to the purpose of the instrument that influence either positively or negatively a group's performance. Given the consequences of using a biased instrument, it is important for counselors to know how to evaluate instruments for possible bias.

Content bias. Instruments may be biased in terms of the content being more familiar or appropriate for one group as compared to another group. As an example, let's imagine that an intelligence test has a question regarding what is the state bird of Wyoming. Many individuals would have difficulty remembering this piece of trivia; however, if you went to school in Wyoming, you could probably answer that the Wyoming state bird is the Meadowlark. Thus, individuals from Wyoming would have an advantage on this intelligence test over individuals from other states. The biased content may be subtler than the Wyoming state bird question. For example, some groups could perceive items as irrelevant or not engaging. Children living below the poverty level may see little relevance in a question concerning how long it will take an airplane to fly from Point A to Point B when these children cannot imagine ever having the financial resources to fly on an airplane. Children may be less likely to engage in questions when the names and circumstances on the test are always associated with the majority culture. Bracken and Barona (1991) found evidence to suggest that children from different cultural backgrounds interpret test items differently.

In evaluating an instrument for content bias, the practitioner needs to examine the procedures used in developing the instrument. Haphazard selection of instrument content may result in an instrument with content bias. There needs to be specific attention to multicultural issues during the initial stages of instrument development. Instrument developers should document in the manual the steps they took to guard against content bias. Care in writing items that appear nonbiased may not be sufficient. A common procedure is to have a panel made up of diverse individuals review the instrument. Nevertheless, content bias can be difficult to uncover because subtle biases may not always appear by simply examining the instrument.

Often statistical methods are employed in order to supplement the review of the content. One statistical method for investigating item bias that has received increasing attention is **differential item functioning** (DIF). Differential item functioning is a method for analyzing the relative difficulty of individual items for different racial or ethnic groups. Although there are different methods for performing differential item functioning, these methods strive to examine differences in performance among individuals who are equal in ability but are from different groups. If an item is found to have unequal probabilities for responding correctly from certain groups with equal ability, then the item may be biased. Sometimes, however, statistical artifacts can result in group differences rather than the item being biased. Although DIF techniques have been very useful in identifying and eliminating individual items on specific instruments, these techniques have not identified common themes or characteristics of items that are prone to bias. Advances are being made in this area, and hopefully research will soon shed light on methods for developing unbiased items.

Internal structure. Another method for detecting possible instrument bias is to examine the internal structure of the instrument. For instance, an instrument's reliability coefficients for one ethnic group could be very high, while for another ethnic group the reliability coefficients could be significantly lower. Thus, an instrument can be a reliable measure for one client but not a reliable measure for another client. Well-developed instruments will investigate this problem and present reliability information for different groups in the manual. Typically, researchers investigate differences between males and females and different ethnic groups. The investigation of differences in reliability among different ethnic groups will depend on the size and representation of the norming group. Hence, if there are problems with the makeup of the norming group in terms of minority participants, then it is difficult to analyze differences in reliability.

Examination of internal structure as related to instrument bias can also involve the factor structure of an instrument. As we saw in Chapters 6 through 11, many instruments and tests used in counseling have subscales (e.g., Verbal and Performances IQs). It is important for researchers to determine if the dimensions or factors underlying the instrument are different for different groups. For example in personality instruments, the factor structure for an ethnic group may not match the subscales of the instrument and it would not be appropriate to interpret those subscales in the typical manner. Practitioners need to examine the research related to the factor structure of an instrument with subscales in order to determine if it is appropriate to interpret the scores of the subscales with clients from diverse backgrounds.

Instrument and criterion relationships. The analyses of possible bias should also include studies related to the relationship between the instrument and the criterion for different groups. As an example, an instrument may be highly related to job performance for one ethnic group but have a low relationship for another ethnic group. It is important to examine the differences among the validity coefficients, not just whether the validity coefficients are statistically significant for one group and not significant for another group. Statistical significance is influenced by sample size and, typically, the sample size is large for Whites or European-Americans and small for Blacks or African-Americans. With correlation, the smaller the sample, the larger the correlation coefficient needs to be in order to be significant. Therefore, the exact same validity coefficients for these two groups could be significant for European-Americans and not significant for African-Americans. Most of the research related to ethnic differences in validity coefficients has compared African-Americans and European-Americans. For some of the more widely used employment selection instruments, Hunter, Schmidt, and Hunter (1979) found that the validity coefficients were not significantly different. In a review of achievement measures, Linn (1978) did not find significant differences between the validity coefficients for these two groups. Very few studies, however, have examined the differences in validity coefficients for Hispanics and other ethnic groups.

Significant differences in validity coefficients can have a notable effect if the instrument is used for selection or predictive purposes. The statistical technique of regression is often used for selection, and when there are different validity coefficients, the instrument can vary in how well it predicts to the criterion for the different groups. If an instrument yields validity coefficients that are significantly different for two or more groups, then this difference is described as **slope bias**. Figure 14.1 reflects slope bias, because, as you can see, the same score on the instrument would predict *different* performance on the criterion depending on whether you were in the green group or the blue group. In this example, a score of 20 by a green individual would predict a grade of a little over a C, whereas for a blue individual a score of 20 would predict a grade between D and F. In cases of slope bias, some experts in the field of assessment have suggested using separate regression equations for the different groups. As we will see in Chapter 15, however, there are certain situations in which legislation has prohibited the use of separate regression equations for different ethnic groups.

Even instruments with the same validity coefficient can predict different criterion scores for members of different groups with the *same score*. If you examine Figure 14.2, the regression lines for the green and the blue groups are parallel, which indicates that the validity coefficients are the same. The lines, however, differ in where they begin on the y-axis; hence, the **intercepts** are different. As we examine the first illustration in Figure 14.2, we see that a score of 20 on the instrument predicts a grade slightly above D for an individual from the blue group and that same score predicts a grade of almost a B for someone from the green group. Thus, using a cutoff score of 20 provides an advantage to

FIGURE 14.1

Slope bias

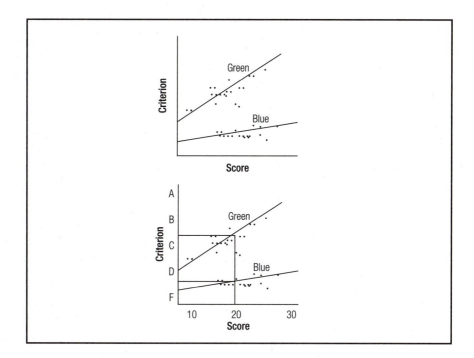

the blue group. As the second illustration in Figure 14.2 reflects, in using the intercept for the blue group, an individual from this group would need a score of almost 30 in order to be predicted to receive a grade of C. Numerous studies have found that there are no intercept differences among ethnic groups on many of the instruments in counseling (Anastasi & Urbina, 1997). Some researchers have found that when there are differences among majority and minority groups, majority group members tend to have higher intercepts than minority members do. Majority groups have been found to have higher intercepts for some instruments that predict college grades (Duran, 1983) and job performance (Hunter, Schmidt, & Hunter, 1979). Thus, in adapting Figure 14.2, the

FIGURE 14.2

Intercept bias

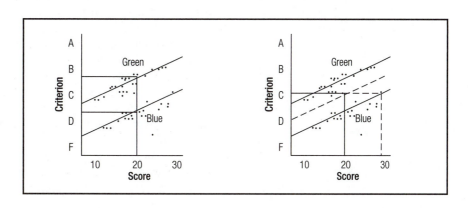

majority group members would be the green group and the minority members would be the blue group. Therefore, these instruments would overpredict minority individual performance rather than underpredict their performance.

The previous section addressed methods for examining whether the instrument is biased. It is possible for an assessment instrument to have culturally sensitive content, almost identical validity coefficients for ethnic groups, and the same intercepts, yet produce very different scores for individuals from different ethnic groups. In the discussion of ability, achievement, and aptitude testing, minority individuals tended to have average scores lower than majority individuals on many of the instruments. Some of these instruments may not be biased, but the result of using these instruments has a disparate or negative impact on some minority individuals.

Differences in Test Performance and Culture

There are various opinions as to the causes for racial differences in test performance. The term *test* is used in this context because most of the debate has concerned differences in ability, achievement, and aptitude testing. It should be noted, however, that occasionally there are also ethnic differences on some personality instruments. Some have argued that the differences are primarily innate and little can be done to remedy this situation (Jensen 1969, 1980). Others have argued that environmental factors are the major reason for the discrepant scores among racial groups. Unequal access to educational and stimulating experiences influences test performance. Those arguing for this perspective contend that tests highlight the unfairness of life, not the unfairness of tests. Helms (1992) proposed that a culturalist perspective provides more insight into differences in ethnic groups, particularly as related to the comparative meaning on cognitive ability tests, when examinees' race or ethnicity is an issue.

Helms (1992) argued that cultural bias and cultural equivalence need to be examined. *Cultural bias* refers to test bias, which is determined using the methods identified previously. *Cultural equivalence* refers to whether the *constructs* have similar meanings within and across cultures. The concept of cultural equivalence being tied to meaning is important, for counselors may not understand that the results could be meaningful in one culture but have a different meaning for individuals from another culture. Thus, an instrument could be measuring intelligence for participants from one ethnic group but not measuring intelligence for another ethnic group. Certainly many, if not most, of the instruments used in counseling were developed by White professionals who were socialized both personally and professionally in the European or European-American culture. Within this culture are values and beliefs that affect assessment, such as competitiveness, individualism, action orientation, and belief in linear problem solving.

For a time, some professionals in assessment focused on developing *culture-free* assessments. In general, experts in the field of assessment concluded that, as of yet, there is *no* culture-free assessment device. Even with nonverbal tests, such as putting puzzles together or deciphering matrices, there are cultural components that influence performance. Because it has been impossible to develop an instrument void of any cultural influences, attempts have been made to develop *culture-fair* instruments. Within the field of assessment, some individuals contend that there are culturally fair instruments, while others suggest that an instrument has yet to be developed that is culturally fair to all individuals.

Recommendations for Practice

Counselors can expect to be involved in either formal or informal assessment of clients from cultures other than their own. The population of the United States is changing and the percentage of minority individuals is increasing. Padilla and Medina (1996) suggested that practitioners may not be aware of how their linguistic, social class, and cultural experiences influence their construction of knowledge, selection of particular tests, and interpretation derived from assessment procedures. Thus, counselors need to find methods for effective cross-cultural assessment. One excellent resource for counselors is the *Multicultural Assessment Standards: A Compilation for Counselors* (Prediger, 1994). This resource is a compilation of standards related to multicultural assessment from five source documents (namely, *Code of Fair Testing Practice in Education, Responsibilities of Users of Standardized Tests* (the RUST statement), *Standards for Educational and Psychological Testing, Multicultural Competencies and Standards: A Call to the Profession,* and *Ethical Standards of the American Counseling Association*). This resource is also being revised in order to reflect changes in standards and ethical codes.

Even though an instrument may be of high quality, that does not mean that it can be used with all ethnic or racial groups. There are unique issues in assessment with clients from diverse cultural backgrounds. Practitioners should *not* attempt to evaluate clients with diverse backgrounds when the clients are outside the counselor's range of academic training or supervised experience. If the counselor is unable to refer or feels that referral would be detrimental to the client, then the counselor needs to gain both knowledge about assessment procedures and information about the client's background characteristics. Culturally, sensitivity assessment cannot be accomplished by following a few guidelines, for it requires careful deliberation concerning a number of factors. The following summary is an attempt to coalesce pertinent information related to culturally sensitive assessment in counseling.

Selection of assessment instruments: content considerations. The counselor needs to clearly identify a client's cultural group and the purpose of the testing or assessment. Once the counselor has acquired this information then he or she should thoroughly review available information in order to determine the appropriate assessment procedures. In evaluating instruments, practitioners need to determine whether a common instrument or different instruments are required for accurate measurement. The counselor, however, should be aware that the use of different instruments for cultural, ethnic, and racial groups may not be effective in correcting for differences. A thorough review performed by the counselor should include evaluating the procedures used by the instrument developers to avoid potentially insensitive content or language. Furthermore, attention should be given to how the instrument handles variation in motivation, working speed, language facility, and individuals' experiential backgrounds, and possible bias in the response to its content. Practitioners also need to consider language and the appropriate language for the assessment. If an instrument is recommended for linguistically diverse populations, then the counselor should expect to find in the manual appropriate information for the proper use and interpretation of that instrument (e.g., illustrations of case studies and examples of interpretative material for diverse clients).

Selection of assessment instruments: norming, reliability, and validity considerations. In using a norm-referenced instrument with any client, a counselor needs to evaluate the suitability of the norming group. The American Counseling Association's *Code of Ethics and Standards of Practice* (ACA, 1995) states that a counselor should be cautious in interpreting the results from clients who are not represented in the norming group on which an instrument was standardized. Priority needs to be given to attempts to ensure fairness to individuals from different races, genders, or ethnic backgrounds (Prediger, 1994). A counselor needs to scrutinize the standardization and norming procedures for relevance to the client or clients. Current norming groups are typically more diverse than previously, with consideration given to representation from ethic and racial groups (Betz, 1990). One also has to be careful with categories for race and ethnicity. People from very similar backgrounds may categorize themselves in very different manners. A self-report of group membership does not provide sufficient information, for the acculturation of individuals often varies greatly even though they may report the same group membership (Betz & Fitzgerald, 1995; Dana, 1993). Often with norm-referenced instruments, information about the ethnicity of the norming group is gathered only by individuals' reporting their racial background.

The clinician should also evaluate the documented evidence related to the instrument appropriateness (e.g., reliability and validity) for individuals with similar characteristics to the client(s). Evaluating instruments involves reviewing the data provided by the publisher on the performance of individuals from different races, genders, and ethnic backgrounds. Counselors also need to consider whether the sample sizes are sufficient for the different groups. Any performance differences found among different groups should be investigated to determine if these differences are caused by inappropriate characteristics of the instrument.

When instruments are used for clinical purposes (e.g., diagnosis, placement in educational programs, treatment selection), then there should be criterion-related validity evidence for populations similar to the client (Moreland, 1996). This is particularly important if the recommendations or decisions are considered to have an actuarial and clinical basis. If there seems to be predictive bias as indicated by differences among groups in the instrument's ability to predict performance, then there also should be investigations into the magnitude of the predictive bias. When instruments suggest or imply career options for clients, counselors also need to examine information related to how the sample distributes in the actual occupational areas in terms of gender and racial or ethnic groups. Due to the limitations of many formal instruments, Goldman (1990, 1992) has championed the use of qualitative techniques with diverse clients.

Administration and scoring of assessment instruments. Participation in assessment can be a new and exciting experience or can stimulate anxiety or frustration for some individuals. A practitioner should consider the effects of examiner-examinee differences in ethnic and cultural background, attitudes, and values based on relevant research. A counselor needs to be able to administer instruments using verbal clarity, calmness, empathy for the examinees, and impartiality toward all being assessed. In addition, unusual circumstances peculiar to the administration and scoring of an instrument should be evaluated (Prediger, 1994).

The examiner's attitudes and nonverbal behaviors during the administration of an instrument can have a subtle influence. The degree of rapport between the administrator and examinee can be particularly important with minority clients influence (Keitel, Kopala, & Adamson, 1996). Methods for establishing rapport will vary depending on the cultural background of the client. Common methods for establishing rapport, such as eye contact and leaning forward, may not be appropriate with clients from diverse backgrounds. For example, Sue and Sue (1977) found that many Asian-American women are uncomfortable with clinician's efforts to make eye contact.

Use/interpretation of assessment results. Culturally skilled counselors understand how race, culture, ethnicity, and so forth may affect assessment in different areas. When using instruments, the counselor needs to examine the possibility that a client's group membership (e.g., socioeconomic status, gender, and subculture) may affect test performance and, consequently, validity. Counselors need to understand the technical aspects and culture limitations of instruments. In interpreting results, knowledge of the instrument needs also to be matched with thorough knowledge about the client.

In interpreting assessment results, counselors must have comprehensive knowledge about each client's culture (Hinkle, 1994; Hood & Johnson, 1997). Knowledge of a culture, however, does not mean viewing any client in a stereotypic manner. Enormous variation exists among individuals from different cultures. Culture is an important facet, but appropriate assessment involves analyzing comprehensive information in order to provide a more holistic view. In working with multicultural clients, there are two areas that are extremely important for counselors to consider, which are the client's level of acculturation and socioeconomic status.

Dana (1993) suggested that an initial step in the process of assessment is to ascertain the extent to which the original culture has been retained as well as the extent to which acculturation to the dominant society and worldview has occurred. Acculturation entails changes in an individual's psychological patterns as a result of contact with a culture different from their original one (Berry, 1980). People vary in terms of the degree of acculturation, and the interpretation of assessment results needs to consider this factor. For example, even though a client may become fluent in English, that does not mean that his or her value system and personal orientation becomes consistent with the dominant European-American culture. Unless the counselor understands the client's level of acculturation, it is not possible to understand how he or she sees the world. Dana (1993) suggested using level of acculturation as a moderator variable in interpreting results.

Another important factor to consider in interpreting assessment results is socioeconomic background. Socioeconomic status is particularly critical because some researchers have found that it has more influence on test performance than either ethnicity or instrument bias (Bond, 1990; Groth-Marnat, 1997). Researchers have found that differences on intelligence tests and on the MMPI dissipate when African-Americans and European-Americans of equal socioeconomic status are compared. Counselors need to be careful that knowledge about a client's culture does not turn into stereotypes. For example, not all African-American clients were raised in poor households. Appropriate multicultural assessment involves considering multiple factors in interpreting the results and incorporating other information in evaluating the usefulness of those results.

Counselors also need to provide an orientation to clients both prior to and after the administration of a test. This orientation needs to include an explanation as to how the results function with other relevant factors. The intent is that clients have a proper perspective on the results in connection with other factors, including recognizing the effects of socioeconomic, ethnic, and cultural factors on test scores. In some situations, clinicians should describe to clients or their parents/guardians the procedures for registering any complaint in order to have problems resolved. Culturally skilled counselors interpret results with knowledge of potential bias, while keeping in mind the cultural and linguistic characteristics of the clients. As the above guidelines suggest, counselors cannot be culturally competent unless they understand the client, the client's culture, and the strengths and limitations of using that assessment device.

Linguistic Background and Appraisal

The issues related to cross-cultural assessment are complex, but the issues increase in complexity when language and nonnative speakers are considered in the assessment process. Language skills almost always have some degree of influence on performance on an assessment device. For example, reading or listening skills are typically needed to hear the instructions for the test or read the instructions. Even with arithmetic or mathematical assessment, most tests require the examinee to read the items. There are cultural differences in terms of language proficiency and these differences in proficiency may introduce irrelevant factors into the assessment process. For some examinees, their results on a test may be more of a reflection of their proficiency with English than their ability in mathematics. These linguistical factors become even more crucial when important decisions are made based on assessment results. Therefore, special attention to language and cultural background often needs to be considered in any assessment.

Clients vary in their abilities with the dominant language in this culture, which often contributes to difficulties in performing culturally fair assessments. Counselors have a responsibility to ensure that all examinees be given the same opportunities to demonstrate their level of competence on the attributes being assessed. In our culture, when English is a client's second language, the counselor needs to consider numerous factors in order to ensure fair assessment. One of the factors to consider is the purpose of the testing or assessment. If the purpose is to evaluate English proficiency, then there may be little need for adaptation of the testing situation. For example, if the successful job performance requires the ability to communicate in English (e.g., technical writer), then it may be legitimate to use a test that assesses ability to write in English. There are, however, a number of occupations for which the ability to communicate in English is not required. It is very rare that a clear distinction can be made concerning the influences of language and how to assess clients appropriately. Take for example, the identification of a learning disability with a child whose dominant language is Spanish. It is sometimes difficult to decipher when the assessment results are related to language issues and when there is evidence of a learning disability. Assessment of individuals in a situation where there is a question of language proficiency requires special attention to administration, scoring, and interpretation.

Instrument translation, adaptation, and modification. Sometimes individuals will consider simply translating an existing instrument into the language of the nonnative speaker in order to assess the person fairly. A simple translation will usually not suffice because there are many issues that need to be attended to in the translation. First, simple translations typically do not take into account different cultural considerations. As Bracken and Barona (1991) documented, there are often problems with translating instruments. First, test directions are often not easy to translate because the directions are often psychotechnical, stilted, and abstract. Second, practitioners rarely translate back to the original after translating the instrument to the second language. This practice can be very helpful in determining if the meaning is retained in the translating process. Third, some of the psychological variables assessed in instruments are not universal across cultures. For example, an instrument could assess ability to make decisions independently, which is a value not held by all cultures. Fourth, even for established instruments, there are no well-established procedures or standards for evaluating translations. In order to translate an instrument, experts would need to consider that the translation is equivalent to the original in terms of content, difficulty level, and reliability. They would also need to study the validity of the translation to see if it could be used in the same circumstances as the original instrument. Test publishers should describe the process of translating an instrument and provide information on the reliability and validity of the translated instrument. Even if care is taken in translating an instrument, one cannot assume that clients' cultural experiences are comparable. For example, an item on an interest inventory on liking to go the opera may have little relevancy for an adolescent from rural Pakistan.

These same difficulties apply to attempts to adapt or modify an assessment for a nonnative speaker. Counselors should not attempt to adapt or modify an assessment. If linguistic modifications are recommended by the publisher, the research supporting the modification and the modification methods should be described in detail in the manual (Prediger, 1994). If the research supports the modifications, the practitioner should follow the procedures unless other research indicates there are procedures that are more appropriate. Potential problems can be avoided if practitioners thoroughly evaluate the existing research on assessment with nonnative speakers.

Issues related to instrument use and interpretation. There are instruments that are available in multiple languages, and with some multilingual individuals, it is difficult to determine which language is appropriate to use in testing. According to the Individuals with Disabilities Education Act (IDEA), which was last reauthorized in 1997, an individual should be assessed in his or her most proficient language. An exception is allowed when the purpose of the assessment is to determine a level of proficiency in a certain language (e.g., English). It is important for counselors to remember that assessing individuals in their most proficient language does not guarantee a comprehensive and fair assessment. Bilingual individuals are likely to be specialized by domain (e.g., they use one language in home and social environments and another language in academic and work environments). Therefore, an assessment in either one of the languages is likely to measure some domains but miss out on others that are primarily related to the other language. Yansen and Shulman (1996) suggested that better information can be gathered if bilingual individuals are assessed in both languages. Interpretation of results from nonnative speakers should be done cautiously. Even with instruments that are designed for cross-cultural assessment, the counselor must are aware of appropriate uses and limitations.

Assessment of Individuals with Disabilities

In assessment, individuals with disabilities may also be adversely affected by certain assessment procedures. For example, if a person has become quadriplegic, it would be difficult to perform the Block Design portion of the WAIS-III because of the limitations with motor dexterity. The likelihood of a counselor having a client with a physical disability is high, as the Center of Disease Control and Prevention

(1994) estimated that one in five individuals over 15 years old in the United States suffers from a physical disability. There are special legal issues related to assessment with individuals with disabilities that will be discussed in Chapter 15.

Assessment of Individuals with Visual Impairments

Many of the assessment tools used in counseling involve reading; yet, for individuals with visual impairments, this is problematic. The most likely solution to this problem is often to have someone read the instrument to him or her. Individuals' reading of the assessment material, however, can vary dramatically in terms of tone, speed, and clarity of speech. The variations in reading can affect the reliability of the instrument and have an impact on individuals' performance. Counselors cannot just randomly adapt an assessment instrument for an individual with a disability, because it will introduce error into the assessment. In order to diminish the amount of error, counselors need to research the procedures for using that specific assessment instrument with an individual with a disability. This step of researching procedures is true for any client with a disability, not just clients with visual impairments. With many well-known instruments, researchers have studied the most effective methods for adapting the instrument in order to eliminate potential sources of error. For example, there are procedures for adapting the WISC-III for individuals with visual impairment that utilize most of the Verbal Subscales. Other instruments have prerecorded tapes that read the instruments in a systematic manner. In addition, many of the personality inventories have Braille or large-print versions.

It is important to remember that vision impairments can vary in severity. If a counselor suspects that a visual impairment might be affecting the assessment process, then he or she should investigate that possibility. Children may not be aware that they have a problem with their vision. Sattler (1993) suggested that the following may indicate a visual problem with children:

- Rubs eyes excessively
- Shuts or covers one eye, tilts head, or leans forward
- Has difficulty in reading or loses place while reading
- Moves head excessively when reading
- Squints eyelids or frowns
- Blinks more than expected or is irritable when doing close visual work
- Avoids close visual work
- Has poor posture while reading
- Has difficulty judging distances
- Complains of dizziness, headaches, or nausea following close visual work
- Has recurring sties
- Reports itching, burning, or scratchy eyes
- Has red-rimmed, encrusted, or swollen eyelids
- Tires easily after visual work

If there is a question about a client's vision, then he or she should be referred to an optometrist or an ophthalmologist.

When clients who have a visual impairment are being assessed in the areas of personality and career interests, it is important that clients answer the questions related to what they enjoy and like to do rather than what they are capable of doing. A problem with many intelligence and general ability tests is the lack of appropriate norms for individuals with severe visual impairments. A recent adaptation of the Stanford-Binet is the Perkins-Binet Tests of Intelligence for the Blind, which is standardized on separate forms for partially sighted and blind children. One of the few instruments developed specifically for visually impaired individuals is the Blind Learning Aptitude Test.

Assessment of Individuals with Hearing Impairments

Assessing individuals with hearing impairments involves a different set of problems than assessing individuals with visual impairments. Hearing has a direct link to language acquisition, and verbal content is embedded in many of the methods by which individuals are assessed. Sometimes in the past, hearing-impaired children were tested using instruments involving reading, without an understanding of the connection between hearing and reading. It is often difficult to decipher aptitude and ability separately from the verbal handicap. In recent years, gains have been made in identifying children with hearing problems earlier and initiating beneficial educational interventions sooner. Nevertheless, in using assessment results in counseling with clients with hearing disabilities, counselors need to consider the magnitude of the hearing loss, the age of onset of the problem, the effects of the loss on language acquisition, and whether the loss is affecting adjustment.

The Wechlser scales have been used extensively with hearing-impaired children. There are also more instruments with norms for individuals with hearing impairments than for those with visual impairments. For example, the WISC-R has established norms for individuals with hearing impairments. The Hiskey-Nebraska Test of Learning Aptitude was developed and standardized for children with hearing impairments, including children who are deaf. The norming group information was gathered in the 1960s, but the instrument has better reliability and validity evidence than many other tools used with individuals with hearing impairments (Sullivan & Burley, 1990).

In terms of assessment in the affective domain, counselors need to ensure that clients with hearing impairments comprehend the questions. Sometimes, particularly with children, they may give the impression they understand what is being discussed when, in fact, they are confused. There are also some indications that individuals with hearing impairments have a tendency to respond in concrete terms to projective techniques or more abstract counseling questions. Counselors may enlist the use of an interpreter or use sign language themselves. There are, however, variations in types of sign languages, and individuals with hearing impairments vary in their proficiency with sign language.

Assessment of Individuals with Motor Disabilities

Imagine for a minute that you are able to understand what is being asked of you on a test, but you are unable to make your body physically respond and complete the required task. Individuals with motor disabilities are often faced with this exact situation, for they may immediately realize how to put the puzzle pieces together but they are unable to do so quickly. The methods used to assess clients with motor impairment, as with all clients, will vary depending on the information needed. Sometimes the intent of the testing is to assess where their strengths and limitations are in order to determine possible careers and to identify areas where accommodations can be made. In cases like this, clients may be compared to a normal sample rather than a special norm, because they will be competing with people without disabilities for jobs. Sometimes examiners will perform certain assessments with clients with motor disabilities twice; once, using the specified time limits and, a second time, without time limits, to determine if they can perform the tasks. A well-written psychological report will identify any departures from the standardized procedures and discuss how the violations will influence the results.

There are a number of methods for assessing intelligence or general ability with individuals with motor disabilities. One commonly used method involves picture vocabulary tests, in which the individual simply points to the correct answer. The pictures eliminate the problems associated with reading, and the pointing is not timed and eliminates many of the problems associated with motor coordination difficulties. The *Peabody Picture Vocabulary Test—Third Edition* (PPVT-III, Dunn & Dunn, 1997) is the most commonly used of these types of instruments. The PPVT-III takes about 11 to 12 minutes to administer. The examinee is presented with a plate with four pictures. The examiner says a stimulus word and the examinee responds by pointing to the appropriate picture. PPVT-III scores are similar to other measures of intelligence, with a mean of 100 and a standard deviation of 15. A measure of expressive vocabulary and word retrieval, the Expressive Vocabulary Test, is also conormed with the PPVT-III to allow for comparisons of receptive and expressive vocabulary.

Sampson (1990) discussed how computer technology can be used to adapt assessment devices so that individuals with disabilities can complete instruments with little outside assistance. Examples of computer technology used are voice inputs, simplified keyboards, pneumatic controls, joysticks, head pointers, and Braille keyboards. These devices can eliminate an intermediary who reads and/or responds to the test items for the examinee. An example of a work samples assessment that has been adapted for the computer is the Pesco 2001.

Assessment of Individuals with Cognitive Impairments

The assessment of individuals with mental retardation falls within the area of assessment of cognitive impairments. Counselors usually do not perform the testing related to the determination of mental retardation, but it is important from them to have an understanding of this area. Rather than viewing mental retardation as a trait, a current view focuses on the interaction between the limitations of the individual and the demands of the environment. The American Association of Mental Retardation (AAMR, 1992) stated that "mental retardation refers to substantial limitations in present functioning. It is characterized by significantly subaverage intellectual functioning, existing concurrently with related limitations in two or more of the following applicable adaptive skill areas: communication, self-care, home living, social skills, community use, self-direction, health and safety, functional academics, leisure, and work" (p. 1). The AAMR's definition also stated that these conditions must be present before the age of 18. The classification system suggested by the American Association of Mental Retardation is listed in Table 14.1. The AAMR's system is different from previously used classifications and the method suggested in DSM-IV, where the categories are mild, moderate, severe, and profound. In examining the current AAMR classification system in Table 14.1, you will notice that the focus is on intensity of support needed rather than on level of retardation.

No matter which classification system is used, the assessment of retardation typically involves an individual test of intelligence (e.g., the WISC-III or the Stanford-Binet) and a measure of adaptive behavior. The *Vineland Adaptive Behavior Scales* are often used by psychologists to measure adaptive behavior. There are three versions of the Vineland that can be used in combination or alone: the Interview Edition, Survey Form (Sparro, Balla, & Cicchetti, 1984a); the Interview Edition, Expanded Form (Sparro, Balla, & Cicchetti, 1984b); and the Classroom Edition (Sparro, Balla, & Cicchetti, 1985). The interviews are semi-structured in nature and are given to either the parents or the caregivers, while the Classroom Edition is a questionnaire completed by a teacher. The major domains assessed in the Vineland are Communication, Daily Living Skills, Socialization, and Motor Skills. Another measure of adaptive behavior is the Adaptive Behavior Scale, in which there is a version for adults and a version for children ages 3 to 18.

Another major area of assessment related to cognitive impairments is *neuropsychological assessment*. Neuropsychological assessment concerns assessing

TABLE 14.1

The American Association of Mental Retardation's (1992) Classification System

Intermittent	Individuals in this category need support on an "as needed basis." This category is characterized by support being needed of an episodic nature, persons not always needing the support(s), or short-term support being needed during life-span transitions. The intermittent support may be of high or low intensity when provided.
Limited	This category is classified by an intensity of support that is characterized as consistent over time. The support can be time limited but it is not of an intermittent nature. The support may require fewer staff members and be less costly than more intense levels of support (e.g., time-limited employment training or transitional support during the school-to-adult transition.).
Extensive	The support is characterized by regular involvement (e.g., daily) in at least some environments (such as home or work). Also, the support is not time limited and can include long-term support.
Pervasive	The support in this category is characterized as consistent and high intensity. The support needs to be provided across environments and be of a life-sustaining nature. Pervasive support usually involves more staff members and intrusion than do extensive or time-limited support.

Reprinted by permission.

the behavioral effects of possible brain injury or damage. Brain damage can result from injury or disease, or it can be organic. Insults to the nervous system are often associated with cognitive dysfunctions, such as memory difficulties, but can also have an effect on personality and temperament. Once again, a counselor will not be performing neuropsychological testing , but a counselor needs an overview of the typical process in order to know when to refer clients for neuropsychological assessment.

Clients who display abrupt mental or behavioral changes should be referred for a neuropsychological assessment. An evaluation is also probably warranted if the changes are more subtle, such as individuals exhibiting mild memory changes, borderline EEG, attention lapses, speech disturbances, and motor dysfunction (Swiercinsky, 1978). It is also wise for a client to be evaluated if there is any suspected trauma to the brain resulting from illness or injury. For instance, clients should be referred for a neurological screening if an injury results in their losing consciousness.

Neuropsychologists often administer a battery of tests to clients, because no one test can detect the diversity of brain dysfunctions. These batteries were designed to systematically assess a broad spectrum of neurological functioning. Two of the most commonly used assessment batteries for neuropsychological testing are the *Halstead-Reitan Neuropsychological Test Battery* and the *Luria-Nebraska Neuropsychological Battery*. The Halstead-Reitan takes about 6 to 8 hours to administer and typically also involves administering either the WISC-III or the WAIS-III. The Luria-Nebraska Neuropsychological Battery takes about two and a half hours to administer and is designed to assess a broad range of neurological impairments.

These specifically designed neuropsychological batteries are not the only methods used in this area. Neuropsychologists will often use individual measures of intelligence or specific subscales (e.g., Digit Span of the WAIS-III) as a part of the assessment process. Another commonly used instrument is the *Bender Visual Motor Gestalt Test,* usually referred to as the Bender-Gestalt Test. The Bender-Gestalt test consists of nine cards, with each card containing an abstract design that the examinee is asked to copy. The Bender-Gestalt may reveal visual-motor difficulties that may be indicative of neurological impairments. There are different methods of administering the Bender-Gestalt, many of them requiring that the examiner show the examinee the card for a specific time period so that the test can also provide information on memory deficits. In addition to neurological assessment, the Bender-Gestalt is also frequently used to assess possible learning disabilities.

Recent medical advances have also contributed to the assessment of brain injury and damage. Techniques such as magnetic resonance imaging (MRI) and positron emission tomography (PET) provide better insight into the brain's functioning then before. These medical techniques, however, cannot provide the entire picture, and often neurologists and neuropsychologists work together in both diagnosing the impairments and determining appropriate treatment. Sometimes the treatment involves counseling, either for the victim of the neurological impairment or the family, in coping with the disability.

Summary   Counselors can expect to work with clients from different cultures than their own and they need to be skilled in cross-cultural assessment. When selecting an instrument, counselors need to consider the client's ethnic or racial background and select an instrument that is appropriate for that client. Counselors also work in locations (e.g., schools) where they do not choose the assessment instruments (e.g., achievement tests) but are the ones responsible for administering and interpreting the results. In both of these situations, counselors would need to evaluate the assessment instruments for possible bias. One area counselors should consider is whether the instrument has been evaluated for possible content bias. Content bias concerns whether the content of the instrument is more familiar or appropriate to one group as compared to another group or groups. Another area counselors should examine is the instrument's internal structure for different ethnic groups. Instruments can differ in the degree to which they are reliable for different groups, and the factor structure may vary depending on the ethnic group. The analyses of possible bias should also include studies related to the relationship between the instrument and the criterion for different groups. It is important to examine differences among the validity coefficients and possible slope bias. Another area to examine is whether there are differences in the intercepts for different ethnic groups.

Some of the instruments counselors use may not be biased but may still produce results that have a disparate or negative impact on some minority individuals. There is debate about whether differences in ability, achievement, and aptitude testing are primarily genetic, social, or cultural. Helms (1992) argued that researchers should also examine cultural equivalence; that is, whether the *constructs* have similar meanings within and across cultures. Presently, it is impossible to develop a culture-free instrument, but many professionals are committed to developing instruments that attempt to be more culturally fair. There are also multicultural assessment standards to which counselors should adhere in order to provide competent services to clients from diverse backgrounds.

Counselors also need to give special consideration to clients with physical disabilities. In assessing clients with disabilities, counselors need to review the research on the most appropriate methods for adapting the assessment for these individuals. A well-written psychological report will identify any departures from the standardized procedures and discuss how the violations will influence the results. The results from any significant departure from standard procedures should be viewed with concern. Assessment with a special population can provide useful information if it is carefully performed and conservatively interpreted.

CHAPTER 15

Ethical and Legal Issues in Assessment

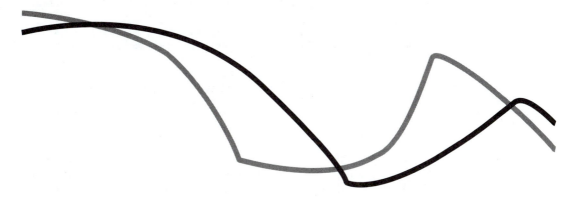

This chapter addresses some of the possible misuses of assessment and methods for ensuring that client appraisals are performed in an ethical and legal manner. Both ethical and legal guidelines influence counseling practice; yet there are differences between these two entities. Laws are related to a body of *rules*, while ethics are a body of *principles* that address proper conduct. Therefore, ethics and laws sometimes focus on different aspects or issues in assessment. The focus of both, however, is to protect people from possible harm from misuses of assessments.

Ethics

Sources for Ethical Decisions

Due to the complexities of appraisal issues in counseling, there are a number of sources that can aid the practitioner in practicing in an ethical manner. Table 15.1 includes a listing of some of the primary resources available to counselors in making ethical decisions. The ethical standards of professional organizations

TABLE 15.1

Consultation resources for ethical practices

American Association of Counseling and Development & Association for Measurement and Evaluation in Counseling and Development (1989). *The responsibility of test users.* Alexandria, VA: Author.

American Counseling Association (1995). *Code of ethics and standards of practice.* Alexandria, VA: Author.

American Education Research Association, American Psychological Association, & National Council on Measurement in Education (1985). *Standards for educational and psychological testing.* Washington, DC: American Psychological Association.

American Psychological Association (1992). Ethical principles of psychologists and code of conduct. *American Psychologist, 47,* 1597–1611.

American Rehabilitation Counseling Association, Commission of Rehabilitation Counselor Certification, and the National Rehabilitation Counseling Association (1995). *Code of professional ethics for rehabilitation counselors.* Chicago: Author

Eyde, L. D., Robertson, G.J., Moreland, K. L., Robertson, A. G., Shewan, C. M., Harrison, P. L., Porch, B. E., Hammer, A. L., & Primoff, E.S. (1993). *Responsible test use: Case studies for assessing human behavior.* Washington, DC: American Psychological Association.

Joint Committee on Testing Practices (1998). *Code of Fair Testing Practices in Education.* Washington, DC: Author. (Mailing Address: Joint Committee on Testing Practices, American Psychological Association, 750 First Avenue, NE, Washington, DC, 20002–4242).

related to counseling and assessment are a primary source. In the American Counseling Association's *Code of Ethics and Standards of Practice* (ACA, 1995), an entire section is devoted to evaluation, assessment, and interpretation (see Appendix C for a copy of this section of the Code of Ethics and Standards of Practice). Other professional organizations have standards that address assessment issues also, such as the American Psychological Association's (1992) *Ethical Principles of Psychologists and Code of Conduct* and the American Rehabilitation Counseling Association, Commission of Rehabilitation Counselor Certification, and the National Rehabilitation Counseling Association's (1995) *Code of Professional Ethics for Rehabilitation Counselors.* These ethical standards and codes establish principles and define ethical conduct for the members of the organizations. Members of these organizations are required to adhere to their ethical standards, which have arisen out of clients being harmed or the potential for clients to be harmed.

Another major resource regarding both ethical and legal questions is the *Standards for Educational and Psychological Testing* (AERA, APA, & NCME, 1985), which is often referred to as the *Standards.* These professional organizations worked together to produce the 1985 version of the *Standards* and are working on a revision that will be published in either 1999 or 2000. The *Standards* serves as a technical guide for testing practices. The current version includes (1) Technical Standards for Test Construction and Evaluation, (2) Professional Standards for Test Use, (3) Standards for Particular Applications (e.g., testing with linguistic minorities or individuals with disabilities), and (4) Standards for Administrative Procedures. The *Standards* provides expectations of professional services and should be reviewed by every practitioner who is involved in any type of assessment. The *Standards* has also been used in legal cases as an indicator of standard procedures within the profession.

The third resource counselors can use concerning ethical behavior is related to the *Standards* and is the *Code of Fair Testing Practices in Education* (Joint Committee on Testing Practices, 1988). The *Code of Fair Testing Practices in Education* is a document adapted from the *Standards*. The *Code* is designed to discuss testing information in a manner that can be understood by the general public. The *Code* addresses four areas: developing/selecting tests, interpreting scores, striving for fairness, and informing test takers. This document is not copyrighted and can be copied and given to clients, parents, or others who might benefit from this knowledge. In addition, the JCTP developed a videotape called the *ABC's of Schools Testing*, which is designed to help parents understand the many uses of testing in schools. A *Leader's Guide* is also available with this tape to assist counselors in working with parents on testing issues.

Another excellent resource related to ethical issues in assessment is *The Responsibilities of Tests Users* (AACD/AMECD, 1989), which is often referred to as the *Rust Statement*. The *Rust Statement* was intended for members of AACD, which is now the American Counseling Association. This statement addressed responsible and proper use of standardized tests. The focus of this document is not on the development of instruments, but rather the proper use of tests and methods for safeguarding against the misappropriate use of tests.

A fifth resource that practitioners find extremely helpful is the casebook *Responsible Test Use: Case Studies for Assessing Human Behavior* (Eyde et al., 1993), which was also developed by a working group of the JCTP. This resource includes 78 cases that illustrate both proper and improper test usages. There are case examples related to topics such as testing special populations, individuals with disabilities, test translations, and reasonable accommodations. This resource is particularly useful in describing real-world situations and applying ethical principles to these actual incidents. The casebook's major emphasis is on the application of basic principles of sound test selection, use, and interpretation.

A number of other resources are in the process of being developed during the writing of this book. For example, the Joint Committee on Testing Practices is in the process of developing a document titled *Test Taker Rights and Responsibilities* that should be published soon. A committee from the American School Counselor Association and the Association for Assessment in Counseling is in the process of developing *Standards for School Counselor Competence in Assessment and Evaluation*. Therefore, numerous resources currently exist to assist the practitioner in ethical assessment, and other resources are being developed to shed light on some of the more complicated issues.

Who Is Responsible for Appropriate Use?

In ethics there are often gray areas; however, the responsibility for test or instrument usage is *not* an equivocal area. It is clear from many ethical sources that the *clinician* is responsible for appropriate use. The *Code of Ethics and Standard of Practice* in E.1.b states, "Counselors are responsible for the appropriate application, scoring, interpretation and use of assessment instruments, whether they score and interpret such tests themselves or use computerized or other services" (p.36). Test publishers have the responsibility to publish the needed information, but the ultimate responsibility lies with the counselor. As the standards indicate, this responsibility includes scoring and interpretation that is performed by a computer. Thus, the practitioners must ensure that the computer programs or other scoring services are reliable, valid, and appropriate.

Part of being a responsible user of tests or other assessment instruments is practicing within one's limits. Instruments can easily be misused by practitioners who are untrained. Once again the ACA standards provide assistance in E.2.a:

> *Limits of Competence.* Counselors recognize the limits of their competence and perform only those testing and assessment services for which they have been trained. They are familiar with reliability, validity, related standardization, error of measurement, and proper application of any technique utilized. Counselors using computer-based test interpretations are trained in the construct being used prior to using this type of computer application. Counselors take reasonable measures to ensure the proper use of psychological assessment techniques by persons under their supervision. (p. 36)

Therefore, counselors must be knowledgeable about the specific instrument before they can give it to a client. Instruments vary in the amount of training and experience that is necessary in order to be competent. Although some publishers require that user qualifications be documented before they will sell an instrument to an individual, the ultimate responsibility still rests with the counselor. The three levels (i.e., Level A, Level B, and Level C) serve as a guideline to practitioners on the types of instruments they can use. Qualified and competent use requires more than having the necessary training, for the practitioner must also be knowledgeable about the specific instrument being used. Sufficient knowledge of an instrument is gained only by thorough examination of the manual and accompanying materials. The counselor must know the limitations of an instrument and for what purposes the instrument is valid.

Counselors have the responsibility of monitoring their own practice and use of assessment. In addition, counselors are professionals and professionals have the responsibility of monitoring their profession. The counselor has the responsibility of monitoring not only his or her own competencies in test usage but also the use of assessment instruments by others. If a counselor becomes aware of another counselor misusing an assessment measure, then the counselor is bound to first discuss the misuse with the other practitioner. If the situation is not remedied at that point, then the counselor should pursue appropriate actions with appropriate professional organizations.

Because assessment can have a profound effect on clients' lives, counselors need to consider clients' rights in this process. Appropriate and ethical assessment considers what is in clients' best interest. In terms of assessment, it is particularly critical that clinicians attend to issues related to the right of privacy, the right to results, the right to confidentiality, and the right to the least stigmatizing label.

Invasion of Privacy

When clients enter counseling, they still retain the right to decide what information to disclose and what information to keep private. In assessment, however, that choice can sometimes be blurred because of the subtleties involved with assessment. An example of how a client's privacy can be unintentionally invaded is illustrated through the case of a client named Claire. Claire's company is paying for career counseling for clients who are being permanently laid off because of downsizing. The counselor's procedure for all of his clients in this situation is to have them take an interest inventory, an abilities assessment, and a values inventory before meeting with the clients. The counselor believes this procedure expedites the process because they can begin counseling with meaningful information already available. Although there are three distinct inventories, the instruments are packaged for easy administration as one with a generic career exploration title. Claire felt some discomfort with many of the questions, but felt compelled to answer; she was not sure of the consequences of not answering all of the questions because the company had arranged the counseling as a part of the terminating process. Claire was receiving some severance pay and was concerned that being seen as not cooperating with the counseling process could affect that agreement. As the clinician was interpreting the result to Claire during the first session, Claire became upset and began to feel as though her privacy had been invaded. Claire is a very spiritual and private woman who believes her values are a private and intensely personal matter. The counselor, in this case, impinged on Claire's right to privacy.

There are two major points clinicians need to consider in assessment in order to avoid invading an individual's privacy: *informed consent* and *relevance*. Informed consent involves informing the client about both the nature of the information being collected and the purpose(s) for which the results will be used. Informed consent is clearly stated in the ACA *Code of Ethics and Standards of Practice* (see E.3.a in Appendix C), and the counselor in Claire's case is not in accordance with those standards. First, Claire was never informed about the nature of the instruments she was taking nor how the information would be used. The instrument that concerned values had a generic career exploration title, so even that didn't indicate to Claire what she was answering. Furthermore, Claire was never given the opportunity to consent or decline to take the assessments. Claire might have declined to take the values inventory if she had previous information on what it measured and how the information was going to be used. The counselor could probably make a case as to the relevance of the values inventory, but he invaded her privacy by not obtaining informed consent prior to her taking the assessments.

Clients need to be informed about any assessment in language that they can understand. Clients also must be given the opportunity to consent to the assessments. There are some exceptions to needing informed consent as covered by the *Standard for Educational and Psychological Testing* (AERA, APA, & NCME, 1985):

Informed consent should be obtained from test takers or their legal representative before testing is done except:

(a) when testing without consent is mandated by law or governmental regulation (e.g., statewide testing programs);

(b) when testing is conducted as a regular part of school activities (e.g., school-wide testing programs and participation by schools in norming or research studies);

(c) when consent is clearly implied (e.g., application for employment or educational admission). (p. 85)

Even when consent is not required, the individual should still be informed concerning the assessment process.

If the client is a minor, the informed consent must be completed by the parent or guardian. Occasionally practitioners will wonder if clients' informed consent should be oral or written. In general, a written informed consent is better; however, if this is taken to an extreme it could affect the counseling process. The decision of whether the informed consent should be written or oral mainly depends on the significance of the assessment situation. If the assessment process and results could have a significant impact on the client, then a written informed consent is wise. On the other hand, there may be times when oral consent is acceptable (e.g., the use of a self-exploration inventory). Many practitioners have general written informed consent forms explaining the counseling process, which the client (or the client's parents or guardian) signs before counseling begins. If counselors have standard instruments that are typically used (e.g., instruments given during the intake process), then the nature of those assessments and how the information is going to be used should be covered in the general informed consent materials. Often practitioners will also cover the possibility of future formal and informal assessment procedures (e.g., interviewing, exercises) in their general informed consent form that clients sign.

As was said earlier, informed consent is only one part of the invasion of privacy issue. The second major concept is relevance. With some instruments, particularly personality instruments, clients may not be aware of the variables or characteristics being measured and, thus, may unintentionally disclose information about themselves. Many of us have limitations or weaknesses that we would rather others didn't have information on. One of the critical questions related to invasion of privacy is whether this assessment is relevant to the counseling. If the assessment is not relevant to the counseling then no purpose is served by uncovering this information. Therefore, the clinician should be able to clearly state the purpose of the assessment and the benefits gained from the process. The practitioner is responsible for identifying and using an assessment tool that does indeed measure that purpose. In selecting a relevant measure, the clinician needs to consider the reliability, validity, psychometric limitation, and appropriateness of the instrument.

The concept of relevance is certainly logical, but it is occasionally unheeded. For example, some practitioners become quite "enthralled" with an instrument and will give it to all their clients whether it is relevant or not. Another more common example of neglecting the concept of relevance is a counselor interviewing a client on an area that is of interest to the counselor but is not relevant to the counseling. Counselors have the responsibility of considering the client's privacy in using any assessment technique. Therefore, the concepts of informed consent and relevance apply to both formal assessment instruments and informal techniques, such as interviewing.

The Right to Results

Not only do clients have the right to have the assessment process explained to them, they also have the right to an explanation of the results. The Informed Consent section (E.3.) of the ACA *Code of Ethics and Standards of Practice* contains the statement, "Regardless of whether the scoring and interpretation are completed by counselors, by assistants, or by computers or other outside services, counselors take reasonable steps to ensure that appropriate explanations are given to the client" (p. 38). This does not mean the client has to be told every result and conclusion; it is the client's welfare that dictates the interpretation of the results. For example, if a diagnostic conclusion would probably increase the anxiety level of the client, then the practitioner may decide that it is in the best interest of the client not to disclose that information at that time. The informed consent will also determine if anyone else may have access to the results (e.g., other family members in a family counseling situation or teachers).

Clients also deserve the interpretation of the assessment results in terms they can understand. Misinterpretation of the results can be enormously painful to individuals. A child of eleven may hear 60% when the result is the 60th percentile. In fact, even some well-educated adults have been known to confuse percentile and percentage. Interpreting results requires well-developed counseling skills. Misinterpretation of results often occurs when the individual is simply given the results without an explanation. As was said in the discussion concerning the interpretation of results in Chapter 5, the counselor should prepare different methods for explaining the results in case the client does not understand the initial explanation.

The Right to Confidentiality

Clients also have the right to have the results kept confidential. Confidentiality means only the counselor and the client (or parents/guardians in the case of a minor) have access to the results. The results can only be released to a third person with the consent of the client. In addition, the release of information needs to be to individuals who have the expertise to competently interpret the information. Exceptions to this are institutions (e.g., schools, court systems) where a number of people may have legitimate reasons for accessing the testing results. In these cases, the informed consent should address the question of who may have access to the results and how they will use these results. As we will see later, there are laws that govern who has access to the information in schools.

Counselors often fail to keep assessment results confidential by acts of carelessness. For example, a school counselor who allows a student aide to file papers that contain achievement results of other students is breaking confidentiality. A marriage and family counselor who provides a summary of the wife's scores on a marital satisfaction inventory to the husband without getting consent to release the information is breaking confidentiality. A counselor in a college counseling center who allows an unmonitored computerized career assessment and information system in the waiting room of the center might also be breaking confidentiality. Some students may have the computer sophistication to retrieve other students' confidential information. Counselors have the responsibility for securing the assessment information, and any limits to confidentiality should be communicated to the client beforehand.

Clinicians also need to understand that client records, including assessment results, could be subpoenaed. Therefore, clinicians want to ensure that assessment records are retained in a professional manner. Counselors cannot predict future court action that may occur and, hence, attendance to detail is important. The case of Carole may illustrate this point. Carole entered counseling when her husband requested a divorce. During this period Carole was saddened and upset by the end of her marriage. The counselor decided to have Carole take a depression inventory to assess the level of depression, which indicated Carole was slightly depressed. The results of the inventory were kept in her file, but the counselor did not record any notes on why the inventory was given. Three years later, Carole was in a car accident, which resulted in Carole's requiring extensive medical care. When Carole sued the driver who caused the accident, the other driver's attorney had the counseling records subpoenaed. This attorney attempted to make the case that Carole's depression, as documented by the assessment results, was at the root of her medical problems. If the counselor had documented that the reason for the depression assessment was because of the divorce, Carole's case in court would have been considerably easier.

Not only is the counselor responsible for keeping the assessment results secure, but the professional is also responsible for keeping the content of the assessment secure. Securing test content is particularly important in the areas of intelligence or general ability, achievement, and aptitude assessment. It can also be important when personality instruments are used for decision making (e.g., employment). Sometimes parents will have concerns and want to preview an instrument their child is going to take. The counselor will need to keep the exact content of the instrument secure and should talk generally about what the test measures. The parents should not be shown the specific questions on the test. Counselors need to be familiar with the instrument's manual in order to know the procedures concerning keeping the instrument secure. For some instruments, like the Medical College Admissions Test, the security procedures are quite elaborate.

The Right to the Least Stigmatizing Label

Sometimes in counseling the purpose of the assessment is diagnosis, which in many ways is applying a label. Standard 16.6 of the *Standards for Education and Psychological Testing* states, "When score reporting includes assigning individuals to categories, the categories chosen should be based on carefully selected criteria. The least stigmatizing labels, consistent with accurate reporting should always be assigned" (p. 86). The least stigmatizing label does not mean that clinicians always use diagnostic codes that are less stigmatizing, because a less stigmatizing code that is inaccurate could prevent the client from receiving the appropriate treatment. Ethical standards also reinforce the importance of proper diagnosis of mental disorders. A diagnostic label, however, can have a significant impact, and practitioners need to carefully reflect on these professional decisions. When clinicians are considering diagnostic categories, they need to incorporate contextual factors such as the clients' cultural and socioeconomic experiences.

In conclusion, the ethical use of assessment interventions is a professional responsibility. Not only is the counselor responsible for her or his own professional conduct, but counselors are also responsible for taking reasonable steps to prevent others from misusing assessment procedures or assessment results. Certainly there have been misuses of assessment devices in the past. If, however, professionals monitor their own and others' use of assessments, then hopefully future misuses will be significantly reduced.

Legal Issues in Assessment

As mentioned earlier, there are principles and ethical standards that direct professional behavior in assessment, and there are also *laws* that need to be adhered to by professionals. Laws emanate from two sources: legislation and litigation. *Legislation* concerns governmental bodies passing laws. For example, many state legislatures have passed bills related to the licensing of Licensed Professional Counselors. *Litigation* is the other way that laws are formed by "rules of law." In this case, the courts interpret the Constitution, federal law, state law, and common law in a particular case, and this ruling then influences the interpretations of the relevant laws. In the area of assessment, both legislation and litigation have had an effect. In the past, most of the legislation and litigation that have influenced assessment concerned employment testing and educational testing. This area, however, is ever evolving and changing because a new law could be passed tomorrow or a court could make an influential decision anytime. Therefore, counselors must continually strive to keep abreast of these evolving legal issues.

Legislation

A number of influential acts of legislation related to assessment have been passed by the Congress of the United States. Most of these laws were not written for the specific purpose of controlling assessment practice, but these laws also contained content and language that is related to testing practice. Because these were federal laws, as compared to state laws, these acts affect the entire country.

Civil Rights Act of 1991. Title VII of the Civil Rights Acts of 1964 and the amendments of this act of 1972 and 1978 outlawed discrimination in employment based on race, color, religion, sex, or national origin. The original legislation created the Equal Employment Opportunity Commission (EEOC), which was charged with developing guidelines that would regulate equal employment. In the 1970s, the EEOC developed very strict guidelines related to the use of employment tests that addressed the type of reliability and validity evidence that needed to be present. During the 1980s, there was considerable controversy about the EEOC, which led in part to the passing of the Civil Rights Act of 1991.

Several controversial court decisions that certain civil rights advocates found disturbing were another possible influence on the passage of the Civil Rights Act of 1991. These decisions in the 1980s were changes from a landmark case of *Griggs v. Duke Power Company* (1971). This case involved African-American employees of a private power company who filed suit against the power company claiming that the criteria for promotion such as requiring a high school diploma and passing scores on the Wonderlic Personnel Test and the Bennett Mechanical Comprehension Test were discriminatory. The Supreme Court ruled in favor of the employees and found that an instrument may not appear biased but may discriminate if it has a disparate or adverse impact. The court also ruled that if there is disparate impact, the employer must show that the hiring procedures are job related and a reasonable measure of job performance. The validity of the two instruments was an issue in this decision, and this case spurred more of a focus on the validity of employment tests in employment decisions.

One of the first cases somewhat divergent from the Griggs case was *Watson v. Fort Worth Bank and Trust* (1988). In this case, the Supreme Court did not rule on behalf of the African-American woman who had been passed over for a supervisory position, and this ruling raised questions about employment selection procedures for supervisory positions. The findings indicated that for supervisory positions the procedures need not have strong validity evidence and that subjectivity enters into these decisions. In *Wards Cove Packing Company v. Antonio* (1989), the Supreme Court ruled on the concept of adverse or disparate impact that some employers thought the court would rule on in the Watson case. In the Wards Cove case, most of the cannery jobs were held by Eskimos and Filipinos whereas the noncannery jobs were held by Whites and European-Americans. The judicial decision in this case shifted the burden to the plaintiff to show that there are problems with the selection procedures. On the basis of this case, plaintiffs would need to show that the instruments were not job related, which is very difficult to do with limited access to human resources or personnel information and records.

The Civil Rights Act of 1991 in many ways codified the principles of *Griggs v. Duke Power Company*. The plaintiff must show that there is an adverse or disparate impact. The burden then shifts to the employer to show that discriminatory hiring procedures are needed because of business necessity and job relatedness (Hagen & Hagen, 1995). Therefore, the Civil Rights Act shifts more of the burden back to the employer and requires that hiring procedures and employment tests be connected to the duties of the job.

Another feature of the Civil Rights Act of 1991 is the ban on separate norms in employment tests. The act specifically states that it is unlawful to adjust the scores of, use different cutoff scores for, or otherwise alter the results of employment-related tests on the basis of race, color, religion, sex, or national origin. Some individuals in the field of assessment believe this portion of the act may have untold ramifications. The focus of the ban was on separate norms used by the U.S. Employment Services (USES) for minority and nonminority job applicants. In the 1980s, the USES sent employers percentile scores from the GATB for employers to use in hiring decisions. A problem was that African-Americans and Hispanics tended to have lower average scores on the GATB and, thus, their percentile scores were not competitive. The USES decided to use separate norms so that African-Americans would be compared to African-Americans. The public outcries, however, led to the ban of separate norms in 1991 (Sackett & Wilk, 1994). Besides the race issue, there are other issues such as the differences between men and women on personality tests. There are some findings that women are more likely to disclose negative information about themselves, which may be problematic when personality instruments are used for hiring. Certainly tests that involve muscular strength or cardiovascular endurance also favor men. The debate around the advantages and disadvantages of separate norms will most likely continue in the coming years. Racial differences in hiring and performance on employment tests are complex and multidimensional issues. Gottfredson (1994) suggested that the approach to these issues needs to be broadened, as employment tests did not cause the racial differences, nor can we expect adjusting or not adjusting the scores to solve these complex problems.

Americans with Disabilities Act of 1990. The Americans with Disabilities Act (ADA) bans discrimination in employment and access to public services, transportation, and telecommunications on the basis of physical and mental disabilities. A disability is defined as (1) a physical or mental impairment that substantially limits one or more life activities and (2) a record of such impairment or the individual is regarded as having such an impairment. ADA came to address testing through the focus on employment and employment testing. The language of the bill, however, is broad and covers multiple testing situations. Under ADA, individuals with disabilities must have tests administered to them using reasonable and appropriate accommodations (Geisinger, 1994). This language raises some troublesome questions related to assessment. First, how are reasonable and appropriate accommodations defined? As of yet, there are no uniform and clear definitions that can guide practitioners in these decisions. In addition, there are thousands of disabilities and a researcher could spend a lifetime developing reasonable and appropriate accommodations for just one instrument. The nonstandard administration of a standardized test leads to another major issue, which is related to how to interpret the results of a nonstandard administration. It is often difficult to determine whether the accommodations met the intent of ADA. The intent of ADA is to make accommodations so that instruments measure the construct and not the disability. Interpreting the results of clients with disabilities involves determining if the accommodations were sufficient or if the results still may be unfairly influenced by the disability. There is also an opposite risk, where the accommodations provide an advantage to the examinee with the disability as compared to those without the disability. Geisinger (1994) suggested that the field should consider new ways of assessing individuals with disabilities in order to develop fair measures and assessment procedures.

Individuals with Disabilities Education Act of 1997. Another piece of legislation that affects assessment and testing of individuals with disabilities is the Individuals with Disabilities Education Act (IDEA), which was last reauthorized in 1997. The original version of this law was the Education for All Handicapped Children Act, also known as Public Law 94-142. Although not related to the topic of this book, the last version of IDEA may provide some interesting opportunities to counsel the families of children with disabilities. In regard to assessment, parental consent is sought in order to perform the evaluation of a child suspected of having a disability. The following, from Part B, Sec. 614., concerns the stipulations for conducting the evaluation:

> (A) use a variety of assessment tools and strategies to gather relevant functional and developmental information, including information provided by the parent, that may assist . . .
> (B) not use any single procedure as the sole criterion for determining whether a child is a child with a disability or determining an appropriate educational program for the child; and
> (C) use technically sound instruments that may assess the relative contribution of cognitive and behavioral factors,

The above stipulations for conducting evaluations are consistent with good test practice and the concepts that have been suggested in this book. Part B, Sec. 614 of the Individuals with Disabilities Education Act also addresses specific matters related to the tests or other evaluation materials used. As this legislation reflects, multicultural issues must be attended to in the process of assessing the child.

> (A) tests and other evaluation materials used to assess a child under this section—
>   (i) are selected and administered so as not to be discriminatory on a racial or cultural basis; and
>   (ii) are provided and administered in the child's native language or other mode of communication, unless it is clearly not feasible to do so; and
> (B) any standardized tests that are given to the child—
>   (i) have been validated for the specific purpose for which they are used;
>   (ii) are administered by trained and knowledgeable personnel; and
>   (iii) are administered in accordance with any instructions provided by the producer of such tests;

The focus of this section of the law is to ensure that children are assessed fairly, in their native language, and with psychometrically sound instruments. The child needs to be assessed in all areas where there is a suspected disability. The determination of whether the child is a child with a disability as defined in this act is determined by a team of professionals that sometimes includes a school counselor. If a disability is found, then the child must be reevaluated at least once every three years in order to determine subsequent educational needs.

Family Educational Rights and Privacy Act. The next piece of legislation in this discussion also concerns education but includes both individuals with disabilities and those without. The Family Educational Rights and Privacy Act (FERPA) of 1974 provided parents and "eligible students" (those over 18) with certain rights regarding the inspection and dissemination of educational records. This law was designed to protect student privacy and applies to all school districts and schools that receive funds from the U.S. Department of Education. FERPA mainly concerns the access of educational records and provides parents with access to their children's educational record. Students over 18 also have access to their own record. It further specifies that the educational record cannot be released without parental permission to anyone other than those who have a *legitimate* educational interest. The contents of the educational record will vary somewhat from school district to school district, but group achievement tests, students' grades, and attendance record are routinely considered part of a students' educational records. Although counseling records kept in a separate locked cabinet and accessible only to the counselor are not considered part of the educational record, bills are being introduced in the U.S. House of Representatives that would require counselors to provide those records to parents.

Another provision in FERPA concerns assessment in the schools. FERPA includes language stating that no student shall be required without parental permission to submit to psychological examination, testing, or treatment that may reveal information concerning mental and psychological problems potentially embarrassing to the student or the student's family. This same issue was addressed in an amendment to Goals 2000: Educate America Act of 1994. This amendment is titled the Protection of Pupil Rights Amendment, but it is often called the Grassley Amendment. The Grassley Amendment has similar language to FERPA except that it specifies written parental consent before minor students are required to participate in any survey, analysis, or evaluation that reveals any information concerning mental and psychological problems potentially embarrassing to the student or his family. Some educational administrators have interpreted this to include self-esteem measures or any exercise that involves self-analysis. Many school districts have adopted the policy that any type of assessment except routine achievement tests requires written parental consent. Therefore, school counselors are encouraged to discuss with an administrator the school district's policy concerning any assessment they may want to initiate. This does not mean that counselors cannot use assessment tools, but in many instances they are advised to secure written parental permission beforehand.

Truth in Testing. This last piece of legislation was passed by the legislature in the State of New York and does not apply nationally. New York passed a Truth in Testing Law mainly in reaction to attacks on Educational Testing Service by Ralph Nader and others. A report by one of Nader's associates, Nairn, criticized the Scholastic Aptitude Test in many areas, alleging it had a propensity to rank people by social class rather than aptitude. His report further purported that the SAT was a poor predictor of college grades and called for a full disclosure of the questions and answers on each SAT. The New York Truth in Testing law requires that testing companies (1) make public their studies on validity, (2) provide a complete disclosure to students about what scores mean and how they were calculated, and (3) upon student request, provide a copy of the questions and the correct answers to the student. Most of the publishers of the test did not object to the first two regulations but argued that the third posed a hardship due to the difficulty of having to compile new questions after each testing. According to Aiken (1997), 24 other states have considered truth in testing legislation but only one, California, has passed a similar law. The California law, the Dunlop Act, is somewhat different and only requires that the questions and answers be sent to the California State Department of Education and not to every student who requests a copy. A court case in New York somewhat related to this is *Sharif v. New York State Department of Education* (1989), in which the judge ruled that the SAT could not be used as the sole criterion for scholarship awards. This is, however, consistent with what the College Entrance Examination Board (1995) suggests should be done when using the Scholastic Assessment Test.

Litigation

In the discussion of the second manner in which laws are established, through litigation, the approach will be somewhat different. Rather than discussing this information court case by court case, the focus will be on areas in appraisal where judicial decisions have been influential.

Test bias and placement. There have been some controversial decisions related to the use of intelligence tests for permanently assigning African-American children to classes for the mentally retarded (Fisher & Sorenson, 1996). In California, there was a substantial overrepresentation of African-American students in these classrooms, and there were concerns that the testing procedures were discriminatory. In the Federal District Court of San Francisco, Judge Peckham found in the case of *Larry P. v. Riles* (1979) that intelligence tests discriminated against Black children and could not be used to test Black children for placement in educable mentally retarded classrooms in California. Less than a year later, Judge Grady in Illinois had a similar case, *Parents in Action on Special Education (PASE) v. Hannon* (1980) but ruled the opposite way, declaring that intelligence tests could be used, when used in conjunction with other criteria. In both cases, the rulings affected only those states, but there was confusion in other states concerning the legality of using intelligence tests with minority children. In a similar case in Georgia, *Georgia NAACP v. State of Georgia* (1985), the ruling was once again that intelligence tests did not discriminate. In 1986, Judge Peckham in California reissued his ban on intelligence tests. Therefore at this time, there was some confusion on whether the courts were ruling for the use of intelligence tests or banning the use of intelligence tests with minority students. However, in 1992 he lifted the ban on intelligence tests after African-American parents sought to have their children tested with intelligence tests in order to identify possible learning disabilities. These cases have resulted in the practice of using other criteria along with intelligence tests in the determination of whether a child has a mental disability.

Minimum competency. During the 1980s, there was an upsurge of interest in competency testing or minimum competency testing. Considerable focus was on the lack of academic skills some students had when graduating from high school. Fisher and Sorenson (1996) indicated the courts have consistently ruled that it is within the Constitution for states to require competency examinations for high school graduation. As with the example of intelligence tests, a judicial controversy in the area of minimum competency centered on discrimination. Although other cases were filed in Florida related to the institution of a minimum competency examination for high school graduation, the case of *Debra P. v. Turlington* was the most influential. The examination was instituted in 1978, and a challenge was filed that year on behalf of all Florida seniors and on behalf of African-American Florida seniors. A federal district court ruled that the exam violated all students' rights to procedural due process and violated the Black students' right to equal protection. The court postponed the use of the examination until the 1982–1983 school year. The reason for the postponement was that Florida schools were segregated until 1971 and the court ruled the Black students had not received an equal education. Starting in the 1982–1983 school year, all seniors would have received all of their education in desegregated schools and, thus, had equal educational opportunities. This case is also important because it raised the question of instructional validity. Instructional validity concerns the evidence that the students were taught the material covered on the test. The court ruled that if the test covers material not taught to the students, then it is unfair and violates the Equal Protection and Due Process clauses of the United States Constitution. This ruling has set a precedent concerning the need for a relationship between the curriculum and the minimum competency examination in each state. Most states do not have a standardized curriculum, which confounds the development of a high school competency examination.

Right to privacy. A recent case has been controversial within the field of assessment: the case of *Soroka et al. v. Dayton-Hudson Company* (1991), which is also known as the Target case. This case involved the use of a personality inventory as an employment screening device for a security officer position at Target Department stores. The plaintiffs complained that the psychological inventory was not job related and, furthermore, offensive and intrusive to the point that it invaded their privacy. Many of the items on the assessment device in question were developed from the original version of the MMPI. The case was to go the California Supreme Court when it was settled out of court. The Appellate Court had previously concluded that the Target preemployment psychological screening instrument did violate the plaintiffs' constitutional right to privacy and the statutory prohibition against improper inquiries and discriminatory conduct by inquiring into religious beliefs and sexual orientation. According to Merenda (1995), many in the testing field reacted negatively to this ruling, believing that the ruling indicated that every question on a personality inventory could be challenged in terms of its relationship to job performance. Merenda argued that the ruling was the result of the instrument's not being developed or scored or interpreted in accordance with professional standards. He concluded that this ruling does *not* mean that offensive items must be stricken from every employment test. There may, however, be other court cases related to this one because the Appellate Court's ruling left some question whether personality inventories as employment hiring tools are an invasion of privacy.

Summary

The topic of this chapter is ethical and legal issues in assessment. Ethics concerns the principles that guide professionals in the performance of duties, while laws are legal rules enforced by governmental entities. There are a number of resources that can assist counselors when they are faced with ethical dilemmas regarding assessment. A primary resource is the *Standards for Educational and Psychological Testing,* which is currently being revised.

In terms of ethical responsibility, the clinician bears the ultimate responsibility for the appropriate use of any instruments. Although test publishers may attempt to restrict the sale of instruments to an untrained individual, the ethical standards clearly indicate that the practitioner must practice within his or her level of competency. Instruments vary in the amount of training and experience that is necessary in order to be competent. Counselors need to ensure that they have been competently trained before giving an instrument to a client. Being competently trained also means having thorough knowledge about the specific instrument being used.

Clients retain the right of privacy when they enter a counseling relationship. Assessments, however, are sometimes subtle and there is a chance that a client's privacy could be invaded. The two keys to not invading a client's privacy are *informed consent* and *relevance*. Not only do clients have the right to be informed about the assessment process, they also have the right to an explanation of the results. Clients also have the right to have the results kept confidential. Confidentiality means only the counselor and the client (or parents/guardians in the case of a minor) have access to the results without written permission to release the results. In terms of diagnosis, the least stigmatizing labels should be assigned that are consistent with accurate reporting.

Laws related to assessment have emerged from both legislation and litigation. Concerning legislation, the Civil Rights Act of 1991, the Americans with Disabilities Act, and the Individuals with Disabilities Education Act have all impacted the practice of assessment. The crux of all of these laws is the use of sound and appropriate instruments with individuals in a manner that is fair and equitable. The Family Educational Rights and Privacy Act governs who has access to educational records and assessment in the schools. Legal cases that have significantly influenced assessment have often focused on discrimination issues. Litigation has primarily involved test bias, minimum-competency examinations, and invasion of privacy. It is important for counselors to stay informed about pending legislation and litigation that could affect assessment in counseling. Litigation and legislation are affected by social factors, and as our society changes in the coming years, there will also be changes in the laws governing appraisal.

CHAPTER 16

Technological Applications and Future Trends

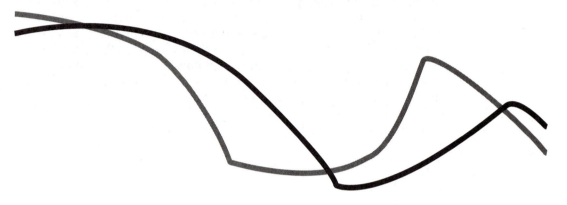

As we approach the end of this book, it may be wise to direct our attention to future trends in appraisal in counseling. In previous chapters, both the history of and current practices in assessment were addressed. This chapter identifies some future trends in assessment that practitioners need to consider when providing counseling services to clients. Many changes have occurred in the area of appraisal in counseling over the last fifty years; however, we can expect even greater changes in the next fifty years. Almost every aspect of our lives is being affected by changes in technology. Certainly the field of assessment has been affected by computers and technology and will be affected by technological change in the future. The intent of this chapter is to examine current trends in terms of the use of computers and technology and to consider future trends in the general field of appraisal.

Technological Applications

Currently in the field of assessment, technology and computers have had a major influence on how assessment services are delivered. Technology and computer applications are not a new phenomenon in this area; the Strong Vocational Interest Blank used electromechanical scoring as early as the 1930s. Computers continued to be used primarily for scoring and sometimes interpretation until the late 1970s and early 1980s. The expansion of computer usage in assessment coincided with the widespread use of microcomputers or personal computers. Computers are now intimately involved in the administration, scoring, and interpretation of many assessment instruments in counseling. Furthermore, professionals are beginning to use the Internet for appraisal activities and it is expected that on-line assessment methods and services will burgeon (Sampson, 1998).

Computer Assessment in Counseling

In terms of computer applications in assessment or appraisal, two terms need to be defined. **Computer-assisted assessment** concerns the use of computers to assist in the administration, scoring, and/or interpretation of any assessment tool. The manner in which the computer assists in the assessment process can vary from simply scoring the instrument to the client's taking the instrument at the computer and the computer then scoring the answers, interpreting the results, and writing a detailed report. In contrast, **computer-adapted assessment** means there is an *interactive* process between the individual and the computer. One example of computer-adapted assessment is sometimes called *item branching*, in which different sets of items or test questions are administered to different individuals and vary according to each individual's responses. As an example, if an answer or answers to test questions indicate a fifth grader is not comprehending material at the fifth grade level, the computer would adapt the questions and select questions at the fourth grade reading level. If another student, however, comprehends the fifth grade reading questions, then the computer would select items at the sixth grade level. This adaptive process is mostly used in achievement tests, but it can be used in other types of assessments. For example, if an individual reports he or she has never experienced any auditory hallucinations or hearing of voices when no one appears to be talking, the computer could then eliminate the items that ask about when the voices are heard and what types of messages the voices are giving. Computer-adapted assessment can be an efficient method because, for most clients, the time needed to complete the instrument is reduced when the computer eliminates inappropriate items. For example, the computer version of the Graduate Record Examination is a computer-adapted assessment, and studies indicate most people spend less time taking it as compared to the paper-and-pencil version of the GRE (Educational Testing Service, 1997).

Issues related to inputting information. Either computer-assisted or computer-adapted assessment involves putting information into the computer and then receiving information from the computer once the computer either scores or interprets the results. When discussing issues related to the inputting of information into computers, the focus tends to be on computer-administered assessment. Many instruments have been adapted from paper-and-pencil formats to also include a computer-administered format. For example, the Beck Depression Inventory-II has both a paper-and-pencil version and a computer-administered version. There are instruments, however, that are only available on the computer, such as some of the computerized career information systems discussed in Chapter 9.

Issues pertinent to computer-administered assessment concern the effects on the results of individual differences in comfort level, amount of experience, and attitudes toward computers. Surveys have indicated that most people have favorable attitudes toward computerized test administration. There are, however, differences in experience level—for example, some clients may think the term *mouse* applies only to an animal while other clients have Carpal Tunnel Syndrome from the extensive use of their computer's keyboard and mouse. Client experience and attitudes toward computerized assessment need to be considered in deciding whether to use a computer-administered instrument and in interpreting the results from such an instrument.

Another issue pertains to the psychometric qualities of a computer-administered instrument. Some people will erroneously view a computer-administered instrument as being scientifically sound simply because it is computerized. In the beginning of computer-administered assessment, there were few investigations into the psychometric qualities of these assessments. With increased usage, professional organizations, such as the American Counseling Association (ACA) and the American Psychological Association (APA), revised their ethical codes or standards to address many of the issues related to computer-assisted assessment (see Appendix C for the ACA *Code of Ethics and Standards of Practice* related to assessment). If the instrument is an adoption of a paper-and-pencil instrument, then the evaluation of the psychometric qualities must include an analysis of the *equivalency* of the two forms of the instrument. Research indicates that the item type or format seems to influence whether the computer-administered version is equivalent to the conventional form of an instrument. Instruments containing multiple-choice or true/false items are more likely to be equivalent (Hoffman & Lundberg, 1976) as compared to matching items or checklist items (Allred & Harris, 1984). Individuals taking a computer-administered matching test tend to have lower scores than those taking the same instrument in the paper-and-pencil format. Also, with checklist items in a computer format, an individual usually has to respond whether or not to check each item. Hence, individuals tend to check more items on a computer-administered version as compared to a paper-and-pencil version.

Another issue is related to differences in levels of self-disclosure and honesty in responses between computer-administered assessment and more conventional methods. Researchers have hypothesized that, with instruments that contain personally sensitive information, computer administration may increase the honesty of the disclosures because the computer may be perceived as offering greater anonymity and less judgmental responses (Lautenschlager & Flaherty, 1990). The opposite can also be hypothesized: that individuals may be more likely to disclose personally sensitive information to a skilled and empathic clinician. The research findings in this area are somewhat mixed. There may be a slight advantage to computer-administered assessment, but the difference between the approaches is often not statistically significant.

Issues related to outputting information. Once the information is inputted, the scores or results that the computer produces are directly tied to the data that are entered. In computer-assisted assessment, the old adage "garbage in/garbage out" certainly applies. Although a computer may accurately score any instrument, if the instrument is lacking in terms of reliability and validity evidence, then it doesn't really matter that the scoring was performed accurately.

In terms of assessment, computer outputs can vary from simple scoring to extended and complex interpretations. Computers are being increasingly used not only to score the results but also to provide interpretative reports. Interpretative reports can be anything from elementary descriptions to complex clinical interpretations involving diagnostic decisions. A counselor using a computer-generated report must evaluate the quality of the report. The interpretative reports can vary in terms of quality, with some being produced by individuals with no counseling or assessment experience. Reports can also be simple cookbook approaches, with a certain score being programmed to indicate a specific implication. Clients are complex human beings and "paint-by-the-numbers approaches" to interpretation are often not particularly useful. In evaluating whether to use a computer-generated report, a counselor should find answers to the following questions:

1. What is the basis for the programming of the report?
2. Who was involved in the writing of this computer program and what are his or her professional credentials?
3. Were the individuals knowledgeable about the instrument and did they have extensive experience in interpreting the results?
4. Is the interpretation based on sound research and validation information?
5. Is there evidence that the computer-generated reports are comparable to clinician-generated reports?
6. Is the interpretative information in the report helpful and appropriate for the client with whom the counselor is working?
7. Is the cost of the computer-generated report (e.g., software, hardware) worth the information produced by the report?
8. Are there supplemental resources such as a hot-line number available for questions?

With the ease of computer-generated reports, clinicians may be lulled into a false sense of security and use the computer-generated results without becoming educated about the instrument. Instruments used in counseling are validated for specific purposes; therefore a counselor cannot in isolation use a general computer-generated report. The American Counseling Association's *Code of Ethics and Standards of Practice* (ACA, 1995) clearly states that clinicians must be

FIGURE 16.1
*Computer-assisted
assessment*

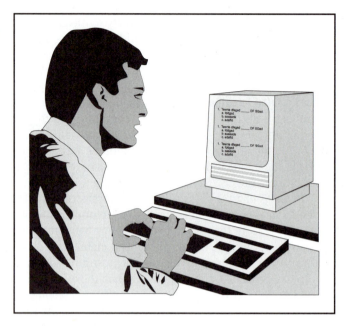

trained in the construct and the specific instrument prior to using a computer-generated report. To use the instrument appropriately and ethically, counselors must be knowledgeable about the instrument. Simply using a computer-generated report without knowledge of the instrument's strengths and limitations is negligent and unprofessional. Computer-generated reports are designed to supplement or complement the clinician's interpretation of the results, not replace them. The *Guidelines for Computer-Based Tests and Interpretations* (American Psychological Association, 1986) indicated that computer-generated interpretative reports should be used only in conjunction with professional judgment and oversight. Sampson (1990) suggested that computer-generated test interpretations are best used as a "second opinion" to confirm or disconfirm hypotheses about clients.

Reviews of the computer-based test interpretation programs could be helpful, but reviews of computer programs are not as easy to access as reviews of more traditional instruments. The publishers of the *Mental Measurement Yearbooks* considered including such reviews, but abandoned that effort (Kramer & Conoley, 1992). Reviews of computer-based test interpretation (CBTI) programs are sometimes published in professional journals such as *Computers in Human Behavior, Computers in Human Services,* and occasionally the *Journal of Counseling and Development.*

Counselors who use computer programs to score and interpret results need to have purchased the appropriate software. As Anderson (1996) pointed out, borrowed or bootlegged software is an infringement on the rights of the copyright holder. There are copyright laws that govern this software and there are penalties for not complying with the licensing agreements. There are also client services issues. A counselor and client may receive inaccurate information from an old or defective product that the counselor continues to let clients use because the counselor who borrowed the software has no connection with the publisher. Anderson (1996) urged counselors to comply with copyright and licensing agreements when they purchase computer software.

There are computer software programs available that combine a number of functions to assist the practitioner. The Psychological Corporation markets a system called OPTAIO, with which clients can take computer-administered instruments that provide both treatment and outcome information. The results of the instruments related to treatment can be integrated into progress notes, clinical reports, and treatment plans. The system also utilizes national norms that provide information on severity and complexity of cases. Furthermore, the system allows for outcome tracking so that the individual practitioner can monitor his or her own effectiveness, or supervisors can review a clinician's performance. It is anticipated that more of these sophisticated and integrated computer programs will be marketed to respond to managed care and other requests for counseling outcome and accountability information.

The use of computers in assessment is expected to increase in the coming years. Computers can be used in a variety of ways related to appraisal in counseling and practitioners are continually identifying additional and novel methods. Computers, however, are not a panacea that solves all the problems and controversies associated with appraisal in counseling. Computer applications in assessment have some advantages, but there are also some disadvantages.

Advantages and disadvantages of computer applications. There are many advantages to computer application in client assessment. Computers can be patient in gathering information and can store substantial amounts of data and information. In addition, because computers can analyze data quickly, there often is a negligible time lag between the administration, scoring, and interpretation of the instrument. Computer applications in assessment have been found to save professionals' time. When computers are used to monitor, score, and interpret results, practitioners can spend more time on other duties. Computers can be programmed to test whether the individual understands the instructions. For example on an analogies test, the computer can determine if the individual understands by giving sample items that involve simple analogies. If the person answers the sample items incorrectly then additional instructions can be provided. Moreover, computers respond to just the information that is entered and do not have any preconceived notions about individuals based on physical appearance or the color of their skin. Computers are unbiased and do not react to the gender, race, age, or demeanor of the individual. If computers are programmed correctly, they do not make scoring errors that often occur when humans do the scoring. The programming can also involve complex scoring and interpretations that the computer can perform in minutes but would take a counselor hours to perform. Examples of instruments that involve complex scoring procedures are the Millon Clinical Multiaxial Inventory and the Strong Interest Inventory.

There are, nonetheless, some disadvantages with computer applications in assessment. When computers administer instruments, frequently the administrations are not observed by professionals. Behavioral observations during the administration of an instrument can provide insight into the client's degree of motivation and level of anxiety. Counselor observations can often supplement instrument results; however, with computer administration these observations are almost always eliminated. There also can be a confidentiality problem if computers retain assessment results and these computers are not closely monitored. A client with sophisticated hacking skills can access other clients' results while appearing to take an instrument on an unmonitored computer. If computers contain any confidential client information, then these machines need to be closely supervised and results kept secure. Other problems related to computer applications in assessment concern the validity of the instruments and the validity of the computerized interpretation. All instruments, whether they are administered on a computer or involve a more traditional format, must be evaluated in terms of their psychometric qualities.

The Internet and Appraisal in Counseling

An extension of computer applications is using the Internet in assessment and appraisal. How the Internet is going to affect counseling and the delivery of counseling services is a hotly debated topic at conferences and on counseling-related list-serves on the Internet. Sampson (1998) projected that the field of assessment is the area in counseling where the Internet will have the most impact. The Internet allows individuals to easily access information from their personal computers, and it is logical to assume that both counselors and clients will want to access assessment information.

The Internet is growing at an astounding rate and, therefore, it is difficult to project how practitioners in the coming years can best utilize it. There already exist a number of ways that counselors can use the Internet in the assessment process. One method is to use the Internet to gather information about possible assessment instruments and techniques. Using one of the common search engines and entering the words "assessment in counseling" produced 631,616 matches. In perusing the matches, we found a multitude of topics, such as overviews of counseling agencies and centers, syllabi for courses in assessment in counseling, overviews of counseling departments' faculty, assessments related to cancer risks, and information on professional organizations. One of the difficulties in using the Internet is sorting through the volumes of information in order to find pertinent and applicable information.

Many times clinicians identify areas where they would like to use a formal instrument to supplement their clinical decision making (e.g., screening tools for groups, suicide potential measures, measures related to certain problems, behavioral checklists). These clinicians, however, often have difficulty identifying potential instruments. The Internet can be an extremely helpful resource in locating possible instruments and getting descriptions of those instruments. Appendix B contains some addresses for Internet sites related to assessment and appraisal in counseling. I have found two of those sites to be particularly helpful in identifying potential instruments. As mentioned in Chapter 5, both through the ERIC Clearinghouse of Assessment and Evaluation (http://ericaenet/testcol.htm) and the Buros Institute of Mental Measurement (http://www.unl.edu/buros) sites, an individual can access the *Test Locator*. A practitioner can enter a descriptor, such as a type of instrument, and the *Test Locator* sorts through 9,500 instruments and provides the counselor with a list of instruments that correspond to the descriptor. The individual can then get descriptions of instruments that seem to have potential. Moreover, from these same sites, the clinician can then use the *Test Review Locator* to get a listing of critiques of the instrument published in the *Mental Measurements Yearbooks, Test In Print,* or *Test Critiques.* These three resources can be found at most local libraries.

Not only can counselors currently get descriptions of counseling assessment instruments, they can also order assessment materials over the Internet. Included in Appendix B are the Internet addresses for many of the larger publishers of assessment instruments used by counselors. Thus, counselors can access information on the costs of potential instruments and order assessment materials. For many of the publishers of psychological assessments, clinicians will first have to submit a user's qualification form that indicates that they have the sufficient background and training to administer the particular instrument they are ordering. A word of caution concerning ordering any materials over the Internet: it is advisable to order materials only through *secured on-line sites*.

People can now take certain instruments on the Internet and it is expected that this practice will grow. Taking instruments on the Internet has some advantages, but it also has the potential to be harmful. Depending on the type of instrument, the Internet could be an easy means for individuals to access the assessment. For example, sites (e.g., schools, colleges, and vocational rehabilitation services) that subscribe to the Alaskan Career Information System can now access it through the Internet. The sites are given a password that they can give to clients who have had an orientation to the system with a counselor. The clients can then access it through the computers provided through the site or in other places, such as their home or in a library. The assessments in this Career Information System are simple and nonthreatening and, thus, many clients can use them unsupervised. Having systems like this on the Internet may allow clients more flexibility in using these simple assessment tools.

There are, however, assessment tools that probably should not be on the Internet unsupervised. Many of the personality instruments discussed in Chapter 10 should not be made available on-line without clinical supervision. The unsupervised use of personality instruments could potentially be harmful. Individuals could easily misinterpret the results and suffer unnecessarily. Many of these instruments were developed by professionals who know the ethical standards and codes and would not allow the inappropriate use of these instruments. Furthermore, these instruments are copyrighted and, hence, others cannot put these exact instruments on the Internet. Sampson (1998) predicted that standard instruments would soon be available over the Internet. In this case, the clinician would be approved by the publisher and pay for a certain number of Internet administrations and scorings or interpretations. Therefore, rather than receiving software for clients to take the instrument on a personal computer, the clinician would receive a password to a cybernet site and the clients would take the instrument at the site. The site would then score the instrument, which would be secured so that it is only accessible to the clinician. This may expedite services to clients, for if a counselor does not have an appropriate instrument in his or her files (or on his or her computer), the client and counselor would not have to wait for the clinician to order materials and for them to be shipped. It may also assist instrument developers and publishers to gather more data related to their instruments, as it would be easy to gather information through the interactive nature of the Internet.

The Internet also holds promise for developing new methods of assessment. One of the possibilities is the integration of interactive video (Sampson, 1998). Interactive video could open new methodologies for assessing multicultural clients and those with literacy deficiencies. Interactive video also may open up new methods for computer analysis of a client's response to projective techniques. The computer would present the stimuli, the client's comments would be fed back to the computer, and themes could then be extracted.

There are, however, substantial risks associated with Internet assessment. One of the greatest risks concerns instruments being developed and marketed by individuals with little or no background in counseling or psychological assessment. Individuals may place more confidence in these results, as compared to magazine personality tests, because by being on the Internet, the instruments have an illusion of technological sophistication. The possibility of making a profit from marketing psychological instruments through the Internet appears to exist. Currently, there are numerous sites that advertise intelligence tests and personality instruments. One problem is that individuals may be taking these instruments and making crucial decisions based on assessments that are low in reliability and have no validation evidence. For example, a depressed client could take a psychometrically unsound instrument that could indicate that she was not depressed. This client may continue to suffer from depression when treatment could have possibly helped her. There are considerable risks associated with the widespread use of invalid instruments over the Internet. Currently, there is no formal or informal oversight of these instruments and they can appear very professional to the layperson

Future Trends and Directions

When we speculate about future trends in assessment in counseling, we would find a crystal ball helpful because there are conflicting opinions concerning those future directions. In the educational community, some individuals will contend that educational reform can best be accomplished by more assessment of students, while others contend that less intrusion and assessment is the wave of the future. Even within counseling, some argue that testing is no longer relevant to counseling practice (Goldman, 1994), while others argue that assessment will continue to play an important role in the services provided to clients (Hood & Johnson, 1997). Certainly social, economic, and political developments have influenced assessment practices in the past and will continue to influence assessment in the future. Current practices and trends in appraisal can also provide some insight into future directions and developments.

Increased Use of Technology

In examining future trends in appraisal in counseling, I would be negligent not to mention again the rapidly evolving influence that technology is having on this field. It may be that our grandchildren will laugh when we tell them how we used to take tests using paper and pencils. The Internet is just beginning to be used in assessment; publishers are beginning to offer testing through the Internet. On the Internet today, individuals can take personality tests, aptitude assessments, and even intelligence tests. Due to the unregulated status of the Internet, there are no controls on who publishes these instruments and whether assessment instruments comply with any established standards. The possibility exists that individuals could take instruments that are unreliable or invalid. Whether professional organizations should monitor the use of psychological assessments on the Internet is the subject of some debate. This certainly is a topic that will be discussed in future professional forums. It is anticipated that in the near future, professional guidelines will be issued that will guide practitioners in the appropriate use of Internet assessment with clients.

The Internet is not the only area related to technology that will influence assessment in counseling, for technological advances may incorporate a wide spectrum of developments. Computer scanners are beginning to be used so that more original works can be entered into the computer. In addition, sophistication in computer programming allows for more intricate and complex scoring. These developments allow for the scoring of less-structured assessments, such as analysis of drawings, essays, or stories. Other technologies, such as the expansion of video analysis, may influence appraisal methods in counseling. In this case, the initial interview could be videotaped and analyzed by computers. There is little doubt that technological applications will be incorporated into assessment procedures; the questions surround what new technologies will be developed in the coming decades.

Alternative Methods for Multicultural Assessment

In many sections of this book, issues related to multicultural assessment have been discussed. As we move to a more global society, the issues in multicultural assessment become even more complex. Developing instruments that may be appropriate for children in Japan, Sri Lanka, Indiana, and Botswana is astoundingly difficult. Yet, as the field of counseling becomes more international, the issues related to multicultural assessment must continue to be studied. One of the issues related to multicultural assessment concerns the development of appropriate norming groups. The determination of whether to use separate norms or combined norms is complex and there are no simple solutions. The counselor must look at the situation and the type of information needed in order to determine the appropriate norming group. In addition, there may be times when an appropriate norming group is not available, and the practitioner must then sort out what information can be appropriately inferred from the client's results. Refinement of testing techniques, such as Item Response Theory, may provide better methods for assessing clients from diverse backgrounds.

Future research may help guide practitioners in the complicated clinical decisions associated with multicultural assessment. Additional research may aid clinicians in understanding different cultures and which instruments provide more valid information. Research may also assist practitioners by identifying other information that is germane to the interpretation of the assessment results of clients from certain cultures. The field must attend to providing practitioners with better methods of assessing all clients.

Expansion of Authentic/Performance Assessment

The movement in the 1990s toward authentic or performance-based assessment is directly related to the concept that better assessment is performed through the gathering of multiple measures of an individual's performance. The intent of these strategies is to assess the individual in a real or authentic manner; hence, the assessment strategy should match the skill or process being measured. In addition, performance-based or authentic assessment employs context-sensitive strategies that focus on higher-order or complex skills. Researchers are beginning to explore methods for evaluating the psychometric qualities of these assessment strategies. It is anticipated that researchers will develop authentic/performance assessments that are standardized. These standardized authentic/performance assessments will be psychometrically sound and have established criteria for evaluating the aspects of the assessment. Attempting to measure in a real or authentic manner does not guarantee that the assessment is valid. In all likelihood, there will be well-established and researched authentic/performance assessments in the future.

Performance or authentic assessment has had a significant influence on assessment in the area of achievement (Baker, O'Neil, & Linn, 1993). This philosophy of assessment may also influence other areas of assessment, such as personality and intelligence. In counseling, it may be helpful to systematically gather context-sensitive or real-life information. For example, in dealing with marital issues a counselor would often find it helpful to observe a disagreement between the couple outside of the counseling office. In many ways, counselors have always attempted to implement authentic or performance assessment. In the future, however, researchers may provide insights into how to systematically use authentic assessment in counseling.

Continued Demands for Accountability Information

Indications are that practitioners will need to provide more accountability information in the future (Whiston, 1996). In all likelihood, administrators, managed health care organizations, school boards, and even clients will increasingly demand proof that the services counselors provide are worth the cost. Researchers are refining methods of outcome assessment and clinicians may be wise to incorporate those methods into their practice. Technology may also change how accountability information is gathered. Some publishers are developing computer-assisted assessment programs that provide treatment planning information and accountability data. The assessment of counseling outcome can not only produce accountability data, but it can also provide information that clinicians can use to increase their own effectiveness.

Rise of New Ethical and Legal Issues

Although it would be desirable to predict that all assessment instruments will be used in an ethical manner in the future, the history of assessment does not support that prediction. Even as far back as 2,000 years ago, there is evidence that there were concerns about the ethical use of the Chinese civil service examination (Bowman, 1989). As technology becomes more intertwined in many types of testing, new ethical issues will probably arise. On-line assessment poses new dilemmas related to confidentiality.

Assessment training and competencies may be a focus of ethical concerns in the coming years. It is anticipated that there will be continued efforts to legally restrict counselors' use of assessment measures. Counselors need to document that they have received adequate training and are competent. There is, however, little research that establishes what constitutes adequate training. Some current research (e.g., Moreland et al., 1995) provides some insight into assessment competencies; yet, additional inquiry is needed in this area. In the future, we may know more about the skills that are necessary in assessing clients effectively.

Summary   This chapter explored current practice in using computers and technologies in assessment and examined future trends and directions in the field. Computers are having a significant influence on current assessment practices. There are two ways that computers are influencing this area. One method is through computer-assisted assessment, in which the computer performs any of the functions related to the administration, scoring, or interpretation of an assessment. The second method is computer-adapted assessment, in which the computer adapts the instrument contingent on the individual's responses while the individual is taking the instrument. The most common example of computer-adapted assessment is item branching, in which items or test questions are dependent on the previous responses.

When we discuss issues related to the inputting of information into computers, the focus tends to be on computer-administered assessment. People generally have positive attitudes toward computer-administered assessment, but there is variation in the amount of experience clients have with computers. The psychometric qualities of any instrument must be evaluated before it is used and this also applies to a computerized instrument. If the instrument is an adoption of a paper-and-pencil instrument, then the equivalence of the two forms must also be evaluated. In terms of assessment, computer outputs can vary from simple scoring to extended and complex interpretations. Computers are being increasingly used not only to score the results but also to provide interpretive reports. A counselor using a computer-generated report must evaluate the quality and content of the report. Practitioners cannot rely just on computer-generated reports; they must also be knowledgeable about the strengths and limitations of the instrument.

In considering using a computer application, clinicians need to consider the advantages and disadvantages of the computer in the assessment process. Computers can save counselors' time and often provide results back to the client immediately. In addition, they can perform complex scoring and interpretation functions quickly, without the errors to which humans are prone. Computers are not biased and they analyze the information without taking into account the individual's race, gender, or sexual orientation. There are also limitations to using computers in appraisal. Some information is often lost in using computers because clients are often not observed by the clinician while the clients are taking computer-administered assessments. Confidentiality issues must also be addressed if assessment information is stored on a computer.

The Internet is another technology-related tool that counselors can use in the assessment process. The Internet can be very useful in identifying possible instruments and getting descriptions of those instruments. In addition, many instruments can be ordered over the Internet by qualified users. There also appears to be potential for innovative methods of assessment through the Internet. The Internet is unmonitored, however, and there are no controls on the quality of the instruments that are accessible. The possibility exists that unsound instruments are being used by people, and the field needs to consider methods to protect the public from fraudulent instruments.

The second segment of this chapter concerned future trends and directions in the field of appraisal. Technological changes will probably affect the delivery of assessment services in the future. Some of those changes may involve the Internet, more sophisticated computer software, and advances in video technology. It is clear that in the coming years, computers and technology will continue to have a significant influence on assessment in counseling. Professionals need to ensure that these technological advances are used in the best interests of clients. It is anticipated that multicultural assessment will be the focus of future research. Given our more global society and the changing demographics in the United States, there will probably be more demands for effective methods of assessing clients from diverse cultures. Authentic or performance-based assessment has had an influence on the assessment of achievement in the 1990s. There is some speculation that this approach will continue to be influential and influence other assessment areas. Some of the ideas from authentic or performance-based assessment may have an influence on the methods used in assessment in counseling. The ethical delivery of assessment services will continue to be a professional issue in the coming decades. Research, we hope, will provide insight into ethical practices and needed competencies.

Concluding Remarks

In this book I have argued that assessment is an integral part of the counseling process and that counselors need to be skilled assessors. To provide effective counseling service, the counselor has to first assess the client. For counselors, competency in both formal and informal assessment techniques is a necessity in today's mental health care environment. In my opinion, formal and informal assessment strategies can complement each other, resulting in more effective assessment. Informal assessments are subject to counselor bias and typically lack reliability and validation evidence. Formal assessment instruments, while typically objective, are often narrow in focus and cannot measure all client factors. The purpose of this book is to assist counseling students, counselors, and others in the helping professions to become skillful consumers of assessment measures. By using assessment measures effectively, practitioners can assist clients in making decisions, solving problems, functioning more effectively, and achieving their potential.

As I close this book, I want to encourage readers to consider their future clients. In terms of assessment skills, each counselor has strengths and limitations and it is important for you to consider what your strengths and limitations are in this area. In considering future directions, you need to consider methods for expanding those strengths and find avenues for remediating those limitations. All of your clients deserve professional and ethical counseling services, which can be facilitated by the development of competent assessment skills. Therefore, I want to encourage you to continue to expand your assessment skills.

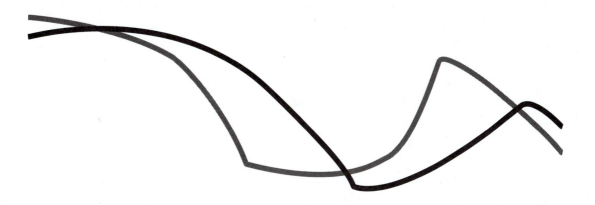

APPENDIX A

Table of Areas under the Normal Curve

z	.00	.01	.02	.03	.04	.05	.06	.07	.08	.09
−3.0	.0013	.0013	.0013	.0012	.0012	.0011	.0011	.0011	.0010	.0010
−2.9	.0019	.0018	.0018	.0017	.0016	.0016	.0015	.0015	.0014	.0014
−2.8	.0026	.0025	.0024	.0023	.0023	.0022	.0021	.0021	.0020	.0019
−2.7	.0035	.0034	.0033	.0032	.0031	.0030	.0029	.0028	.0027	.0026
−2.6	.0047	.0045	.0044	.0043	.0041	.0040	.0039	.0038	.0037	.0036
−2.5	.0062	.0060	.0059	.0057	.0055	.0054	.0052	.0051	.0049	.0048
−2.4	.0082	.0080	.0078	.0075	.0077	.0071	.0069	.0068	.0066	.0064
−2.3	.0107	.0104	.0102	.0099	.0096	.0094	.0091	.0089	.0087	.0084
−2.2	.0139	.0136	.0132	.0129	.0125	.0122	.0119	.0116	.0113	.0110
−2.1	.0179	.0174	.0170	.0166	.0162	.0158	.0154	.0150	.0146	.0143
−2.0	.0228	.0222	.0217	.0212	.0207	.0202	.0197	.0192	.0188	.0183
−1.9	.0287	.0281	.0274	.0268	.0262	.0256	.0250	.0244	.0239	.0233
−1.8	.0359	.0351	.0344	.0336	.0329	.0322	.0314	.0307	.0301	.0294
−1.7	.0446	.0436	.0427	.0418	.0409	.0401	.0392	.0384	.0375	.0367
−1.6	.0548	.0537	.0526	.0516	.0505	.0495	.0485	.0475	.0465	.0455
−1.5	.0668	.0655	.0643	.0630	.0618	.0606	.0594	.0582	.0571	.0559
−1.4	.0808	.0793	.0778	.0764	.0749	.0735	.0721	.0708	.0694	.0681
−1.3	.0968	.0951	.0934	.0918	.0901	.0885	.0869	.0853	.0838	.0823
−1.2	.1151	.1131	.1112	.1093	.1075	.1056	.1038	.1020	.1003	.0985
−1.1	.1357	.1335	.1314	.1292	.1271	.1251	.1230	.1210	.1190	.1170
−1.0	.1587	.1562	.1539	.1515	.1492	.1469	.1446	.1423	.1401	.1379
−0.9	.1841	.1814	.1788	.1762	.1736	.1711	.1685	.1660	.1635	.1611
−0.8	.2119	.2090	.2061	.2033	.2005	.1977	.1949	.1922	.1894	.1867
−0.7	.2420	.2389	.2358	.2327	.2296	.2266	.2236	.2206	.2177	.2148
−0.6	.2743	.2709	.2676	.2643	.2611	.2578	.2546	.2514	.2483	.2451
−0.5	.3085	.3050	.3015	.2981	.2946	.2912	.2877	.2843	.2810	.2776
−0.4	.3446	.3409	.3372	.3336	.3300	.3264	.3228	.3194	.3156	.3121
−0.3	.3821	.3783	.3745	.3707	.3669	.3632	.3594	.3557	.3520	.3483
−0.2	.4207	.4168	.4129	.4090	.4052	.4013	.3974	.3936	.3897	.3859
−0.1	.4602	.4562	.4522	.4483	.4443	.4404	.4364	.4325	.4286	.4247
−0.0	.5000	.4960	.4920	.4880	.4840	.4801	.4761	.4721	.4681	.4641
0.0	.5000	.5040	.5080	.5120	.5160	.5199	.5239	.5279	.5319	.5359
0.1	.5398	.5438	.5478	.5517	.5557	.5596	.5636	.5675	.5714	.5753
0.2	.5793	.5832	.5871	.5910	.5948	.5987	.6026	.6064	.6103	.6141
0.3	.6179	.6217	.6255	.6293	.6331	.6368	.6406	.6443	.6480	.6517
0.4	.6554	.6591	.6628	.6664	.6700	.6736	.6772	.6808	.6844	.6879
0.5	.6915	.6950	.6985	.7019	.7054	.7088	.7123	.7157	.7190	.7224

z	.00	.01	.02	.03	.04	.05	.06	.07	.08	.09
0.6	.7257	.7291	.7324	.7357	.7389	.7422	.7454	.7486	.7517	.7549
0.7	.7580	.7611	.7642	.7673	.7704	.7734	.7764	.7794	.7823	.7852
0.8	.7881	.7910	.7939	.7967	.7995	.8023	.8051	.8078	.8106	.8133
0.9	.8159	.8186	.8212	.8238	.8264	.8289	.8315	.8340	.8365	.8389
1.0	.8413	.8438	.8461	.8485	.8508	.8531	.8554	.8577	.8599	.8621
1.1	.8643	.8665	.8686	.8708	.8729	.8749	.8770	.8790	.8810	.8830
1.2	.8849	.8869	.8888	.8907	.8925	.8944	.8962	.8980	.8997	.9015
1.3	.9032	.9049	.9066	.9082	.9099	.9115	.9131	.9147	.9162	.9177
1.4	.9192	.9207	.9222	.9236	.9251	.9265	.9279	.9292	.9306	.9319
1.5	.9332	.9345	.9357	.9370	.9382	.9394	.9406	.9418	.9429	.9441
1.6	.9452	.9463	.9474	.9484	.9495	.9505	.9515	.9525	.9535	.9545
1.7	.9554	.9564	.9573	.9582	.9591	.9599	.9608	.9616	.9625	.9633
1.8	.9641	.9649	.9656	.9664	.9671	.9678	.9686	.9693	.9699	.9706
1.9	.9713	.9719	.9726	.9732	.9738	.9744	.9750	.9756	.9761	.9767
2.0	.9772	.9778	.9783	.9788	.9793	.9798	.9803	.9808	.9812	.9817
2.1	.9821	.9826	.9830	.9834	.9838	.9842	.9846	.9850	.9854	.9857
2.2	.9861	.9864	.9868	.9871	.9875	.9878	.9881	.9884	.9887	.9890
2.3	.9893	.9896	.9898	.9901	.9904	.9906	.9909	.9911	.9913	.9916
2.4	.9918	.9920	.9922	.9925	.9927	.9929	.9931	.9932	.9934	.9936
2.5	.9938	.9940	.9941	.9943	.9945	.9946	.9948	.9949	.9951	.9952
2.6	.9953	.9955	.9956	.9957	.9959	.9960	.9961	.9962	.9963	.9964
2.7	.9965	.9966	.9967	.9968	.9969	.9970	.9971	.9972	.9973	.9974
2.8	.9974	.9975	.9976	.9977	.9977	.9978	.9979	.9979	.9980	.9981
2.9	.9981	.9982	.9982	.9983	.9984	.9984	.9985	.9985	.9986	.9986
3.0	.9987	.9987	.9987	.9988	.9988	.9989	.9989	.9989	.9990	.9990

Web Sites of Assessment-Related Organizations and Instrument Sources

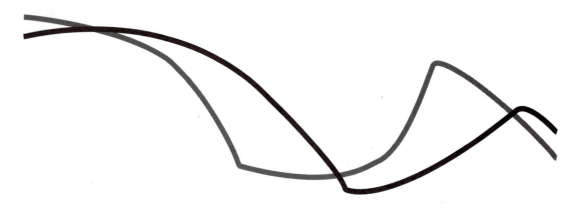

American Association for Marriage and Family Therapists   http://www.amft.org/
  The site for the American Association for Marriage and Family Therapists.

American College Testing Program   http://www.act.org/
  The site for the American College Testing Program's assessment services and on-line registration.

American Counseling Association   http://www.counseling.org/
  The site of the American Counseling Association.

American Guidance Service   http://www.agsnet.com/
  A publisher of educational assessments, clinical instruments, and instructional materials.

American Psychological Association   http://www.apa.org/
  The site of the American Psychological Association, which provides methods for searching for information related to psychology.

Armed Services Vocational Aptitude Battery   http://www.dmdc.osd.mil/asvab/
  A site where information related to the ASVAB and career exploration can be downloaded.

Behavior Data Systems   http://www.bdsltd.com/bdsltd/front.html
  A publisher of computerized assessments in the area of drug or alcohol abuse, substance abuse disorders, and chemical dependency.

Buros Institute of Mental Measurements   http://www.unl.edu/buros/
>An excellent source for identifying possible instruments and gathering information about those instruments.

College Board   http://www.collegeboard.org/
>Provides information on the College Board and students can register for the SAT.

Consulting Psychologists Press, Inc.   http://www.cpp-db.com/
>A publisher that distributes a number of personality and career instruments.

Cresst   http://www.cresst96.cse.ucla.edu/index.htm
>Site for the National Center for Research on Evaluation, Standards, and Student Testing (CRESST), which is funded to perform research related to important topics in K–12 educational testing.

CTB/McGraw-Hill   http://www.ctb.com/
>A publisher of tests such as the TerraNova and the Comprehensive Test of Basic Skills.

Educational Testing Service   http://www.ets.org/
>A publisher of instruments such as the SAT, the GRE, and the TOEFL.

ERIC Clearinghouse on Assessment and Evaluation   http://www.ericae.net/
>An excellent sit for identifying possible instruments and getting information about those instruments.

Frequently Asked Questions on Psychological Assessment   http://www.apa.org/science/index.htm
>A site developed by the American Psychological Association that answers many of the typical questions related to assessment.

Harcourt Brace Educational Measurement   http://www.hbem.com/
>A subsidiary of Harcourt Brace & Company that specializes in educational assessment instruments.

Individuals with Disabilities Education Act   http://www.edlaw.net/public/ptabcont.html
>Provides information related to this legislation.

Mental Health Net—Professional Resources Index   http://www.cmhc.com/prof.htm
>A site that provides information on other on-line information sources related to mental health counseling.

National Association of Testing Directors   http://www.natd.org/
>This organization is charged with providing information on testing and the Web site has resources related to testing.

National Computer Systems, Inc.   http://www.ncs.com/
>A company that provides software, systems, and services for the collection, management, and interpretation of psychological data.

National Council on Meaurement in Education   http://www.assessment.iupui.edu/NCME/NCME.html
>A professional organization that is committed to the continual improvement of testing and measurement practices in education.

Pesco International   http://www.pesco.org/
  A publisher of career assessment and job placement tools.
PRO-ED Publishing   http://www.proedinc.com/frame1603031.html
  PRO-ED publishes, produces, and sells books, tests, curricular materials,
  journals, and therapy materials. Publications include *A Consumer's Guide
  to Tests in Print, Tests, and Test Critiques.*
Psychological Assessment Online   http://wso.net/assessment/
  A site designed to provide comprehensive information on on-line psy-
  chological assessment. The site provides basic information on the types
  of psychological assessments and resources that are available on-line.
Psychological Assessment Resources, Inc.   http://www.parinc.com/
  A publisher of psychological assessment instruments related to
  counseling, personality, career, and other areas.
Psychological Assessment—A Brief Guide   http://www.ourworld.compuserve.
  com/homepages/inkblot/
  A brief guide that explains different types of assessments (e.g., Projective
  Personality Tests, Objective Personality Tests).
PsychQuest Psychological Assessment Services   http://www.psychquest.com/
  An organization that provides psychological assessment services
  specifically for those located in health care or medical contexts.
Riverside Publishing   http://www.riverpub.com/
  A publisher of both educational and clinical assessment instruments.
SASSI Institute   http://www.sassi.com/
  A publisher of instruments related to substance abuse.
Sigma Assessment Systems, Inc.   http://www.mgl.ca/~sigma/
  A publisher that focuses on personality and career assessment instruments.
Teacher/Pathfinder Organization on Assessment   http://www.teacherpathfinder.
  org/School/Assessment/assessment.html
  A site that has many resources related to assessment in the schools (e.g.,
  Alternative Assessment Essays, Assessment and Accountability Program).
Tests Materials Resource Book Online   http://www.psychtest.com/
  A Canadian organization that provides services on the selection and
  purchasing of commercially published standardized tests.
The Psychological Corporation   http://www.psychcorp.com/
  A subsidiary of Harcourt Brace & Company that primarily publishes
  assessment instruments for psychologists (e.g., WAIS-III).

American Counseling Association's Code of Ethics and Standards of Practice

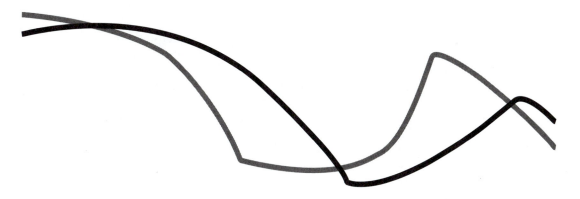

Section E: Evaluation, Assessment, and Interpretation

E.1. General

a. *Appraisal Techniques.* The primary purpose of educational and psychological assessment is to provide measures that are objective and interpretable in either comparative or absolute terms. Counselors recognize the need to interpret the statements in this section as applying to the whole range of appraisal techniques, including test and nontest data.

b. *Client Welfare.* Counselors promote the welfare and best interests of the client in the development, publication, and utilization of educational and psychological assessment techniques. They do not misuse assessment results and interpretations and take reasonable steps to prevent others from misusing the information these techniques provide. They respect the client's right to know the results, the interpretations made, and the bases for their conclusions and recommendations.

E.2. *Competence to Use and Interpret Tests*

a. *Limits of Competence.* Counselors recognize the limits of their competence and perform only those testing and assessment services for which they have been trained. They are familiar with reliability, validity, related standardization, error of measurement, and proper application of any technique utilized. Counselors using computer-based test interpretations are trained in the construct being measured and the specific instrument being used prior to using this type of computer application. Counselors take reasonable measures to ensure the proper use of psychological assessment techniques by persons under their supervision.

b. *Appropriate Use.* Counselors are responsible for the appropriate application, scoring, interpretation, and use of assessment instruments, whether they score and interpret such tests themselves or use computerized or other services.

c. *Decisions Based on Results.* Counselors responsible for decisions involving individuals or policies that are based on assessment results have a thorough understanding of educational and psychological measurement, including validation criteria, test research, and guidelines for test development and use.

d. *Accurate Information.* Counselors provide accurate information and avoid false claims or misconceptions when making statements about assessment instruments or techniques. Special efforts are made to avoid unwarranted connotations of such terms as IQ and grade equivalent scores. (See C.5.c.)

E.3. *Informed Consent*

a. *Explanation to Clients.* Prior to assessment, counselors explain the nature and purposes of assessment and the specific use of results in language the client (or other legally authorized person on behalf of the client) can understand, unless an explicit exception to this right has been agreed upon in advance. Regardless of whether scoring and interpretation are completed by counselors, by assistants, or by computer or other outside services, counselors take reasonable steps to ensure that appropriate explanations are given to the client.

b. *Recipients of Results.* The examinee's welfare, explicit understanding, and prior agreement determine the recipients of test results. Counselors include accurate and appropriate interpretations with any release of individual or group test results. (See B.1.a. and C.5.c.)

E.4. *Release of Information to Competent Professionals*

a. *Misuse of Results.* Counselors do not misuse assessment results, including test results, and interpretations, and take reasonable steps to prevent the misuse of such by others. (See C.5.c.)

b. *Release of Raw Data.* Counselors ordinarily release data (e.g. protocols, counseling or interview notes, or questionnaires) in which the client is identified only with the consent of the client or the client's legal representative. Such data are usually released only to persons recognized by counselors as competent to interpret the data. (See B.1.a.)

E.5. *Proper Diagnosis of Mental Disorders*

a. *Proper Diagnosis.* Counselors take special care to provide proper diagnosis of mental disorders. Assessment techniques (including personal interview) used to determine client care (e.g., focus of treatment, type of treatment, or recommended follow-up) are carefully selected and appropriately used. (See A.3.a. and C.5.c.)

b. *Cultural Sensitivity.* Counselors recognize that culture affects the manner in which clients' problems are defined. Clients' socioeconomic and cultural experience is considered when diagnosing mental disorders.

E.6. *Test Selection*

a. *Appropriateness of Instruments.* Counselors carefully consider the validity, reliability, psychometric limitations, and appropriateness of instruments when selecting tests for use in a given situation or with a particular client.

b. *Culturally Diverse Populations.* Counselors are cautious when selecting tests for culturally diverse populations to avoid inappropriateness of testing that may be outside of socialized behavior or cognitive patterns.

E.7. *Conditions of Test Administration*

a. *Administration Conditions.* Counselors administer tests under the same conditions that were established in their standardization. When tests are not administered under standard conditions or when unusual behavior or irregularities occur during the testing session, those conditions are noted in interpretation, and the results may be designated as invalid or of questionable validity.

b. *Computer Administration.* Counselors are responsible for ensuring that administration programs function properly to provide clients with accurate results when a computer or other electronic methods are used for test administration. (See A.12.b.)

c. *Unsupervised Test-Taking.* Counselors do not permit unsupervised or inadequately supervised use of tests or assessments unless the tests or assessments are designed, intended, and validated for self-administration and/or scoring.

d. *Disclosure of Favorable Conditions.* Prior to test administration, conditions that produce most favorable test results are made known to the examinee.

E.8. Diversity in Testing

Counselors are cautious in using assessment techniques, making evaluations, and interpreting the performance of populations not represented in the norm group on which an instrument was standardized. They recognize the effects of age, color, culture, disability, ethnic group, gender, race, religion, sexual orientation, and socioeconomic status on test administration and interpretation and place tests results in proper perspective with other relevant factors. (See A.2.a.)

E.9. Test Scoring and Interpretation

a. *Reporting Reservations.* In reporting assessment results, counselors indicate any reservations that exist regarding validity or reliability because of the circumstances of the assessment or the inappropriateness of the norms for the person tested.

b. *Research Instruments.* Counselors exercise caution when interpreting the results of research instruments possessing insufficient technical data to support respondent results. The specific purposes for the use of such instruments are stated explicitly to the examinee.

c. *Testing Services.* Counselors who provide test scoring and test interpretation services to support the assessment process confirm the validity of such interpretations. They accurately describe the purpose, norms, validity, reliability, and applications of the procedures and any special qualifications applicable to their use. The public offering of an automated test interpretations service is considered a professional-to-professional consultation. The formal responsibility of the consultant is to the consultee, but the ultimate and overriding responsibility is to the client.

E.10. Test Security

Counselors maintain the integrity and security of tests and other assessment techniques consistent with legal and contractual obligations. Counselors do not appropriate, reproduce, or modify published tests or parts thereof without acknowledgment and permission from the publisher.

E.11. Obsolete Tests and Outdated Test Results

Counselors do not use data or test results that are obsolete or outdated for the current purpose. Counselors make every effort to prevent the misuse of obsolete measures and test data by others.

GLOSSARY

Achievement test An assessment in which the person has "achieved" either knowledge, information, or skills through instruction, training or experience. Achievement tests measure acquired knowledge and do not make any predictions about the future.

Age norms Age norms are often based on the typical or average score of that age group and the scores are then extrapolated to provide age-equivalent scores. Other times, age norms are used where there are appropriate successive age groups and scores are based on comparisons of students who are at different age levels.

Alternate form reliability A reliability coefficient is estimated by examining the relationship between two alternate, or parallel, forms of an instrument. The reliability coefficient indicates the extent to which the two forms are consistent or reliable in measuring that specific content.

Aptitude test A test that provides a prediction about the individual's future performance or ability to learn based on his or her performance on the test. Aptitude tests often predict either future academic or vocational/career performance.

Authentic assessments Performance assessments that involve the performance of "real" or authentic applications rather than proxies or estimators of actual learning.

Barnum effect A personality description that appears to be authentic but is written so vaguely that it applies to everyone.

Bias testing A term that refers to the degree to which construct-irrelevant factors systematically affect a specific group's performance.

Coefficient of determination This statistic estimates the percent of shared variance between two sets of variables that have been correlated. The coefficient of determination (r^2) is calculated by squaring the correlation coefficient.

Cognitive instruments Tests that assess cognition. The cognitive domain typically involves skills of perceiving, processing, concrete and abstract thinking, and remembering. The three types of cognitive tests are intelligence or general ability tests, achievement tests, and aptitude tests.

Computer-adapted assessment A term that applies to an interactive process between the individual and the computer during the assessment.

Computer-assisted assessment An assessment in which computers are used to assist in the administration, scoring, or interpretation of the assessment.

Concurrent validity A type of criterion-related validity in which there is no delay between the time the instrument is administered and the time the criterion information is gathered.

Content-related validity One of the three major categories of validity, in which the focus is on whether the instrument's content adequately represents the domain being assessed. Evidence of content-related validity is particularly important in achievement tests.

Construct validity One of the three types of validity that is broader than either content- or criterion-related validity. Construct validity is concerned with the extent to which the instrument measures some psychological trait or construct. This type of validation involves the gradual accumulation of evidence.

Convergent evidence Validation evidence that indicates the measure is positively related with other measures of the construct.

Correlation A statistic that provides an indication of the degree to which two sets of scores are related. A *correlation coefficient* (r) can range from -1.00 to $+1.00$ and, thus, provides an indicator of both the strength and direction of the relationship. A correlation of $+1.00$ represents a perfect positive relationship; a correlation of -1.00 represents a perfect negative or inverse relationship. A correlation coefficient of .00 indicates the absence of a relationship.

Criterion-referenced instrument Instruments designed to compare an individual's performance to a stated criterion or standard. Often criterion-referenced instruments provide information on specific knowledge or skills and on whether the individual has "mastered" that knowledge or skill. The focus is on what the person knows rather than how he or she compares to other people.

Criterion-related validity One of the three types of validity in which the focus is the extent to which the instrument confirms (concurrent validity) or predicts (predictive validity) a criterion measure.

Cronbach's Alpha Also known as *coefficient alpha,* it is one of the methods of estimating reliability through the examination of the internal consistency of the instrument. This method is appropriate when the instrument is *not* dichotomously scored, such as an instrument that uses a Likert-scale.

Crystallized abilities (Gc) A factor theorized to be part of intelligence that includes acquired skills and knowledge. Crystallized abilities are thought to be influenced by cultural, social, and educational experiences.

Differential item functioning (DIF) A statistical method for investigating item bias that examines differences in performance among individuals who are equal in ability but are from different groups (e.g., different ethnic groups).

Discriminant evidence Validation evidence that indicates the measure is not related to measures of different psychological constructs.

Domain sampling theory Another term for generalizability theory.

Expectancy table A method of providing criterion-related validity evidence that involves charting performance on the criterion based on the instrument's score. It is often used to predict who would be expected to fall in a certain criterion category (e.g., who is likely to succeed in graduate school) and to determine cutoff scores.

False negative In decision theory, a term used to describe when the assessment procedure is incorrect in predicting a negative outcome on the criterion.

False positive In decision theory, a term used to describe when the assessment procedure is incorrect in predicting a positive outcome on the criterion.

Fluid abilities (Gf) A factor theorized to be part of intelligence and related to the abilities to respond to and solve entirely new kinds of problems. These abilities are thought to be influenced by genetic factors.

Frequency distribution A chart that summarizes the scores on an instrument and the frequency or number of people receiving that score. Scores are often grouped into intervals to provide an easy-to-understand chart that summarizes overall performance.

Frequency polygon A graphic representation of the frequency of scores. The number or frequency of individuals receiving a score or falling within an interval of scores is plotted with points that are connected by straight lines.

Generalizability theory An alternative model to the true score model of reliability. The focus of this theory is on estimating the extent to which specific sources of variation under defined conditions influence scores on an instrument.

Grade equivalent norms Norms that are typically used in achievement tests and pro-vide scores in terms of grade equivalents. In some instruments, grade equivalent scores are not validated on each specific grade but are extrapolated scores based on group performance at each grade level.

Group separation table Another term for an expectancy table.

Heritability index (h²) An estimate of the amount of variation of a trait (e.g., intelligence) that is due to genetic influences.

Histogram A graphic representation of the frequency of scores in which columns are utilized.

Interval scale A type of measurement scale in which the units are in equal intervals. Many of the statistics used to evaluate an instrument's psychometric qualities require an interval scale.

Ipsative Interpretation One in which the format of the item requires the individual to make choices (i.e., forced-choice), so that an individual's score on one variable is affected by his or her scores on other variables measured.

Item analysis A set of procedures used to evaluate individual items on an assessment instrument. The most common item analysis techniques are item difficulty and item discrimination.

Item difficulty An item analysis method in which the difficulty of individual items is determined. The most common item difficulty index (*p*) is the percentage of people who get the item correct.

Item discrimination A form of item analysis that examines the degree to which an individual item discriminates on some criterion. For example, in achievement testing, item discrimination would indicate whether the item discriminates between people who know the information and people who do not.

Item response theory A measurement approach in which the focus is on each item and on establishing items that measure the individual's ability or level of a latent trait. This approach involves examining the item characteristic function and the calibration of each individual item.

Kuder-Richardson formulas   Two formulas (KR 20 and KR 21) that were developed to estimate reliability. Both of these methods are measures of internal consistency. KR 20 has been shown to approximate the average of all possible split-half coefficients. KR 21 is easier to compute, but the items on the instrument must be homogeneous.

Latent trait theory   Another term for item response theory.

Learning disabilities   A general term referring to a group of disorders that are related to significant difficulties in the acquisition and use of listening, speaking, reading, writing, reasoning, and mathematical abilities.

Mean   The arithmetic average of the scores. It is calculated by adding the scores together and dividing by the number in the group.

Median   The middle score, with 50% of the scores falling below it and 50% of the scores falling above it.

Mode   The most frequent score in a distribution.

Multitrait-multimethod matrix   A matrix that includes information on correlations between the measure and traits that it should be related to and traits that it should not theoretically be related to. The matrix also includes correlations between the measure of interest and other same-methods measures and measures that use different assessment methods.

Nominal scale   A scale of measurement characterized by assigning numbers to name or represent mutually exclusive groups (e.g., 1 = male, 2 = female).

Normal curve   A bell-shaped, symmetrical, and unimodal curve. The majority of cases are concentrated close to the mean, with 68% of the individual scores falling between one standard deviation below the mean and one standard deviation above the mean.

Normal distribution   A distribution of scores with certain specific characteristics.

Norm-referenced instruments   Ones in which the interpretation of performance is based on the comparison of an individual's performance with that of a specified group of people.

Objective assessment   Instruments that require little or no judgment on the part of the individual scoring the assessment. In *subjective assessment,* the scoring of the instrument involves judgment. A multiple-choice test with a fixed scoring key is an example of an objective assessment.

Ordinal scale   Type of measurement scale in which the degree of magnitude is indicated by the rank ordering of the data.

Percentile rank   A ranking that provides an indication of the percent of scores that fall at or below a given score. For example: "Mary's percentile of 68 means that if there were 100 people who had taken this instrument, 68 of them would have a score at or below Mary's."

Performance assessments   An alternate method of assessing individuals, other than through multiple-choice types of items, in which the focus is on evaluating the performance of tasks or activities.

Power test   Tests that have items that vary in difficulty. The focus is not on the speed at which the individual completes the items but rather on the difficulty of the items answered correctly. Often the items are arranged in order of difficulty, with the easier items placed at the beginning and the most difficult items at the end of the test.

Predictive validity   A type of criterion-related validity in which there is a delay between the time the instrument is administered and the time the criterion information is gathered.

Projective techniques   A type of personality assessment that provides the client with a relatively ambiguous stimulus, thus encouraging a nonstructured response. The assumption underlying these techniques is that the individual will project his or her personality into the response. The interpretation of projective techniques is subjective and requires extensive training in the technique.

Psychological report   A summary of a client's assessment results that is geared toward other professionals. Typical reports include background information, behavioral observations, test results and interpretations, recommendations, and a summary.

Psychosocial interview   A detailed interview that gathers background information and information about the client's current psychological and social situation.

Range   Range is a measure of variability that provides an indication of the difference between the highest and the lowest scores.

Ratio scale   A scale of measurement that has both interval data and a meaningful zero (e.g., weight, height). Because ratio scales have a meaningful zero, ratio interpretations can be made.

Raw scores   Raw scores are the unadjusted scores on an instrument before they are transformed into standard scores. An example of a raw score is the number of answers an individual gets correct on an achievement test.

Regression equation   An equation that describes the linear relationship between the predictor variable(s) and the criterion variable. These equations are often used to determine if it is possible to predict to the criterion based on the instrument's scores.

Reliability   Concerns the degree to which a measure or a score is free of unsystematic error. In classical test theory, it is the ratio of true variance to observed variance.

Selected-response item format   A method of writing an item in which the individual is provided with a choice of answers and needs to select an answer from those provided alternatives.

Semi-structured interview   An interview that is a combination of a structured and unstructured format in which there are a set of established questions and the clinician can also ask additional questions for elaboration or to gather additional information.

Sequential processing   The use of mental abilities to arrange stimuli in sequential, or serial, order in order to process the information.

Simultaneous processing   The use of mental abilities to integrate information in a unified manner, with the individual integrating fragments of information in order to comprehend the whole.

Skewed distributions   Distributions in which the majority of scores are either high or low. Skewed distributions are not asymmetrical and the mean, mode, and median are different. In *positively skewed distributions,* the majority of scores are on the lower end of the distribution; in *negatively skewed distributions,* the majority of scores are on the upper end of the distribution.

Slope bias   A term referring to a situation in which a test yields significantly different validity coefficients for different groups, resulting in different regression lines.

Spearman-Brown formula   A formula for correcting a split-half reliability coefficient that estimates what the coefficient would be if the original number of items were used.

Split-half reliability   One of the internal consistency measures of reliability in which the instrument is administered once and then split into two halves. The scores on the two halves are then correlated to provide an estimate of reliability. Often the split-half reliability coefficients are corrected using the Spearman-Brown formula. This formula adjusts the coefficient for using only half of the total number of items to provide an estimate of what the correlation coefficient would be if the original number of items were used.

Standard deviation   The most common statistic used to describe the variability of a set of measurements. It is the square root of the variance.

Standard error of difference A measure used by a counselor to examine the difference between two scores and determine if there is a significant difference.

Standard error of estimate One that indicates the margin of expected error in the individual's predicted criterion score as a result of imperfect validity.

Standard error of measurement This deviation provides an indication of what an individual's true score would be if he or she took the instrument repeated times. Counselors can use standard error of measurement to determine the range of scores 68%, 95%, or 99.5% of the time.

Standard score A general term that refers to transformed raw scores that have set standard deviations and means. The base of the standard scores is the z score, which expresses the individual's distance from the mean in terms of the standard deviation of the distribution. For example, if an individual has a z score of 1.00, he or she is one standard deviation above the mean, and if an individual has a z score of −2.00, he or she is two standard deviations below the mean.

Standardized test An instrument having established materials and fixed directions for administration and scoring. The instrument was developed according to certain standards. (Sometimes standardization will also refer to the establishment of norms for the instrument.)

Structured interview An interview that is conducted using a predetermined set of questions that is asked in the same manner and sequence for every client.

Structured personality instruments Formalized assessments in which clients respond to a fixed set of questions or items.

Test-retest reliability One in which the reliability coefficient is obtained by correlating a group's performance on the first administration of an instrument with the same group's performance on the second administration of that same instrument.

Unstructured interview An interview in which the clinician gears the questions toward each individual client and there is no established set of questions.

Validity coefficient The correlation between the scores on an instrument and the criterion measure.

Validity generalization A term applied to findings indicating that the validity of cognitive ability tests can be generalized and that cognitive ability is highly related to job performance.

Variance The average of the squared deviation from the mean. It is a measure of variability and its square root is the standard deviation of the set of measurements.

z scores Standard scores that serve as the base for all other standard scores. The mean for z scores is always 0 and the standard deviation is 1. Often z scores are used with instruments that have a normal distribution and provide a simple method of reflecting the score's place along the distribution.

REFERENCES

Achenbach, T. M. (1997). *Child Behavioral Checklist for ages 4–18*. Itasca, IL: Riverside Publishing.

ACT (1997). *ACT Assessment user handbook 1997–1998*. Iowa City, IA: Author.

Adair, F. L. (1984). Review of the Coopersmith Self-Esteem Inventories. In D. J. & R. C. Sweetlands (Eds.), *Test critiques* (pp. 226–232). Kansas City, MO: Test Corporation of America.

Agresi, A., & Finlay, B. (1997). *Statistical methods for the social sciences*. Englewood Cliffs, NJ: Prentice-Hall.

Aiken, L. R. (1996). *Personality assessment: Methods and practices* (2nd ed.). Seattle: Hogrefe & Huber.

Aiken, L. R. (1997). *Psychological testing and assessment* (9th ed.). Boston: Allyn and Bacon.

Airasian, P. W. (1994). *Classroom assessment* (2nd ed.). New York: McGraw-Hill.

Allred, L. J., & Harris, W. G. (1984). *The non-equivalence of computerized and conventional administration of the Adjective Checklist*. Unpublished manuscript, Johns Hopkins University.

American Association of Counseling and Development & Association for Measurement and Evaluation in Counseling and Development (1989). *The responsibility of test users*. Alexandria, VA: Author.

American Association of Mental Retardation (1992). *Mental retardation: Definition, classification, and systems of supports* (9th ed.). Washington, DC: Author.

American Counseling Association (1995). *Code of ethics and standards of practice*. Alexandria, VA: Author.

American Education Research Association, American Psychological Association, & National Council on Measurement in Education (1985). *Standards for educational and psychological testing*. Washington, DC: American Psychological Association.

American Psychiatric Association (1994). *Diagnostic and statistical manual of mental disorders* (4th ed.). Washington, DC: Author.

American Psychological Association (1992). Ethical principles of psychologists and code of conduct. *American Psychologist, 47,* 1597–1611.

American Psychological Association, Committee on Professional Standards and Committee on Psychological Tests and Assessment (1986). *Guidelines for computer-based tests and interpretation*. Washington, DC: Author.

American Rehabilitation Counseling Association, Commission of Rehabilitation Counselor Certification, & the National Rehabilitation Counseling Association (1995). *Code of professional ethics for rehabilitation counselors.* Chicago: Author.

Anastasi, A. (1981). Coaching, test sophistication, and developed abilities. *American Psychologist, 36,* 1086–1093.

Anastasi, A. (1985). Review of Kaufman Assessment Battery for Children. In J. V. Mitchell (Ed.), *The ninth mental measurements yearbook* (pp. 769–771). Highland Park, NJ: Gryphon.

Anastasi, A. (1988). *Psychological testing* (6th ed.). New York: Macmillan.

Anastasi, A. (1992). What counselors should know about the use and interpretation of psychological tests. *Journal of Counseling & Development, 70,* 610–616.

Anastasi, A. (1993). A century of psychological testing: Origins, problems and progress. In T. K. Fagen & G. R. VandenBos (Eds.), *Exploring applied psychology: Origins and critical analyses* (pp. 3–36). Washington, DC: American Psychological Association.

Anastasi, A., & Urbina, S. (1997). *Psychological testing* (7th ed.). Upper Saddle River, NJ: Prentice-Hall.

Anderson, B. S. (1996). *The counselor and the law* (4th ed.). Alexandria, VA: American Counseling Association.

Anderson, W. (1995). Ethnic and cross-cultural differences on the MMPI-2. In J. C. Duckworth & W. P. Anderson, *MMPI and MMPI-2 interpretation manual for counselors and clinicians* (pp. 382–395). Bristol, PN: Accelerated Press.

Archer, R. P. (1992). Review of the Minnesota Multiphasic Personality Inventory-2. In J. C. Conoley & J. J. Kramer (Eds.), *Eleventh mental measurements yearbook* (pp. 558–562). Lincoln, NB: The University of Nebraska Press.

Archer, R. P., & Krishnamurthy, R. (1996). The Minnesota Multiphasic Personality Inventory-Adolescent. In C. S. Newmark (Ed.), *Major psychological assessment instruments* (pp. 59–107). Boston: Allyn and Bacon.

Archer, R. P., Maruish, M., Imhof, E. A., & Piotrowski, C. (1991). Psychological test usage with adolescent clients: 1990 survey findings. *Professional Psychology: Research and Practice, 22,* 247–252.

Athanasou, J. A., & Cooksey, R. W. (1993). Self-estimates of vocational interests. *Australian Psychologist, 28,* 118–127.

Austin, J. T. (1994). Test review: Minnesota Multiphasic Personality Inventory-2. *Measurement and Evaluation in Counseling and Development, 27,* 178–185.

Baghurst, P. A., McMichael, A. J., Wigg, N. R., Vimpani, G. V., Robertson, E. F., Roberts, R. J., & Ton, S. L. (1992). Environmental exposure to lead and children's intelligence at the age of seven years, the Port Pirie cohort study. *New England Journal of Medicine, 327,* 1279–1284.

Baker, E. L., O'Neil, H. F., & Linn, R. L. (1993). Policy and validity prospects for performance-based assessment. *American Psychologist, 48,* 1210–1218.

Baldwin, A. L., Kalhorn, J., & Breese, F. H. (1945). Patterns of parent behavior. *Psychological Monographs, 58* (Whole No. 268).

Bandura, A. (1977). Self-efficacy: Toward a unifying theory of behavioral change. *Psychological Review, 84,* 191–215.

Bayley, N., & Oden, M. H. (1955). The maintenance of intellectual ability in gifted adults. *Journal of Gerontology, 10,* 91–107.

Beck, A. T., & Steer, R. A. (1991). *Beck Scale for Suicide Ideation.* San Antonio, TX: Psychological Corporation.

Beck, A. T., & Steer, R. A. (1993). *Beck Hopeless Scale.* San Antonio, TX: Psychological Corporation.

Beck, A. T., Steer, R. A., & Brown, G. K. (1996). *Beck Depression Inventory-II.* San Antonio, TX: Psychological Corporation.

Bennett, G. K., Seashore, H. G., & Wesman, A. G. (1990). *Differential Aptitude Tests, Fifth Edition.* San Antonio, TX: Psychological Corporation.

Ben-Porath, Y. F. (1997). Use of personality assessment instruments in empirically guided treatment planning. *Psychological Assessment, 9,* 361–367.

Benziman, H., & Toder, A. (1993). The psychodiagnostic experience: Reports of subjects. In B. Nevo & R. S. Jager (Eds.), *Educational and psychological testing: The test taker's outlook* (pp. 287–299). Toronto: Hogrefe & Huber.

Berk, R. A. (1984). Selecting the index of reliability. In R. A. Berk (Ed.), *A guide to criterion-reference test construction* (pp. 231–266). Baltimore, MD: Johns Hopkins University Press.

Berlin, I. N. (1987). Suicide among American Indian adolescents: An overview. *Suicide and Life Threatening Behavior, 17*(3), 218–232.

Berry, J. W. (1980). Acculturation as varieties of adaptation. In A. M. Padilla (Ed.), *Acculturation: Theory, models and some new findings* (pp. 9–25). Boulder, CO: Westview Press.

Betsworth, D. G., & Fouad, N. A. (1997). Vocational interests: A look at the past 70 years and a glance at the future. *The Career Development Quarterly, 46,* 23–41.

Betz, N. E. (1988). The assessment of career development and maturity. In W. B. Walsh & S. H. Osipow (Eds.), *Career decision making* (pp. 77–136). Hillsdale, NJ: Erlbaum.

Betz, N. E. (1990). Contemporary issues in testing use. In C. E. Watkins & V. L. Campbell (Eds.), *Testing in counseling practice* (pp. 419–450). Hillsdale, NJ: Erlbaum.

Betz, N. E. (1992). Career assessment: A review of critical issues. In S. D. Brown & R. W. Lent (Eds.), *Handbook of counseling psychology* (2nd ed., pp. 453–484). New York: Wiley.

Betz, N. E., & Fitzgerald, L. F. (1987). *The career psychology of women.* Orlando, FL: Academic Press.

Betz, N. E., & Fitzgerald, L. F. (1995). Career assessment and intervention with racial and ethnic minorities. In F. T. L. Leong (Ed.), *Career development and vocational behavior of racial and ethnic minorities* (pp. 263–280). Mahwah, NJ: Erlbaum.

Beutler, L. E., & Clarkin, J. F. (1990). *Systematic treatment selection.* New York: Brunner/Mazel.

Beutler, L. E., & Harwood, T. M. (1995). How to assess clients in pretreatment planning. In J. N. Butcher (Ed.), *Clinical personality assessment: Practical approaches* (pp. 59–77). New York: Oxford University Press.

Bjorklund, D. F. (1995). *Children's thinking: Developmental function and individual differences.* Pacific Grove, CA: Brooks/Cole.

Bolton, B. (1994). General Aptitude Test Battery. In J. T. Kapes, M. M. Mastie, & E. A. Whitfield (Eds.), *A counselor's guide to career assessment instruments* (pp. 115–123). Alexandria, VA: National Career Development Association.

Bond, L. (1989). The effects of special preparation on measures of scholastic ability. In R. L. Linn (Ed.), *Educational measurement* (3rd ed., pp. 429–444). New York: Macmillan.

Bond, L. (1990). Understanding the Black-White student gap on measures of qualitative reasoning. In F. C. Serafica, A. I. Schwebel, R. K. Russes, P. D. Issac, & L. B. Myers (Eds.), *Mental health of ethnic minorities* (pp. 89–107). New York: Praeger.

Borman, W. C. (1991). Job behavior, performance, and effectiveness. In M. D. Dunnette & L. C. Houghs (Eds.), *Handbook of industrial and organizational psychology* (2nd ed., Vol. 2, pp. 271–326). Palo Alto, CA: Consulting Psychology Press.

Bornstein, R. F., Rossner, S. C., Hill, E. L., & Stephanian, M. L. (1994). Face validity and fakability of objective and projective measures of dependency. *Journal of Personality Assessment, 63,* 363–386.

Botwin, M. D. (1995). Review of the Revised NEO Personality Inventory. In J. C. Conoley & J. J. Kramer (Eds.), *Twelfth mental measurements yearbook* (pp. 862–863). Lincoln, NB: The University of Nebraska Press.

Boughner, S. R., Hayes, S. F., Bubenzer, D. L., & West, J. D. (1994). Use of standardized assessment instruments by marital and family therapists: A survey. *Journal of Marital and Family Therapy, 20,* 69–75.

Bowen, M. (1978). *Family therapy in clinical practice.* New York: Jason Aronson.

Bowman, M. L. (1989). Testing individual differences in ancient China. *American Psychologist, 41,* 1059–1068.

Boyle, G. J. (1990). Stanford-Binet IV Intelligence Scale: Is its structure supported by LISREL congeneric factor analyses. *Personality and Individual Differences, 11,* 1175–1181.

Bracken, B. A., & Barona, A. (1991). State of the art procedures for translating, validating and using psychoeducational tests in cross-cultural assessment. *School Psychology International, 12,* 119–132.

Braden, J. P. (1995). Review of the Wechsler Intelligence Scale for Children, Third Edition. In J. C. Conoley & J. J. Kramer (Eds.), *Twelfth mental measurements yearbook* (pp. 1098–1103). Lincoln, NB: The University of Nebraska Press.

Bray, D. W. (1982). The assessment center and the study of lives. *American Psychologist, 37,* 180–189.

Brooke, S. L., & Ciechalski, J. C. (1994). Minnesota Importance Questionnaire. In J. T. Kapes, M. M. Mastied, & E. A. Whitfield (Eds.), *A counselors' guide to career assessment instruments* (pp. 222–225). Alexandria, VA: National Career Development Association.

Brown, L., Sherbenou, R. J., & Johnsen, S. K. (1997). *Test of Nonverbal Intelligence, Third Edition.* Los Angeles: Western Psychological Services.

Bruhn, A. R. (1989). *The Early Memories Procedure.* 32 pages. Available from author.

Bruhn, A. R. (1995). Early memories in personality assessment. In J. N. Butcher (Ed.), *Clinical personality assessment: Practical approaches.* New York: Oxford University Press.

Bubenzer, D. L., Zimpfer, D. G., & Mahrle, C. L. (1990). Standardized individual appraisal in agency and private practice: A survey. *Journal of Mental Health Counseling, 12,* 51–66.

Buck, J. (1948). The H-T-P. *Journal of Clinical Psychology, 4,* 151–159.

Buck, J. (1992). *The House-Tree-Person projective drawing technique: Manual and interpretive guide.* (Revised by W. L. Warren). Los Angeles: Western Psychological Services.

Burnett, P. (1987). Assessing marital adjustment and satisfaction: A review. *Measurement and Evaluation in Counseling, 20,* 113–121.

Burns, R. (1982). *Self-growth in families: Kinetic Family Drawings (K-F-D) research and application.* New York: Brunner/Mazel.

Burns, R. (1987). *Kinetic-House-Tree-Person Drawings (K-H-T-P).* New York: Brunner/Mazel.

Burns, R., & Kaufman, S. (1970). *Kinetic Family Drawings (K-F-D): An introduction to understanding children through kinetic drawings.* New York: Brunner/Mazel.

Burns, R., & Kaufman, S. (1972). *Action, styles, symbols in Kinetic Family Drawings (K-F-D).* New York: Brunner/Mazel.

Busch, J. C. (1995). Review of the Strong Interest Inventory (Fourth Edition). In J. C. Conoley & J. J. Kramer (Eds.), *Twelfth mental measurements yearbook* (pp. 997–999). Lincoln, NB: The University of Nebraska Press.

Butcher, J. N. (1990). *The MMPI-2 in psychological treatment.* New York: Oxford University Press.

Butcher, J. N. (1995). Clinical personality assessment: An overview. In J. N. Butcher (Ed.), *Clinical personality assessment: Practical approaches,* 3–9. New York: Oxford University Press.

Butcher, J. N., Dahlstrom, W. G., Graham, J. R., Tellegen, A., & Kraemmer, B. (1989). *Minnesota Multiphasic Personality Inventory-2 (MMPI-2): Manual for administration and scoring.* Minneapolis, MN: University of Minnesota Press.

Butcher, J. N., & Williams, C. L. (1992). *Essentials of MMPI-2 and MMPI-A interpretation.* Minneapolis, MN: University of Minnesota Press.

Butcher, J. N., Williams, C. L., Graham, J. R., Archer, R., Tellegen, A., Ben-Porath, Y. S., & Kraemmer, B. (1992). *MMPI-A manual for administration, scoring, and interpretation.* Minneapolis, MN: University of Minnesota Press.

Campbell, D. P. (1992). *Career Interest and Skills Survey Manual.* Minneapolis, MN: National Computer Systems.

Campbell, D. T., & Fiske, D. W. (1959). Convergent and discriminant validation by the multi-trait multi-method matrix. *Psychological Bulletin, 56,* 81–105.

Campbell, J. P. (1994). Alternative models of job performance and their implications for selection and classification. In M. G. Rumsey, C. B. Walker, & J. H. Harris (Eds.), *Personnel selection and classification* (pp. 33–51). Hillsdale, NJ: Erlbaum.

Campbell, V. L. (1990). A model for using tests in counseling. In C. E. Watkins & V. L. Campbell (Eds.), *Testing in counseling practice* (pp. 1–7). Hillsdale, NJ: Erlbaum.

Caprara, G. V., Barbaranelli, C., & Comfrey, A. L. (1995). Factor analysis of the NEO-PI Inventory and the Comfrey Personality Scales in an Italian sample. *Personality and Individual Differences, 18,* 193–200.

Carter, B., & McGoldrick, M. (1988). Overview: The changing family cycle—A framework for family therapy. In B. Carter & M. McGoldrick (Eds.), *The changing family life cycle: A framework for family therapy* (2nd ed., pp. 3–28). New York: Gardner.

Cattell, R. B. (1971). *Abilities: Their structure, growth, and action.* Boston: Houghton Mifflin.

Cattell, R. B (1979). Are culture fair intelligence tests possible and necessary? *Journal of Research and Development in Education, 12*(2), 3–13.

Cattell, R. B., Cattell, A. K., & Cattell, H. E. (1993). *Sixteen Personality Factor Questionnaire, Fifth Edition.* Champaign, IL: Institute for Personality and Ability Testing.

Ceci, S. J. (1990). *On intelligence—more or less: A bio-ecological treatise on intellectual development.* Englewood Cliffs, NJ: Prentice-Hall.

Ceci, S. J. (1991). How much does school influence general intelligence and its cognitive components: A re-assessment of the evidence. *Developmental Psychology, 27,* 703–723.

Ceci, S. J. (1993). Contextual trends in intellectual development. *Developmental Review, 13,* 403–435.

Centers for Disease Control and Prevention (1994). Prevalence of disabilities and associated health conditions, 1972–1991. *Journal of the American Medical Association, 272,* 1735–1737.

Chipuser, H. M., Rovine, M., & Plomin, R. (1990). LISREL modeling: Genetic and environmental influences on IQ revisited. *Intelligence, 14,* 11–29.

Cicchetti, D. V. (1994). Guidelines, criteria, and rules of thumb for evaluating normed and standardized assessment instruments in psychology. *Psychological Assessment, 6,* 284–290.

Clair, D., & Pendergast, D. (1994). Brief psychotherapy and psychological assessment: Entering a relationship, establishing a focus, and providing feedback. *Professional Psychology: Research and Practice, 25,* 46–49.

Clark, D. C., & Fawcett, J. (1992). Review of empirical risk factors for evaluation of the suicidal patient. In B. Bongar (Ed.), *Suicide: Guidelines for assessment, management, and treatment* (pp. 16–48). New York: Oxford University Press.

Clawson, T. W. (1997). Control of psychological testing: The threat and a response. *Journal of Counseling and Development, 76,* 90–93.

Cohen, R. J., Swerdlik, M. E., Smith, D. K. (1992). *Psychological testing and assessment: An introduction to tests and measurement* (2nd ed.). Mountain View, CA: Mayfield.

College Entrance Examination Board (1995). *Counselor's handbook for the SAT program.* Princeton, NJ: Author.

Conners, C. K. (1996). *Conners' Revised Scales—Revised.* North Tonawanda, NY: Multi-Health Systems.

Conoley, C. W. (1994). Review of the Beck Depression Inventory. In J. C Impara & L. L. Murphy (Eds.), *Buros desk reference: Psychological assessment in the schools* (pp. 309–311). Lincoln, NB: Buros Institute.

Conoley, C. W., & Impara, J. C. (1998). *The thirteenth mental measurements yearbook.* Lincoln, NB: Buros Institute.

Cormier, S., & Cormier, B. (1998). *Interviewing strategies for helpers: Fundamental skills and cognitive behavioral interventions.* Pacific Grove, CA: Brooks/Cole.

Costa, P. T., & McCrae, R. R. (1992). *Revised NEO Personality Inventory (NEO-PI-R) and NEO Five-Factor Inventory (NEO-FFI) professional manual.* Odessa, FL: Psychological Assessment Resources.

Coupland, S. K., Serovic, J. & Glenn, J. E. (1995). Reliability in constructing genograms: A study among marriage and family therapy doctoral students. *Journal of Marital and Family Therapy, 21,* 251–263.

Craig, R. J. (1993). *The Millon Clinical Multiaxial Inventory: A clinical research information synthesis.* Hillsdale, NJ: Erlbaum.

Crites, J. O. (1978). *Administration and use manual* (2nd ed.). Monterey, CA: CTB/McGraw-Hill.

Crocker, L., & Angina, J. (1986). *Introduction to classical and modern test theory.* Fort Worth, TX: Harcourt Brace Jovanovich.

Cromwell, R., Fournier, D., & Kvebaek, D. (1980). *The Kvebaek Family Sculpture Technique: A diagnostic and research tool in family therapy.* Jonesboro, TN: Pilgramage.

Cronbach. L. J. (1951). Coefficient alpha and internal structure of tests. *Psychometika, 16,* 297–334.

Cronbach, L. J. (1990). *Essentials of psychological testing* (5th Ed.). New York: HarperCollins.

Cronbach, L. J., & Gleser, G. C. (1965). *Psychological tests and personnel decisions* (2nd ed.). Champaign, IL: University of Illinois Press.

Cronbach, L. J., Gleser, G. C., Rajaratnam,N., & Nanda, H. (1972). *The dependability of behavioral measurements.* New York: Wiley.

CTB/McGraw-Hill (1996). *TerraNova prepublication technical bulletin.* Monterey, CA: Author.

CTB/McGraw-Hill (1997a). *Teacher's guide to TerraNova.* Monterey, CA: Author.

CTB/McGraw-Hill (1997b). *The one and only: TerraNova* [Brochure]. Monterey, CA: Author.

Cull, J. G., & Gill, W. S. (1992). *Suicide Probability Scale.* Los Angeles: Western Psychological Services.

Cummings, J. A. (1995). Review of the Woodcock-Johnson Psycho-Educational Battery-Revised. In J. C. Conoley & J. J. Kramer (Eds.), *Twelfth mental measurements yearbook* (pp. 1113–1116). Lincoln, NB: The University of Nebraska Press.

Dahlstrom, W. G. (1995). Pigeons, people, and pigeon holes. *Journal of Personality Assessment, 64,* 2–20.

Dana, R. H. (1993). *Multicultural assessment perspectives for professional psychology.* Boston: Allyn and Bacon.

Daniels, M. H. (1994). Self-Directed Search. In J. T. Kapes, M. M. Mastied, & E. A. Whitfield (Eds.), *A counselors' guide to career assessment instruments* (pp. 206–212). Alexandria, VA: National Career Development Association.

Dawes, R. M. (1994). *House of cards: Psychology and psychotherapy built on myths.* New York: Free Press.

Dawes, R. M., Faust, D., Meehl, P. E. (1989). Clinical and actuarial judgment. *Science, 243,* 1668–1674.

Day, S. X., & Rounds, J. (1998). Universality of vocational interest structure among racial and ethnic minorities. *American Psychologist, 53,* 728–736.

Deary, I. J. (1995). Auditory inspection time and intelligence: What is the causal direction? *Developmental Psychology, 31,* 237–250.

Deffenbacher, J. L. (1980). Worry and emotionality in test anxiety. In I. G. Sarason (Ed.), *Test anxiety: Theory, research, and application* (pp. 111–128). Hillsdale, NJ: Erlbaum.

Deffenbacher, J. L. (1992). Counseling for anxiety management. In S. D. Brown & R. W. Lent (Eds.)., *Handbook of Counseling Psychology* (2nd ed., pp. 719–756). New York: Wiley.

Dendata, K. M., & Diener, D. (1986). Effectiveness of cognitive/relaxation therapy and study-skills training in reducing self-reported anxiety and improving academic performance of test anxious students. *Journal of Counseling Psychology, 33,* 131–135.

Derogatis, L. R. (1993). *The Brief Symptom Inventory (BSI) administration, scoring, and procedures-II.* Minneapolis, MN: National Computer Systems.

Derogatis, L. R. (1994). *Administration, scoring, and procedures manual for the SCL-90-R* (3rd ed). Minneapolis, MN: National Computer Systems.

DeRosa, A. P., & Patalano, R. (1991). Effects of familiar proctor on fifth and sixth grade students' test anxiety. *Psychological Reports, 68,* 103–113.

DiClemente, C. C., Prochaska, J. O., Fairhurst, S. K., Velicer, W. F., Velasquez, M. M., & Rossi, J. S. (1991). The process of smoking cessation: An analysis of precontemplation, contemplation, and preparation stages of change. *Journal of Consulting and Clinical Psychology, 59,* 295–304.

Digman, J. M. (1990). Personality structure: Emergence of the Five-Factor Model. *Annual Review of Psychology, 41,* 417–440.

Digman, J. M., & Takemoto-Chock, N, K, (1981). Factors in the natural language of personality: Re-analysis, comparison, and interpretation of six major studies. *Multivariate Behavioral Research, 16,* 149–170.

Dixon, D. N., & Glover. J. A. (1984). *Counseling: A problem solving approach.* New York: Wiley.

Doll, E. J. (1989). Review of the Kaufman Test of Educational Achievement. In J. C. Conoley & J. J. Kramer (Eds.), *Tenth mental measurements yearbook.* Lincoln, NB: University of Nebraska Press.

Donlon, T. F. (Ed.) (1984). *The College Board technical handbook for the Scholastic Aptitude Test and achievement testing.* New York: College Board Publications.

Dorr, D. (1981). Conjoint psychological testing in marriage therapy: New wine in old skins. *Professional Psychology, 12,* 549–555.

Druckman, J. M., Fournier, D. F, Robinson, R., & Olsen, D. H. (1980). *Effectiveness of five types of premarital preparation programs.* Minneapolis, MN: PREPARE-ENRICH, Inc.

Drummond, R. J. (1996). *Appraisal procedures for counselors and helping professionals* (3rd ed.). Englewood Cliffs, NJ: Merrill.

Duckworth, J. (1990). The counseling approach to the use of testing. *The Counseling Psychologist, 18,* 198–204.

Duckworth, J. C., & Anderson, W. P. (1997). *MMPI and MMPI-2: Interpretation manual for counselors and clinicians.* Muncie, IN: Accelerated Press.

Duley, S. M., Cancelli, A. A., Kratochwill, T. R., Bergan, J. R., & Meredith, K. E. (1983). Training and generalization of motivational analysis interview assessment skills. *Behavioral Assessment, 5,* 281–293.

Dunn, L. M., & Dunn, L. M. (1997). *Examiner's Manual for the Peabody Picture Test Third Edition.* Circle Pines, MN: American Guidance Service.

Duran, R. P. (1983). *Hispanics' education and background: Predictors of college achievement.* New York: College Entrance Examination Board.

Educational Testing Service (1997). *GRE 1997–98 Guide to the use of scores.* Princeton, NJ: Author.

Elliot, C. D. (1990). *Differential Ability Scales introductory and technical manual—DAS.* San Antonio, TX: The Psychological Corporation.

Elmore, P. B., & Bradley, R. W. (1994). Armed Services Vocational Aptitude Battery (ASVAB) Career Exploration Program. In J. T. Kapes, M. M. Mastie, & E. A. Whitfield (Eds.), *A counselor's guide to career assessment instruments* (pp. 71–77). Alexandria, VA: National Career Development Association.

Elmore, P. B., Ekstrom, R., & Diamond, E. E. (1993). Counselors' test use practices: Indicators of the adequacy of measurement training. *Measurement and Evaluation in Counseling and Development, 26,* 116–124.

Elmore, P. B., Ekstrom, R., Diamond, E. E., & Whittaker, S. (1993). School counselors' test use patterns and practices. *The School Counselor, 41,* 73–80.

Elmore, P. B., Ekstrom, R., Shafer, W., & Webster, B. (1998, January). *School counselors' activities and training in assessment and evaluations.* Presented at the Assessment '98, assessment for Change—Changes in Assessment, St. Petersburg, FL.

Embretson, S. E. (1996). The new rules of measurement. *Psychological Assessment, 8,* 341–349.

Epstein, J. H. (1985). Review of the Piers-Harris Children's Self-Concept Scale. In J. V. Mitchell (Ed.), *Ninth mental measurements yearbook* (pp. 1167–1169). Highland Park, NJ: Gryphon.

Eyde, L. D., Robertson, G. J., Moreland, K. L., Robertson, A. G., Shewan, C. M., Harrison, P. L., Porch, B. E., Hammer, A. L., & Primoff, E. S. (1993). *Responsible test use: Case studies for assessing human behavior.* Washington, DC: American Psychological Association.

Fine, S. F., & Glasser, P. H. (1996). *The first helping interview: Engaging the client and building trust.* Thousand Oaks, CA: Sage.

Finn, S. E., & Tonsager, M. E. (1992). Therapeutic effects of providing MMPI-2 test feedback to college students awaiting therapy. *Psychological Assessment, 4,* 278–287.

Finn, S. E., & Tonsager, M. E. (1997). Information-gathering and therapeutic models of assessment: Complementary paradigms. *Psychological Assessment, 9,* 374–385.

Fisher, C. F., & King, R. M. (1995). *Authentic assessment: A guide to implementation.* Thousand Oaks, CA: Corwin.

Fisher, L., & Sorenson, G. P. (1996). *School law for counselors, psychologists, and social workers.* White Plains, NY: Longman.

Fitts, W. H., & Warren, W. L. (1997). *Tennessee Self-Concept Scale: Second Edition (TSCS:2).* Los Angeles: Western Psychological Services.

Flanagan, D. P. (1995). Review of the Kaufman Adolescent and Adult Intelligence Test. In J. C. Conoley & J. J. Kramer (Eds.), *Twelfth mental measurements yearbook* (pp. 527–530). Lincoln, NB: The University of Nebraska Press.

Fletcher, J. M., Shaywitz, S. E., Shankweiler, D. P., Katz, L., Liberman, I. Y., Stuebing, K. K., Francis, D. J., Fowler, A. E., & Shaywitz, B. A. (1994). Cognitive profiles of reading disability: Comparisons of discrepancy and low achievement definitions. *Journal of Educational Psychology, 25,* 6–23.

Flynn, J. R. (1984). The mean IQ of Americans: Massive gains 1932 to 1978. *Psychological Bulletin, 95,* 29–51.

Flynn, J. R. (1987). Massive IQ gains in 14 nations: What IQ tests really measure. *Psychological Bulletin, 101,* 171–191.

Flynn, J. R. (1991). *Asian-Americans: Achievement beyond IQ.* Hillsdale, NJ: Erlbaum.

Fong, M. L. (1993). Teaching assessment and diagnosis within a DSM-III-R framework. *Counselor Education and Supervision, 32,* 276–286.

Fong, M. L. (1995). Assessment and DSM-IV diagnosis of personality disorders: A primer for counselors. *Journal of Counseling and Development, 73,* 635–639.

Forrest, L., & Brooks, L. (1993). Feminism and career assessment. *Journal of Career Assessment, 1,* 233–245.

Fortier, L. M., & Wanlass, R. L. (1984). Family crisis following the diagnosis of a handicapped child. *Family Relations, 33,* 13–24.

Fouad, N., Harmon, L. W., & Borgen, F. H. (1997). The structure of interests in employed adult members of U.S. racial/ethnic minority groups and nonminority groups. *Journal of Counseling Psychology, 44,* 339–345.

Fowers, B. J. (1983). *PREPARE as a predictor of marital satisfaction.* Unpublished master's thesis, University of Minnesota, St. Paul, MN 55108.

Franklin, M. R., & Stillman, P. L. (1982). Examiner error in intelligence testing: Are you a source? *Psychology in the Schools, 19,* 563–569.

Fredman, N., & Sherman, R. (1987). *Handbook of measurements for marriage and family therapy.* New York: Brunner/Mazel.

Fuchs, D., & Fuchs, L. S. (1986). Test procedure bias: A meta-analysis of examiner familiarity effects. *Review of Educational Research, 56,* 243–262.

Fuqua, D. R., & Newman, J. L. (1994). Campbell Interest and Skill Survey (CISS). In J. T. Kapes, M. M. Mastie, & E. A. Whitfield (Eds.), *A counselor's guide to career assessment instruments* (pp. 138–143). Alexandria, VA: National Career Development Association.

Gardner, H. (1993). *Frames of mind: The theory of multiple intelligences* (10th anniversary ed.). New York: Basic Books.

Garis, J. W., & Niles, S. G. (1990). The separate and combined effects of SIGI and DISCOVER and a career planning course on undecided university students. *Career Development Quarterly, 39,* 261–274.

Garrison, C. A. (1992). Demographic predictors of suicide. In R. W. Maris, A. L. Berman, & J. T. Maltsberger (Eds.), *Assessment and prediction of suicide* (pp. 484–498). New York: Guilford.

Gati, I. (1994). Computer-assisted career counseling: Dilemmas, problems, and possible solutions. *Journal of Counseling and Development, 73,* 51–56.

Geisinger, K. F. (1994). Psychometric issues in testing students with disabilities. *Applied Measurement in Education, 72,* 121–140.

Gelso, C. J., & Carter, J. A. (1994). Components of psychotherapy relationship: Their interaction and unfolding during treatment. *Journal of Counseling Psychology, 41,* 296–306.

Gergen, K. J. (1985). The social constructionist movement in modern psychology. *American Psychologist, 34,* 127–140.

Glass, G. V., McGaw, B., & Smith, M. L. (1981). *Meta-analysis in social science research.* Thousand Oaks, CA: Sage.

Glutting, J. J., & Kaplan, D. (1990). Stanford-Binet Intelligence Scale: Fourth Edition: Making the case for reasonable interpretation. In C. R. Reynolds & R. W. Kamphaus (Eds.), *Handbook of psychological and educational assessment of children* (pp. 277–295). New York: Guilford.

Goldberg, L. R. (1992). The development of markers of the Big-Five factor structure. *Psychological Assessment, 4,* 26–42.

Goldberg, L. R. (1994). The structure of phenotypic personality traits. *American Psychologist, 48,* 26–34.

Goldman, L. (1990). Qualitative assessment. *The Counseling Psychologist, 18,* 205–213.

Goldman, L. (1992). Qualitative assessment: An approach for counselors. *Journal of Counseling & Development, 70,* 616–621.

Goldman, L. (1994). The marriage is over . . . for most of us. *Measurement and Evaluation in Counseling and Development, 26,* 217–218.

Goodyear, R. K. (1990). Research on the effects of test interpretation: A review. *The Counseling Psychologist, 18,* 240–257.

Goodyear, R. K., & Lichtenberg, J. W. (1999). A scientist-practitioner perspective on test interpretation. In J. W. Lichtenberg, & R. K. Goodyear (Eds.), *Scientist-practitioner perspectives on test interpretation* (pp. 1–14). Boston: Allyn and Bacon.

Gordon, H. W., & Lee, P. (1986). A relationship between gonadotroins and visuospatial function. *Neuropsychologia, 24,* 563–576.

Gottfredson, L. S. (1994). The science and politics of race-norming. *American Psychologist, 49,* 955–963.

Gough, H. G., & Bradley, P. (1996). *CPI manual* (3rd ed.). Palo Alto, CA: Consulting Psychologists Press.

Graduate Record Examination Board (1997). *GRE 1997–1998 guide to the use of scores.* Princeton, NJ: Educational Testing Service.

Graham, J. R. (1990). *MMPI-2: Assessing personality and psychopathology.* New York: Oxford University Press.

Greene, R. L., & Banken, J. A. (1995). Assessing alcohol/drug abuse problems. In J. N. Butcher (Ed.), *Clinical personality assessment: Practical approaches* (pp. 460–474). New York: Oxford University Press.

Greenspan, S. I., & Greenspan, N. T. (1981). *The clinical interview of the child.* New York: McGraw-Hill.

Gregory, S., & Lee, S. (1986). Psychoeducational assessment of racial and ethnic minority groups: Professional implications. *Journal of Counseling & Development, 14,* 635–637.

Gronlund, N. E. (1998). *Assessment of student achievement* (6th ed.). Boston: Allyn and Bacon.

Groth-Marnat, G. (1997). *Handbook of psychological assessment* (3rd ed.). New York: Wiley.

Guilford, J. B. (1967). *The nature of human intelligence.* New York: McGraw-Hill.

Guilford, J. B. (1988). Some changes in the structure of the intellect model. *Educational and Psychological Measurement, 48,* 1–4.

Hackett, G., & Lonberg, S. D. (1993). Career assessment for women: Trends and issues. *Journal of Career Assessment, 3,* 197–216.

Hackett, G., & Watkins, C. E. (1995). Research in career assessment: Abilities, interests, decision making, and career development. In W. B. Walsh & S. H. Osipow (Eds.), *Handbook of vocational psychology: Theory, research, and practice* (2nd ed., pp. 181–216). Mahwah, NJ: Erlbaum.

Hagen, J. W., & Hagen, W. W. (1995). What employment counselors need to know about employment discrimination and the Civil Rights Act of 1991. *Journal of Employment Counseling, 32,* 2–10.

Hallahan, D. P., & Kauffman, J. M. (1997). *Exceptional learners: Introduction to special education.* Boston: Allyn and Bacon.

Hambleton, R. K., Swaminathan, H., & Rogers, J. H. (1991). *Fundamentals of Item Response Theory.* Thousand Oaks, CA: Sage.

Handler, L. (1996). The clinical use of figure drawings. In C. S. Newmark (Ed.), *Major psychological assessment instruments* (2nd ed., pp. 206–293). Boston: Allyn and Bacon.

Hanson, W. E., & Claiborn, C. D. (1998). Providing test feedback to clients: What really matters. In C. Claiborn (Chair), *Test interpretation in counseling—Recent research and practice.* Symposium conducted at the conference of the American Psychological Association, San Francisco.

Hanson, W. E., Claiborn, C. D., & Kerr, B. (1997). Differential effects of two test-interpretation styles in counseling: A field study. *Journal of Counseling Psychology, 44,* 400–405.

Harmon, L. W. (1994). Career Decision Scale (CDS). In J. T. Kapes, M. M. Mastie, & E. A. Whitfield (Eds.), *A counselor's guide to career assessment instruments* (pp. 258–262). Alexandria, VA: National Career Development Association.

Harmon, L. W., Hansen, J. C., Borgen, F. H., & Hammer, A. L. (1994). *Strong Interest Inventory: Applications and technical guide.* Palo Alto, CA: Consulting Psychologists Press.

Harren, V.A., Buck, J. N., & Daniels, H. (1985). *Assessment of Career Decision Making.* Los Angeles: Western Psychological Press.

Hartigan, J. A., & Wigdor, A. K. (1989). *Fairness in employment testing: Validity generalization minority issues and the General Aptitude Test Battery.* Washington, DC: National Academy Press.

Haynes, S., Follingstad, T., & Sullivan, J. (1979). Assessment of marital satisfaction and interaction. *Journal of Consulting and Clinical Psychology, 47,* 789–791.

Hebree, R. (1988). Correlates, causes, effects, and treatment of test anxiety. *Review of Educational Research, 58,* 47–77.

Hedges, L. V., & Olkin, I. (1985). *Statistical methods for meta-analysis.* Orlando, FL: Academic Press.

Helms, J. E. (1992). Why is there no study of cultural equivalence in standardized cognitive ability testing? *American Psychologist, 47,* 1083–1101.

Heppner, P. P., & Claiborn, C. D. (1989). Social influence research in counseling: A review and critique. *Journal of Counseling Psychology, 36,* 365–387.

Herman, D. O. (1985). Review of the Career Decision Scale. In J. V. Mitchell (Ed.), *Ninth mental measurements yearbook* (pp. 270–271). Highland Park, NJ: Gryphon.

Hernstein, R. J., & Murray, C. A. (1994). *The bell curve: Intelligence and class structure in American life.* New York: Free Press.

Herr, E. L., & Ashby, J. S. (1994). Kuder Occupational Interest Survey, Form DD (KOIS). In J. T. Kapes, M. M. Mastie, & E. A. Whitfield (Eds.), *A counselor's guide to career assessment instruments* (pp. 194–199). Alexandria, VA: National Career Development Association.

Herr, E. L., & Cramer, S. H. (1992). *Career guidance and counseling through the life span: Systematic approaches.* New York: HarperCollins.

Hersh, J. B. (1971). Effects of referral information on testers. *Journal of Consulting and Clinical Psychology, 37,* 116–122.

Highlen, P. S., & Hill, C. E. (1984). Factors affecting change in individual counseling. In S. D., Brown, & R. W. Lent (Eds.), *Handbook of counseling psychology* (pp. 334–396). New York: Wiley.

Hines, M. (1990). Gonadal hormones and human cognitive development. In J. Balthazart (Ed.), *Hormones, brains, and behaviors in vertebrates: 1. Sexual differentiation, neuroanatomical aspects, neurotransmitters, and neuropeptides* (pp. 51–63). Basel, Switzerland: Karger.

Hinkle, J. S. (1994). Practitioners and cross-cultural assessment: A practical guide to information and training. *Measurement and Evaluation in Counseling and Development, 27,* 103–115.

Hoffman, K. I., & Lundberg, G. D. (1976). A comparison of computer monitored group tests and paper-and-pencil tests. *Educational and Psychological Measurement, 36,* 791–809.

Hogan, R., Hogan, J., & Roberts, B. W. (1996). Personality measurement and employment: Questions and answers. *American Psychologist, 51,* 469–477.

Hoge, R. D. (1985). The validity of direct observation measures of pupil classroom behavior. *Review of Educational Research, 55,* 469–483.

Hohenshil, T. H. (1993). Teaching the DSM-III-R in counselor education. *Counselor Education and Supervision, 32,* 267–275.

Hohenshil, T. H. (1996). Editorial: Role of assessment and diagnosis in counseling. *Journal of Counseling and Development, 75,* 64–67.

Holland, J. L. (1985). *Making vocational choices: A theory of vocational personalities and work environments* (2nd ed.). Englewood Cliffs, NJ: Prentice-Hall.

Holland, J. L. (1997). *Making vocational choices: A theory of vocational personalities and work environments* (3rd ed.). Odessa, FL: Psychological Assessment Resources.

Holland, J. L., Daiger, D., Power, P. G. (1980). *My vocational situation.* Odessa, FL: Psychological Assessment Resources.

Holland, J. L., Fritzsche, B. A., & Powell, A. B. (1994). *The Self-Directed Search (SDS) technical manual—1994 edition.* Odessa, FL: Psychological Assessment Resources.

Honzik, M. P. (1967). Environmental correlates of mental growth: Predictions from the family setting at 21 months. *Child Development, 38,* 323–337.

Hood, A. B., & Johnson, R. W. (1997). *Assessment in counseling: A guide to the use of psychological assessment procedures* (2nd ed.). Alexandria, VA: American Counseling Association.

Horn, J. L. (1985). Remodeling old models of intelligence: G-Gc theory. In B. B. Wolman (Ed.), *Handbook of intelligence* (pp. 267–300). New York: Wiley.

Horn, J. L., & Noll, J. (1997). Human cognitive capabilities: Gf-Gc theory. In D. P. Flanagan, J. L. Genshaft, & P. L. Harrison (Eds.), *Contemporary intellectual assessment: Theories, tests, and issues* (pp. 53–91). New York: Guilford.

Hummel, T. J. (1998). The usefulness of tests in clinical decisions. In J.W. Lichtenburg & R. K. Goodyear (Eds.), *Scientist-Practitioner perspectives on test interpretation* (pp. 59–112). Boston: Allyn and Bacon.

Hunter, J. E. (1980). *Validity generalization for 12,000 jobs: An application of synthetic validity and validity generalization to the General Aptitude Test Battery (GATB)*. Washington, DC: U.S. Department of Labor.

Hunter, J. E. (1982). *The dimensionality of the General Aptitude Test Battery and the dominance of general factors over specific factors in the prediction of job performance*. Washington, DC: U.S. Department of Labor.

Hunter, J. E. (1986). Cognitive ability, cognitive aptitudes, job knowledge, and job performance. *Journal of Vocational Behavior, 29,* 340–362.

Hunter, J. E., & Schmidt, F. L. (1983). Quantifying the effects of psychological interventions on employee performance and work-force productivity. *American Psychologist, 38,* 473–478.

Hunter, J. E., Schmidt, F. L., & Hunter, R. (1979). Differential validity of employment tests by race: A comprehensive review and analysis. *Psychological Bulletin, 86,* 721–735.

Hyde, J., Fennema, E., & Lamon, S. J. (1990). Gender differences in mathematics performance: A meta-analysis. *Psychological Bulletin, 107,* 139–155.

Impara, J. C., & Plake, B. S. (1998). *Thirteenth mental measurements yearbook*. Lincoln, NB: Buros Institute.

Ivey, A. E. (1994). *Intentional interviewing and counseling: Facilitating client development in a multicultural society* (3rd ed.). Pacific Grove, CA: Brooks/Cole.

Ivey, A. E., Ivey, M. B., & Simek-Morgan, L. (1993). *Counseling and psychotherapy: A multicultural perspective* (3rd ed.). Boston: Allyn and Bacon.

Jackson, D. N. (1996a). *Jackson Personality Inventory-Revised*. Port Huron, MI: Sigma Assessment Systems.

Jackson, D. N. (1996b). *Jackson Vocational Interest Survey*. Port Huron, MI: Sigma Assessment Systems.

Jackson, D. N. (1996c). *Personality Research Form manual*. Port Huron, MI: Sigma Assessment Systems.

Jastak, J. F., & Jastak, S. (1979). *Wide Range Interest-Opinion Test*. Wilmington, DL: Jastak Associates.

Jensen, A. R. (1969). How much can we boost IQ and scholastic achievement? *Harvard Educational Review, 39,* 1–23.

Jensen, A. R. (1972). *Genetics and education*. New York: Harper & Row.

Jensen, A. R. (1980). *Bias in mental testing*. New York: Free Press.

Jensen, A. R. (1985). The nature of black-white differences on various psychometric tests: Spearman's hypothesis. *The Behavioral and Brain Sciences, 8,* 192–263.

Jepsen, D. A. (1994). Jackson Vocational Interest Survey. In J. T. Kapes, M. M. Mastied, & E. A. Whitfield (Eds.), *A counselors' guide to career assessment instruments* (pp. 183–189). Alexandria, VA: National Career Development Association.

Jeske, R. J. (1985). Review of the Piers-Harris Children's Self-Concept Scale. In J. V. Mitchell (Ed.), *Ninth mental measurements yearbook* (pp. 1169–1170). Highland Park, NJ: Gryphon.

Johansson, C. B. (1984). *Manual for the Career Assessment Inventory* (2nd ed.). Minneapolis, MN: National Computer Systems.

Johansson, C. B. (1986). *Manual for the Career Assessment Inventory: The enhanced version*. Minneapolis, MN: National Computer Systems.

Joint Committee on Testing Practices (1988). *Code of Fair Testing Practices in Education*. Washington, DC: Author. (Mailing Address: Joint committee on Testing Practices, American Psychological Association, 750 First Avenue, NE, Washington, DC, 20002-4242).

Jones, A. S., & Gelso, C. J. (1988). Differential effects of style of interpretation: Another look. *Journal of Counseling Psychology, 35,* 363–369.

Juni, S. (1995). Review of the Revised NEO Personality Inventory. In J. C. Conoley & J. J. Kramer (Eds.), *Twelfth mental measurements yearbook* (pp. 863–868). Lincoln, NB: The University of Nebraska Press.

Kahne, J. (1996). The politics of self-esteem. *American Educational Research Journal, 33,* 3–22.

Kamphaus, R. W. (1993). *Clinical assessment of children's intelligence: A handbook for professional practice*. Boston: Allyn and Bacon.

Kapes, J. T., Borman, C. A., & Frazier, F. D. (1989). An evaluation of SIGI and DISCOVER microcomputer-based career guidance systems. *Measurement and Evaluation in Counseling and Development, 22,* 126–136.

Kaplan, R. M., & Saccuzzo, D. P. (1997). *Psychological testing: Principles, applications, and issues* (4th ed.). Pacific Grove, CA: Brooks/Cole.

Kaufman, A. S. (1990). *Assessing adolescents and adults in intelligence*. Boston: Allyn and Bacon.

Kaufman, A. S. (1994). *Intelligent testing with the WISC-III*. New York: Wiley.

Kaufman, A. S., & Kaufman, N. L. (1983a). *Kaufman Assessment Battery for Children: Administration and scoring manual.* Circle Pines, MN: American Guidance Service.

Kaufman, A. S., & Kaufman, N. L. (1983b). *Kaufman Assessment Battery for Children: Interpretive manual.* Circle Pines, MN: American Guidance Service.

Kaufman, A, S., & Kaufman, N. L. (1985). *Kaufman Test of Educational Achievement.* Circle Pines, MN: American Guidance Service.

Kaufman, A, S., & Kaufman, N. L. (1993). *Kaufman Adolescent and Adult Intelligence Test Manual.* Circle Pines, MN: American Guidance Service.

Kavale, K. A. (1995). Setting the record straight on learning disability and low achievement: The tortuous path of ideology. *Learning Disabilities Research and Practice, 10,* 145–152.

Keitel, M. A., Kopala, M., & Adamson, W. S. (1996). Ethical issues in multicultural assessment. In L. A. Suzuki, P. J. Meller, & J. G. Ponterotto (Eds.), *Handbook of multicultural assessment: Clinical, psychological, and educational applications* (pp. 29–50). San Francisco: Jossey-Bass.

Kelley, T. L. (1939). The selection of upper and lower group. *Journal of Educational Psychology, 30,* 17–24.

Kent, N., & Davis, D. R. (1957). Discipline in the home and intellectual development. *British Journal of Medical Psychology, 30,* 27–33.

Kessler, R. C., McGonagle, K. A., Zhao, S., Nelson, C. B., Hughes, M., Eshleman, S., Wittchen, H., & Kendler, K. S. (1994). Lifetime and 12-month prevalence of DSM-III psychiatric disorders in the United States. *Archives of General Psychiatry, 51,* 8–19.

Keyser, D. J., & Sweetland, R. C. (Eds.) (1994). *Test critiques: Volume X.* Austin, TX: PRO-ED.

Kinston, W., Loader, P., & Sullivan, J. (1985). *Clinical assessment of family health.* London: Hospital for Sick Children, Family Studies Group.

Kivlighan, D. M., & Shapiro, R. M. (1987). Holland type as a predictor of benefit from self-help career counseling. *Journal of Counseling Psychology, 34,* 326–329.

Knapp-Lee, L., Knapp, L., & Knapp, R. (1990). A complete career guidance program: The COPSystem. In M. L. Savickas & W. B. Walsh (Eds.), *Handbook of career counseling theory and practice* (pp. 241–283). Palo Alto, CA: Davies-Black.

Knoff, H. M., & Prout, H. T. (1993). *Kinetic drawing system for family and school: A handbook* (5th ed.). Los Angeles: Western Psychological Services.

Koppitz, E. (1968). *Psychological evaluation of children's figure drawings.* New York: Grune & Stratton.

Koppitz, E. (1984). *Psychological evaluation of figure drawings by middle school pupils.* New York: Grune & Stratton.

Kovacs, M. (1992). *Children's Depression Inventory.* North Tonawanda, NY: Multi-Health Systems.

Kramer, J. J., & Conoley, J. C. (Eds.) (1992). *Eleventh mental measurements yearbook.* Lincoln, NE: Buros Institute.

Krivasty, S. E., Magoon, T. M. (1976). Differential effects of three vocational counseling treatments. *Journal of Counseling Psychology, 23,* 112–117.

Kuder, F., & Zytowski, D. G. (1991). *Kuder Occupational Interest Survey Form DD general manual* (3rd ed.). Monterey, CA: CTB/ McGraw-Hill.

L'Abate, L. (1994). *Family evaluation: A psychological approach.* Thousand Oaks, CA; Sage.

Lachar, D., & Gruber, C. P. (1995). *Personality Inventory for Youth (PIY) manual: Technical guide.* Los Angeles: Western Psychological Services.

LaCrosse, M. B. (1980). Perceived counselor social influence and counseling outcome: Validity of the Counselor Rating Form. *Journal of Counseling Psychology, 27,* 320–327.

Lambert, M. J. (1983). Introduction to assessment of psychotherapy outcome. Historical perspectives and current issues. In M. J. Lambert, E. R., Christiensen, & S. S. Dejulio (Eds.), *The assessment of psychotherapy outcome* (pp. 3–32). New York: Wiley.

Lambert, M. J., & Hill, C. E. (1994). Assessing psychotherapy outcomes and processes. In A. E. Bergin & S. L. Garfield (Eds.), *Handbook of psychotherapy and behavior change* (pp. 72–113). New York: Wiley.

Lambert, M. J., Ogles, B. M., & Masters, K. S. (1992). Choosing outcome assessment devices: An organizational and conceptual scheme. *Journal of Counseling and Development, 70,* 527–532.

Last, J., & Bruhn, A.R. (1991). *The Comprehensive Early Memories Scoring System-Revised.* 17 pages. Available from the second author.

Latcher, D., & Gruber, C. P. (1995). *Personality Inventory for Youth (PIY).* Los Angeles: Western Psychological Services.

Lautenschlager, G. J., & Flaherty, V. L. (1990). Computer administration of questions: More desirable or more social desirability? *Journal of Applied Psychology, 75,* 310–314.

Lee, S. W., & Stefany, E. F. (1995). Review of the Woodcock-Johnson Psycho-Educational Battery-Revised. In J. C. Conoley & J. J. Kramer (Eds.), *Twelfth mental measurements yearbook* (pp. 1116–1117). Lincoln, NB: The University of Nebraska Press.

Lent, R. W., Brown, S. D., & Hackett, G. (1994). Toward a unifying social cognitive theory of career and academic interest, choice, and performance. *Journal of Vocational Behavior, 45,* 79–122.

Lent, R. W., & Hackett, G. (1987). Career self-efficacy: Empirical status and future directions. *Journal of Vocational Behavior, 30,* 347–382.

Lenz, J. G., Reardon, R. C., & Sampson, J. P. (1993). Holland's theory and effective use of computer-assisted career guidance systems. *Journal of Career Development, 19,* 245–253.

Lerner, B. (1981). The minimum competence testing movement: Social, scientific, and legal implications. *American Psychologist, 36,* 1056–1066.

Lichtenberg, J. W., & Hummel, T. J. (1998). The communication of probablistic information through test interpretation. In C. Claiborn (Chair), *Test inerpretation in counseling—Recent research and practice.* Symposium conducted at the conference of the American Psychological Association, San Francisco.

Lindzey, G. (1959). On the classification of projective techniques. *Psychological Bulletin, 56,* 158–168.

Linn, R. L. (1978). Single-group validity, differential validity, and differential prediction. *Journal of Applied Psychology, 63,* 507–512.

Linn, R. L., Baker, E. L., & Dunbar, S. B. (1991). Complex, performance-based assessment: Expectations and validation criteria. *Educational Researcher, 20,* 15–21.

Linn, R. L., & Burton, E. (1994). Performance-based assessments: Implications of task specificity. *Educational Measurement: Issues and Practice, 13,* 5–8, 15.

Locke, H., & Wallace, K. (1959). Short marital adjustment and predictions tests: Their reliability and validity. *Marriage and Family Living, 2,* 251–255.

Loehlin, J. C. (1989). Partitioning environmental and genetic contributions to behavioral development. *American Psychologist, 10,* 1285–1292.

Loehlin, J. C., Lindzey, G., & Spuhler, J. N. (1975). *Race differences in intelligence.* San Francisco: Freeman.

Long, K. A., Graham, J. R., & Timbrook, R. E. (1994). Socioeconomic status and MMPI-2 interpretation. *Measurement and Evaluation in Counseling and Development, 27,* 159–177.

Lord, F. M. (1980). *Applications of item response theory to practical testing problems.* Hillsdale, NJ: Erlbaum.

Lubin, B. (1994). *State Trait-Depression Adjective Check Lists.* Odessa, FL: Psychological Assessment Resources.

Luria, A. R. (1966). *Human brain and psychological processes.* New York: Harper & Row.

Lyddon, W. J., & Alford, D. J. (1993). Constructivist assessment: A developmental-epistemic perspective. In G. J. Neimeyer (Ed.). *Constructivist assessment: A casebook* (pp. 31–57). Thousand Oaks, CA: Sage.

Mabry, L. (1995). Review of the Wide Range Achievement Test 3. In J. C. Conoley & J. J. Kramer (Eds.), *Twelfth mental measurements yearbook* (pp. 1108–1110). Lincoln, NB: The University of Nebraska Press.

Machover, K. (1949). *Personality projection in the drawings of the human figure. A method of personality investigation.* Springfield, IL: Charles C. Thomas.

Manuele-Adkins, C. (1989). Review of The Self-Directed Search. In J. C. Conoley & J. J. Kramer (Eds.), *Tenth mental measurements yearbook* (pp. 738–740). Lincoln, NB: University of Nebraska Press.

Masters, M. S., & Sanders, B. (1993). Is the gender difference in mental rotation disappearing? *Behavior Genetics, 23,* 337–341.

Mayfield, D. G., McLeod, G., & Hall, P. (1974). The CAGE questionnaire: Validation of a new alcoholism screening instrument. *American Journal of Psychiatry, 131,* 1121–1123.

McConnaughy, E. A., DiClemente, C. C., Prochaska, J. O., & Velicer, W. F. (1989). Stages of change in psychotherapy: A follow-up report. *Psychotherapy, 26,* 494–503.

McConnaughy, E. A., Prochaska, J. O., & Velicer, W. F. (1983). Stages of change in psychotherapy: Measurement and sample profiles. *Psychotherapy: Theory, Research, and Practice, 20,* 368–375.

McCrae, R. R., & Costa, P. T. (1987). Validation of the five-factor model of personality across instruments and observers. *Journal of Personality and Social Psychology, 52,* 81–90.

McCrae, R. R., & Costa P. T. (1997). Personality trait structure as a human universal. *American Psychologist, 52,* 509–516.

McCrae, R. R., & John, O. P. (1992). An introduction to the five-factor model and its applications. *Journal of Personality, 60,* 175–215.

McGoldrick, M., & Gerson, R. (1985) *Genograms in family assessment.* New York: Norton.

McGue, M., Bouchard, T. J., Jr., Iacono, W. G., & Lykken, D. T. (1993). Behavioral genetics of cognitive ability: A life-span perspective. In R. Ploomin & G. E. McClearn (Eds.), *Nature, nurture, & psychology* (pp. 59–76). Washington, DC: American Psychological Association.

McIntosh, J. L. (1992). Methods of suicide. In R. W. Maris, A. L. Berman, & J. T. Maltsberger (Eds.), *Assessment and prediction of suicide* (pp. 381–397). New York: Guilford.

McMichael, A. J., Baghurst, P. A., Wigg, N. R., Vimpani, G. V., Robertson, E. F., & Roberts, R. J. (1988). Port Pirie cohort study: Environmental exposure to lead and children's abilities at the age of four years. *New England Journal of Medicine, 319,* 468–475.

McNamara, K. (1992). Depression assessment and intervention: Current status and future direction. In S. D. Brown & R. W. Lent (Eds.), *Handbook of counseling psychology* (2nd ed., pp. 691–718). New York: Wiley.

McShane, D., & Cook, V. J. (1985). Transcultural intellectual assessment: Performance by Hispanics on the Wechsler scales. In B. B. Wolman (Ed.), *Handbook of intelligence: Theories, measurements, and applications* (pp. 737–785). New York: Wiley.

McShane, D. A., & Plas, J. M. (1984). The cognitive functioning of American Indian children: Moving from the WISC to the WISC-R. *School Psychology Review, 13,* 61–73.

Meehl, P. E. (1954). *Clinical versus statistical prediction: A theoretical analysis and a review of the evidence.* Minneapolis, MN: University of Minnesota Press.

Meehl, P. E. (1956). Wanted: A good cookbook. *American Psychologist, 11,* 263–272.

Mehrens, W. A. (1994). Kuder General Interest Survey (KGIS). In J. T. Kapes, M. M. Mastie, & E. A. Whitfield (Eds.), *A counselor's guide to career assessment instruments* (pp. 189–193). Alexandria, VA: National Career Development Association.

Merenda, P. F. (1995). Substantive issues in the Soroka v. Dayton-Hudson case. *Psychological Reports, 77,* 595–606.

Merrens, M. R., & Richards, W. S. (1970). Acceptance of generalized versus "bona fide" personality interpretations. *Psychological Reports, 27,* 691–694.

Messick, S. (1995). Validity of psychological assessment: Validation of inferences from persons' responses and performances as scientific inquiry into score meaning. *American Psychologist, 50,* 741–749.

Millon, T. (1969). *Modern psychological pathology: A biosocial approach to maladaptive learning and functioning.* Philadelphia: Saunders.

Millon, T. (1994). *Millon Index of Personality Styles (MIPS) manual.* San Antonio, TX: Psychological Corporation.

Millon, T., Millon, C., & Davis, R. (1994a). *Millon Adolescent Clinical Inventory.* Minneapolis, MN: National Computer Systems.

Millon, T., Millon, C., & Davis, R. (1994b). *MCMI-III manual: Millon Clinical Multiaxial Inventory-III.* Minneapolis, MN: National Computer Systems.

Minuchin, S. (1974). *Families and family therapy.* Cambridge, MA: Harvard University Press.

Mitchell, R. R., & Friedman, H. (1994). *Sandplay: Past, present, and future.* New York: Routledge.

Mohr, D. C. (1995). Negative outcome in psychotherapy: A critical review. *Clinical Psychology: Science and Practice, 2,* 1–27.

Moore, R. D., Bone, L. R., Geller, G., Mamon, J. A., Stokes, E. J., & Levine, D. M. (1989). Prevalence of detection, and treatment of alcoholism in hospitalized patients. *Journal of the American Medical Association, 261,* 403–407.

Moos, R. H. (1973). Conceptualizing human environments. *American Psychologists, 28,* 652–665.

Moos, R. H., & Moos, B. S. (1994). *Family Environment Scale manual: Develpment, application, research.* Palo Alto, CA: Consulting Psychologists Press.

Moreland, K. L. (1996). Persistent issues in multicultural assessment of social and emotional functioning. In L. A. Suzuki, P. J. Meller, & J. G. Ponterotto (Eds.), *Handbook of multicultural assessement: Clinical, psycho-*

logical, and educational applications (pp. 51–76). San Francisco: Jossey-Bass.

Moreland, K. L., Eyde, L. D., Robertson, G. J., Primoff, E. S., & Most, R. B. (1995). Assessment of test user qualifications: A research-based measurement procedure. *American Psychologist, 50,* 14–23.

Morera, O. F., Johnson, T. P., Freels, S., Parsons, J., Crittenden, K. S., Flay, B. R., & Warnecke, R. B. (1998). The measure of stages of readiness to change: Some psychometric considerations. *Psychological Assessment, 10,* 182–186.

Morris, T. M. (1990). Culturally sensitive family assessment: An evaluation of the Family Assessment Device with Hawaiian-American and Japanese-American families. *Family Process, 29,* 105–116.

Morrison, J. (1995). *DSM-IV made easy: The clinician's guide to diagnosis.* New York: Guilford.

Munoz-Sandoval, A. F., Cummins, J., Alvarado, C. G., & Ruef, M. L. (1998). *Bilingual Verbal Ability Tests.* Itasca, IL: Riverside.

Munroe, R. L. (1955). *Schools of psychoanalytic thought.* New York: Oxford University Press.

Murphy, E., & Meisgeier, C. (1987). *Murphy-Meisgeier Type Indicatory for Children.* Palo Alto, CA: Consulting Psychologists Press.

Murray, H. A. (1943). *Thematic Apperception Test.* Cambridge, MA: Harvard University Press.

Myers, I. S. (1962). *Manual for the Myers-Briggs Type Indicator.* Princeton, NJ: Educational Testing Service.

Myers, I. B., & McCaulley, M. H. (1985). *Manual: A guide to the the development and used of the Myers-Briggs Type Indicator.* Palo Alto, CA: Consulting Psychologists Press.

Myers, I. B., with Myers, P. B. (1980). *Gifts differing.* Palo Alto, CA: Consulting Psychologists Press.

National Institute of Mental Health (1998). *Suicide facts* [On-line]. Available: http://www.nimh.nih.gov/research/suifact.htm.

Neisser, U., Boodoo, G., Bouchard, T. J., Boykin, A. W., Brody, N., Ceci, S. J., Halpern, D. F., Loehlin, J. C., Perloff, R., Sternberg, R. J., & Urbina, S. (1996). Intelligence: Knowns and unknowns. *American Psychologist, 51,* 77–98.

Nelson, R. O. (1983). Behavioral assessment: Past, present, and future. *Behavioral Assessment, 5,* 196–206.

Nevill, D. D., & Super, D. E. (1986). *The Salience Inventory: Theory, application, and research.* Palo Alto, CA: Consulting Psychologists Press.

Nevill, D. D., & Super, D. E. (1989). *The Values Scale: Theory, application, and research.* Palo Alto, CA: Consulting Psychologists Press.

Newman, M. L., & Greenway, P. (1997) Therapeutic effects of providing MMPI-2 test feedback to clients at a university counseling service: A collaborative approach. *Psychological Assessment, 9,* 122–131.

Newmark, C. S., & McCord, D. M. (1996). The Minnesota Multiphasic Personality Inventory- 2. In C. S. Newmark (Ed.), *Major psychological assessment instruments* (2nd ed., pp. 1–58). Boston: Allyn and Bacon.

Nichols, D. S. (1992). Review of the Minnesota Multiphasic Personality Inventory-2. In J. C. Conoley & J. J. Kramer (Eds.), *Eleventh mental measurements yearbook* (pp. 562–565). Lincoln, NB: The University of Nebraska Press.

Nicholson, C. L., & Hibpshman, T. H. (1990). *Slosson Intelligence Test for Children and Adults, Revised.* East Aurora, NY: Slosson Educational Publications.

Niles, S. G., & Garis, J. W. (1990). The effects of a career planning course and a computer-assisted career guidance program (SIGI PLUS) on undecided university students. *Journal of Career Development, 16,* 237–248.

Oetting, E. R., & Beauvais, F. (1990). Adolescent drug use: Findings of national and local surveys. *Journal of Consulting and Clinical Psychology, 58,* 385–394.

Okun, B. F. (1997). *Effective helping: Interviewing and counseling techniques* (5th ed.). Pacific Grove, CA: Brooks/Cole.

Oliver, L. W., & Spokane, A. R. (1988). Career-intervention outcome: What contributes to client gain? *Journal of Counseling Psychology, 35,* 447–462.

Olson, D. H. (1983). *Inventories of premarital, marital, parent-child, and parent-adolescent conflict.* St. Paul, MN: University of Minnesota, Department Family Social Science.

Olson, D. H., Fournier, D. G., & Druckman, J. M. (1996). *PREPARE.* Minneapolis, MN: Life Innovations, Inc.

Olson, D. H., Portner, J., & Lavee, Y. (1985). *FACES III: Family Adaptability and Cohesion Evaluations Scales.* St. Paul, MN: Family Social Science.

Olson, D. H., & Ryder, R. (1978). *Marital and Family Interaction Coding System (MFICS): Abbreviated coding manual.* St. Paul, MN: University of Minnesota, Department Family Social Science.

Oosterhof, A. (1994). *Classroom application of educational measurement* (2nd ed.). Merrill: New York.

Orlinsky, D. E., Grawe, K., & Parks, B. K. (1994). Process and outcome in psychotherapy: NOCH EINMAL. In A. E. Bergin & S. L. Garfield (Eds.), *Handbook of psychotherapy and behavior change* (pp. 72–113). New York: Wiley.

Osborne, W. L., Brown, S., Niles, S., & Miner, C. U. (1997). *Career development, assessment and counseling: Applications of the Donald E. Super C-DAC approach.* Alexandria, VA: American Counseling Association.

Osipow, S. H. (1987). *Career Decision Scale manual.* Odessa, FL: Psychological Assessment Resources.

Osipow, S. H. (1991). Developing instruments for use in counseling. *Journal of Counseling and Development, 70,* 322–326.

Osterlind, S. J. (1989). *Constructing test items.* Boston: Kluwer.

Ownby, R. L. (1997). *Psychological reports: A guide to report writing in professional psychology* (3rd ed.). New York: Wiley.

Padilla, A. M., & Medina, A. (1996). Cross-cultural sensitivity in assessment: Using test in culturally appropriate ways. In L. A. Suzuki, P. J. Meller, & J. G. Ponterotto (Eds.), *Handbook of multicultural assessment: Clinical, psychological, and educational applications* (pp. 3–28). San Francisco: Jossey-Bass.

Page, E. B. (1985). Review of Kaufman Assessment Battery for Children. In J. V. Mitchell (Ed.), *Ninth mental measurements yearbook* (pp. 773–777). Highland Park, NJ: Gryphon.

Parsons, F. (1909). *Choosing a vocation.* Boston: Houghton Mifflin.

Pearlman, K., Schmidt, F. L., & Hunter, J. E. (1980) Validity generalization results for tests used to predict training success and job proficiency. *Journal of Applied Psychology, 65,* 373–406.

Pedersen, P. B. (1991). Multiculturalism as a generic approach to counseling. *Journal of Counseling & Development, 70,* 6–12.

Piaget, J. (1972). *The psychology of intelligence.* Totowa, NJ: Littlefield Adams.

Piers, E. V. (1984). *Piers-Harris Children's Self-Concept Scale: Revised manual 1984.* Los Angeles: Western Psychological Services.

Pinkney, J. W., & Bozik, C. M. (1994). Career Development Inventory. In J. T. Kapes, M. M. Mastie, & E. A. Whitfield (Eds.), *A counselor's guide to career assessment instruments.* (pp. 264–267). Alexandria, VA: National Career Development Association.

Piotrowski, C., & Keller, J. (1989). Psychological testing in outpatient mental health facilities: A national study. *Professional Psychology: Research and Practice, 20,* 423–425.

Pittenger, D. J. (1993). The utility of the Myers-Briggs Type Indicator. *Review of Educational Research, 63,* 467–488.

Ponterotto, J. G., Pace, J. A., & Kaven, K. (1989). A counselor's guide to the assessment of depression. *Journal of Counseling and Development, 67,* 301–309.

Powers, D. E. (1993). Coaching for the SAT: A summary of the summaries and an update. *Educational Measurement Issues and Practice, 12*(2), 24–30.

Poznanski, E. O., & Mokros, H. B. (1996). *Children's Depression Rating Scale, Revised.* Los Angeles: Western Psychological Services.

Prediger, D. J. (1994). Multicultural assessment standards: A compilation for counselors. *Measurement and Evaluation in Counseling and Development, 27,* 68–73.

Prediger, D. J., & Swaney, K. B. (1992). *Career counseling validity of the Discover's job cluster scales for the revised ASVAB score report* (Report No. 92–2). Iowa City, IA: American College Testing Program.

Prochaska, J. O., & DiClemente, C. C. (1992). Stages of change in modification of problem behaviors. In M. Hersen, R. M. Eisler, & P. M. Miller (Eds.), *Progress in behavior modification* (pp. 184–214). Sycamore, IL: Sycamore Press.

Prochaska, J. O., DiClemente, C. C., & Norcross, J. C. (1992). In search of how people change: Applications to addictive behaviors. *American Psychologist, 47,* 1102–1114.

Pryor, R. G. L., & Taylor, N.B. (1986). On combining scores from interest and values measures in counseling. *Vocational Guidance Quarterly, 34,* 178–187.

Psychological Corporation (1991). *Differential Aptitude Tests (5th ed.) Career Interest Inventory counselors' manual.* San Antonio, TX: Author.

Quay, H. C., & Peterson, D. P. (1987). *Revised Problem Behavior Checklist.* Coral Gables, FL: Authors.

Rahdert, E. R. (1997). *Adolescent Assessment Referral Manual* (NIH No. 27189–8252). Rockville, MD: National Institute of Drug Abuse.

Raven, J. C., Court, J. H., & Raven, J. (1983). *Manual for Raven's Progressive Matrices and Vocabulary Scales-Standard progressive matrices.* London: Lewis.

Reid, W. H., & Wise, M. G. (1995). *DSM-IV training guide.* New York: Brunner/Mazel.

Reynolds, W. M. (1987). *Reynolds Adolescent Depression Scale.* Odessa, FL: Psychological Assessment Resources.

Reynolds, W. M. (1988). *Suicidal Ideation Questionnaire.* Odessa, FL: Psychological Assessment Resources.

Reynolds, W. M. (1989). *Reynolds Child Depression Scale.* Odessa, FL: Psychological Assessment Resources.

Reynolds, W. M. (1991). *Adult Suicidal Ideation Questionnaire.* Odessa, FL: Psychological Assessment Resources.

Reynolds, C. R., Chastain, R. L., Kaufman, A. S., & McLean, J. E. (1987). Demographic characteristics and IQ among adults: Analysis of the WAIS-R standardization sample as a function of the stratification variables. *Journal of School Psychology, 25,* 323–342.

Reynolds, W. M., & Kobak, K. A. (1995). *Hamilton Depression Inventory.* Odessa, FL: Psychological Assessment Resources.

Reynolds, W. M., & Mazza, J. J. (1992). *Suicidal Behavior History Form.* Odessa, FL: Psychological Assessment Resources.

Rohrbraugh, M., Rogers, J. C., & McGoldrick, M. (1992). How do experts read family genograms. *Family Systems Medicine, 10,* 79–89.

Rosenthal, R. (1991). *Meta-analtyic procedures for social research.* Thousand Oaks, CA: Sage.

Rosenthal, R., & Jacobsen, L. (1968). *Pygmalion in the classroom.* Hew York: Holt, Rinehart & Winston.

Rosenzweig, S. (1977). *Manual for the Children's Form of the Rosenzweig Picture-Frustration Study.* St. Louis, MO: Rana House.

Rosenzweig, S. (1978a). *Adult Form supplement for the basic manual of the Rosenzweig Picture-Frustration Study.* St. Louis, MO: Rana House.

Rosenzweig, S. (1978b). *The Rosenzweig Picture-Frustration Study: Basic Manual.* St. Louis, MO: Rana House.

Rosenzweig, S. (1988). Revised norms for the Children's Form of the Rosenzweig Picture-Frustration Study, with updated reference list. *Journal of Clinical Child Psychology, 17,* 326–328.

Rotter, J. B., & Rafferty, J. E. (1992). *Rotter Incomplete Sentence Blank, Second Edition.* San Antonio, TX: The Psychology Corporation.

Rounds, J. B. (1990). The comparative and combined utility of work value and interest data in career counseling with adults. *Journal of Vocational Behavior, 37,* 32–45.

Rounds, J. B., & Tinsley, H. E. A. (1984). Diagnosis and treatment of vocational problems. In S. D. Brown & R. W. Lent (Eds.), *Handbook of counseling psychology* (pp. 137–177). New York: Wiley.

Rounds, J., & Tracey, T. J. (1996). Cross-cultural structural equivalence of RIASEC models and measures. *Journal of Counseling Psychology, 43,* 310–330.

Ryan, J., Prefitera, A., & Powers, L. (1983). Scoring reliability on the WAIS-R. *Journal of Consulting and Clinical Psychology, 51,* 149–150.

Sackett, P. R., & Wilk, S. L. (1994). Within-group norming and other forms of scoring adjustment in preemployment testing. *American Psychologist, 49,* 929–954.

Sampson, J. P. (1986). Computer-assisted testing and assessment: Matching the tool to the task. *Measurement and Evaluation in Counseling and Development, 19,* 60–61.

Sampson, J. P. (1990). Computer-assisted testing and the goals of counseling psychology. *The Counseling Psychologist, 18,* 227–239.

Sampson, J. P. (1998, January). Assessment and the Internet. Paper presented at the Assessment '98 Conference, St. Petersburg, FL.

Sandoval, J. (1995). Review of the Wechsler Intelligence Scale for Children, Third Edition. In J. C. Conoley & J. J. Kramer (Eds.), *Twelfth mental measurements yearbook* (pp. 1103–1105). Lincoln, NB: The University of Nebraska Press.

Sarason, I. G. (1984). Stress, anxiety, and cognitive inter-ference: Reactions to tests. *Journal of Personality and Social Psychology, 46,* 929–938.

Sarason, I. G., & Sarson, B. R. (1990). Test anxiety. In H. Leitenberg (Ed.), *Handbook of social evaluation and anxiety* (pp. 475–495). New York: Plenum.

SASSI Institute (1996). *The reliability and validity of the SASSI-2. A summary.* Bloomington, IN: Author.

Sattler, J. M. (1993). *Asssessment of children* (3rd ed. revised reprint). San Diego, CA: Jerome M. Sattler Publisher.

Sattler, J. M., Hillix, W. A., & Neher, L. A. (1970). Halo effect in examiner scoring of intelligence test re-sponses. *Journal of Consulting and Clinical Psychology, 34,* 172–176.

Sattler, J. M., & Wingert, B. M. (1970). Intelligence test-ing procedures as affected by expectancy and I.Q. *Journal of Clinical Psychology, 26,* 446–448.

Saunders, B. T., & Vitro, F. T. (1971). Examiner ex-pectancy and bias as a function of the referral process in cognitive assessment. *Psychology in the Schools, 8,* 168–171.

Savickas, M. L. (1990). The use of career choice process scales in counseling practice. In M. L. Savickas & W. B. Walsh (Eds.), *Handbook of career counseling theory and practice* (pp. 373–417). Palo Alto, CA: Davies-Black.

Scarr, S. (1992). Developmental theories for the 1990s: Developmental and individual differences. *Child De-velopment, 63,* 1–19.

Scarr, S. (1993). Biological and cultural diversity: The legacy of Darwin for development. *Child Development, 64,* 1333–1354.

Schaefer, C. E., Gitlin, K., & Sandgrund, A. (Eds.). (1991). *Play diagnosis and assessment.* New York: Wiley.

Schaie, K. W., & Strother, C. R. (1968). A cross-sequential study of age changes in cognitive be-havior. *Psychological Bulletin, 70,* 671–680.

Schmidt, F. L., & Hunter, J. E. (1977). Development of a general solution to the problem of validity generaliza-tion. *Journal of Applied Psychology, 62,* 529–540.

Schmidt, F. L., Hunter, J. E., & Caplan, J. R. (1981). Valid-ity generalization results for two jobs in the petroleum business. *Journal of Applied Psychology, 66,* 261–273.

Schroeder, H. E., & Kleinsaser, L. D. (1972). Examiner bias: A determinant of children's verbal behavior on the WISC. *Journal of Consulting and Clinical Psychology, 39,* 451–454.

Schwab, D. P., & Packard, G. L. (1973). Response set distortion on the Gordon Personal Inventory and the Gordon Personal Profile in the selection context: Some implications for predicting employee behavior. *Journal of Applied Psychology, 58,* 372–374.

Seipp, B. (1991). Anxiety and academic performance: A meta-analysis. *Anxiety Research, 4,* 27–41.

Sexton, T. L., & Whiston, S. C. (1994). The status of the counseling relationship: An empirical review, theoreti-cal implications, and research direction. *The Counsel-ing Psychologist, 22,* 5–78.

Sexton, T. L., Whiston, S. C., Bleuer, J. C., & Walz, G. R. (1997). *Integrating outcome research into counseling practice and training.* Alexandria, VA: American Coun-seling Association.

Skinner, H. A., Steinhauer, P. D., & Santa-Barbara, J. (1995). *The Family Assessment Measure.* North Tonawanda, NY: Multi-Health Systems.

Slaney, R. B., & MacKinnion-Slaney, F. (1990). The use of vocational card sorts in career counseling. In M. L. Savickas & W. B. Walsh (Eds.), *Handbook of career counseling theory and practice* (pp. 317–371). Palo Alto, CA: Davies-Black.

Slaney, R. B., & Suddarth, B. H. (1994). The Values Scale (VS). In J. T. Kapes, M. M. Mastie, & E. A. Whitfield (Eds.), *A counselor's guide to career assessment instru-ments* (pp. 236–240). Alexandria, VA: National Career Development Association.

Snyder, C. R. (1997). *Marital Satisfaction Inventory, re-vised manual.* Los Angeles: Western Psychological Services.

Snyder, C. R., Shenkel, R. J., & Lowery, C. R. (1977). Acceptance of personality interpretations: The "Bar-num effect" and beyond. *Journal of Consulting and Clin-ical Psychology, 45,* 104–114.

Sokol, M. S., & Pfeffer, C. R. (1992). Suicidal behavior of children. In B. Bongar (Ed.), *Suicide: Guidelines for as-sessment, management, and treatment* (pp. 69–83). New York: Oxford University Press.

Spanier, G. B. (1976). Measuring dyadic adjustment: New scales for assessing the quality of marriage or similar dyads. *Journal of Marriage and the Family, 38,* 15–28.

Sparro, S. S., Balla, D. A., & Cicchetti, D. V. (1984a). *Vineland Adaptive Behavior Scales: Interview Edition, Survey Form.* Circle Pines, MN: American Guidance Services.

Sparro, S. S., Balla, D. A., & Cicchetti, D. V. (1984b). *Vineland Adaptive Behavior Scales: Interview Edition, Ex-panded Form.* Circle Pines, MN: American Guidance Services.

Sparro, S. S., Balla, D. A., & Cicchetti, D. V. (1985) *Vineland Adaptive Behavior Scales: Classroom Edition.* Circle Pines, MN: American Guidance Services.

Spearman, C. (1927). *The abilities of man.* New York: Macmillan.

Spokane, A. R. (1991). *Career interventions.* Englewood Cliffs, NJ: Prentice-Hall.

Spokane, A. R., & Jacob, E. J. (1996). Career and voca-tional assessment 1993–1994: A biennial review. *Jour-nal of Career Assessment, 4,* 1–32.

Sporakowski, M. J., (1995). Assessment and diagnosis in marriage and family counseling. *Journal of Counseling & Development, 74,* 60–64.

Steer, R. A., & Clark, D. A. (1997). Psychometric characteristics of the Beck Depression Inventory-II. *Measurement and Evaluation in Counseling and Development, 30,* 128–136.

Stelmachers, Z. T. (1995). Assessing suicidal clients. In J. N. Butcher (Ed.), *Clinical personality assessment: Practical approaches* (pp. 367–379). New York: Oxford University Press.

Sternberg, R. J. (1985). *Beyond I.Q.: A triarchic theory of human intelligence.* New York: Cambridge University Press.

Sternberg, R. J. (1988). *The triarchic mind: A new theory of human intelligence.* New York: Viking.

Straabs, G. V. (1991). *The Scenotest.* Toronto: Hegrefe & Huber.

Stratton, K., Howey, C., & Battaglia, F. (1996). *Fetal alcohol syndrome: Diagnosis, epidemiology, prevention, and treatment.* Washington, DC: National Academy Press.

Straus, M., & Brown, B. (1978). *Family measurement techniques: Abstracts of published instruments, 1935–1974.* Minneapolis, MN: University of Minnesota Press.

Strickler, L. J. (1969). "Test-wiseness" on personality scales. *Journal of Applied Psychology Mongraph, 53*(3).

Stuart, R. B., & Jacobsen, B. (1987). *Couple's Pre-Counseling Inventory, Revised Edition.* Champaign, IL: Research Press.

Subich, L. M. (1996). Addressing diversity in the process of career assessment. In M. L. Savickas & W. B. Walsh (Eds.), *Handbook of career counseling theory and practice* (pp. 277–289). Palo Alto, CA: Davies-Black.

Subkoviak, M. J. (1984). Estimating the reliability of mastery-nonmastery classifications. In A. S. Bellack & M. Hersen (Eds.), *A guide to criterion-referenced test construction* (pp. 267–291). Baltimore: Johns Hopkins University Press.

Sue, D. W., & Sue, D. (1977). Barriers to effective cross-cultural counseling. *Journal of Counseling Psychology, 24,* 420–429.

Sullivan, P. M., & Burley, S. K. (1990). Mental testing of the hearing impaired child. In C. R. Reynolds & R. W. Kamphaus (Eds.), *Handbook of psychological and educational assessment of children: Intelligence and achievement* (pp. 761–788). New York: Guilford.

Sundberg, N. D. (1994). Review of the Beck Depression Inventory. In J. C Impara & L. L. Murphy (Eds.), *Buros desk reference: Psychological assessment in the schools* (pp. 311–313). Lincoln, NB: Buros Institute.

Super, D. E. (1980). A life-span approach to career development. *Journal of Vocational Behavior, 16,* 282–298.

Super, D. E., Thompson, A. S., Lindeman, R. H., Jor-daan, J. P., & Myers, R. A. (1988a). *Adults Career Concerns Inventory.* Palo Alto, CA: Consulting Psychologists Press.

Super, D. E., Thompson, A. S., Lindeman, R. H., Jor-daan, J. P., & Myers, R. A. (1988b). *Career Development Inventory.* Palo Alto, CA: Consulting Psychologists Press.

Swanson, J. L. (1995). The process and outcome of career counseling. In W. B. Walsh & S. H. Osipow (Eds.), *Handbook of vocational psychology: Theory, research, and practice* (pp. 217–259). Hillsdale, NJ: Erlbaum.

Sweetland, R. C., & Keyser, D. J. (Eds.) (1991). *Tests* (3rd ed.). Austin,TX: PRO-ED.

Swenson, C. H. (1968). Empricial evaluations of human figure drawings: 1957–1966. *Psychological Bulletin, 70,* 20–44.

Swiercinsky, D. (1978). *Manual for the adult neurological evaluation.* Springfield, IL: Thomas.

Taylor, R. M., & Morrison, L. D. (1996). *Taylor-Johnson Temperament Analysis test manual.* Thousand Oaks, CA: Sigma Assessment Systems.

Thompson, B., & Snyder, P. A. (1998). Statistical significance and reliability analyses in recent *Journal of Counseling and Development* research articles. *Journal of Counseling and Development, 76,* 436–441.

Thorndike, R. L. (1990). Would the real factors of the Stanford-Binet Fourth Edition please come forward? *Journal of Psychoeducational Assessment, 8,* 223–230.

Thorndike, R. L., Hagen, E. P., & Sattler, J. M. (1986a). *The Stanford-Binet Intelligence Scale: Fourth edition, guide for administering and scoring.* Chicago: Riverside.

Thorndike, R. L., Hagen, E. P., & Sattler, J. M. (1986b). *The Stanford-Binet Intelligence Scale: Fourth edition, technical manual.* Chicago: Riverside.

Thurstone, L. L. (1938). Primary mental abilities. *Psychometric Monographs,* No. 1.

Timbrook, R. E., & Graham, J. R. (1994). Ethnic differences on the MMPI-2? *Psychological Assessment, 6,* 212–217.

Topman, R. M., Kleijn, W. C., van der Ploeg, H. K., & Masset, E. A. (1992). Test anxiety, cognitions, study habits and academic performance: A prospective study. In K. A. Hagtvet & T. B. Johnsen (Eds.), *Advances in test anxiety research: Volume 7.* Amsterdam: Swets & Zeitlinger.

Touliatos, J., Perlmutter, B. F., & Straus, M. A. (Eds.) (1990). *Handbook of family measurement techniques.* Thousand Oaks, CA: Sage.

Tracey, T. J., & Rounds, J. (1998). Inference and attribution errors in test interpretation. In J. W. Lichtenburg & R. K. Goodyear (Eds.), *Scientist-practitioner perspectives on test interpretation* (pp. 113–131). Boston: Allyn and Bacon.

Transberg, M., Slane, S., & Ekeberg, S. E. (1993). The relation between interest congruence and satisfaction: A meta-analysis. *Journal of Vocational Behavior, 42,* 253–264.

Tuddenham, R. D., Blumenkrantz, J., Wilken, W. R. (1968). Age changes on AGCT: A longitudinal study of average adults. *Journal of Consulting and Clinical Psychology, 32,* 659–663.

Ulrich, R. E., Stachnik, T. J., & Stainton, N. R. (1963). Student acceptance of generalized personality interpretations. *Psychological Report, 13,* 831–834.

U. S. Bureau of Census (1990). *Statistical abstract for 1990.* Washington, DC: Author.

U. S. Department of Defense (1995). *ASVAB 18/19: Educator and counselor guide* (DOD Publication No. 1304.12). Washington, DC: U.S. Government Printing Office.

U. S. Department of Labor (1970). *Manual of the USES General Aptitude Test Battery, Section III: Development.* Washington, DC: U.S. Government Printing Office.

Vacc, N. A., & Hinkle, J. S. (1994). Career Assessment Inventory-Enhanced Version and Vocational Version (CAI-EV/CAI-VV). In J. T. Kapes, M. M. Mastie, & E. A. Whitfield (Eds.), *A counselor's guide to career assessment instruments* (pp. 144–150). Alexandria, VA: National Career Development Association.

Vacc, N. A., & Juhnke, G. A. (1997). The use of structured clinical interviews for assessment in counseling. *Journal of Counseling and Development, 75,* 470–480.

van der Linden, W. J., & Hambleton, R. K. (1997). Item response theory: Brief history, common models, and extensions. In W. J. van der Linden & R. K. Hambleton (Eds.), *Handbook of modern item response theory* (pp. 1–28). New York: Springer.

Vernon, P. E. (1950). *The structure of human abilities.* New York: Wiley.

Vondracek, F. W. (1991). Osipow on the Career Decision Scale: Some comments. *Journal of Counseling and Development, 70,* 327.

Vondracek, F. W., Hostetler, M., Schulenber, J. E., & Shimuzu, K. (1990). Dimensions of career indecision. *Journal of Counseling Psychology, 37,* 98–106.

Waiswol, N. (1995). Projective techniques as psychotherapy. *American Journal of Psychotherapy, 49,* 244–259.

Ward, A. W. (1995). Review of the Wide Range Achievement Test 3. In J. C. Conoley & J. J. Kramer (Eds.), *Twelfth mental measurements yearbook* (pp. 1110–1111). Lincoln, NB: The University of Nebraska Press.

Warren, W. L. (1994). *Revised Hamilton Rating Scale for Depression.* Los Angeles: Western Psychological Services.

Watkins, C. E., Campbell, V. L., & Nieberding, R. (1994). The practice of vocational assessment by counseling psychologists. *The Counseling Psychologist, 22,* 115–128.

Watts-Jones, D. (1997). Toward an African American genogram. *Family Process, 36,* 375–383.

Wechsler, D. (1989). *Wechsler Preschool and Primary Scale of Intelligence-Revised.* San Antonio, TX: The Psychological Corporation.

Wechsler, D. (1991). *Wechsler Intelligence Scale for Children-Third Edition.* San Antonio, TX: The Psychological Corporation.

Wechsler, D. (1992). *Wechsler Individual Achievement Test.* San Antonio, TX: The Psychological Corporation.

Wechsler, D. (1997). *Wechsler Adult Intelligence Scale-Third Edition.* San Antonio, TX: The Psychological Corporation.

Weiss, D. J., Dawis, R. V., & Lofquist, L. H. (1981). *Minnesota Importance Questionnaire.* Minneapolis, MN: Vocational Psychology Research.

Weiss, L. G., Preifitera, A., & Roid, G. (1993). The WISC-III and the fairness of predicting achievement across ethnic and gender groups. In B. A. Bracken (Ed.), *Monograph series advances in psychoeducational assessment: Wechsler Intelligence Scale for Children: Third Edition; Journal of Psychoeducational Assessment* (pp. 114–124). Brandon, VT: Clinical Psychology Publishing.

Westbrook, B. W., Sanford, E., Gilleland, K., Fleenor, J., & Merwin, J. (1988). Career maturity in grade 9: The relationship between accuracy of self-appraisal and ability to appraise the career-relevant capabilities of others. *Journal of Vocational Behavior, 32,* 269–283.

Whiston, S. C. (1990). Evaluation of the Adult Career Concerns Inventory. *Journal of Counseling & Development, 69,* 78–80.

Whiston, S. C. (1996a). The relationship among family interaction patterns and career indecision and career decision-making self-efficacy. *Journal of Career Development, 23,* 137–149.

Whiston, S. C. (1996b). Accountability through action research: Research methods for practitioners. *Journal of Counseling & Development, 74,* 616–623

Whiston, S. C., & Sexton, T. L. (1998). A review of school counseling outcome research: Implications for practice. *Journal of Counseling & Development, 76,* 412–426.

Whiston, S. C., Sexton, T. L., & Lasoff, D. L. (1998). Career-intervention outcome: A replication and extension of Oliver and Spokane. *Journal of Counseling Psychology, 45,* 150–165.

Widiger, T. A. (1992). Review of the NEO Personality Inventory. In J. C. Conoley & J. J. Kramer (Eds.), *Eleventh mental measurements yearbook* (pp. 605– 606). Lincoln, NB: The University of Nebraska Press.

Wigdor, A. K., & Green, B. F. (1991a). *Performance assessment for the workplace: Vol. 1.* Washington, DC: National Academy Press.

Wigdor, A. K., & Green, B. F. (1991b). *Performance assessment for the workplace: Vol. 2. Technical issues.* Washington, DC: National Academy Press.

Wiggins, J. S. (1966). Social desirability estimation and "faking good" well. *Educational and Psychological Measurement, 26,* 329–341.

Wiggins, J. S. (1989). Review of the Myers-Briggs Type Indicator. In J. C. Conoley & J. J. Kramer (Eds.), *Tenth mental measurements yearbook* (pp. 536–538). Lincoln, NB: University of Nebraska Press.

Wilkinson, G. S. (1993). *Wide Range Achievement Test 3.* Willmington, DE: Jastak Associates/Wide Range Inc.

Williams, S. K. (1978). The vocational card sort: A tool for vocational exploration. *The Vocational Guidance Quarterly, 48,* 237–243.

Willson, V. L., & Stone, E. (1994). Differential Aptitude Tests. In J. T. Kapes, M. M. Mastie, & E. A. Whitfield (Eds.), *A counselor's guide to career assessment instruments* (pp. 90–98). Alexandria, VA: National Career Development Association.

Wirt, R. D., Lachar, D., Klinedinst, J. E., Seat, P. D., & Broen W. E. (1982). *Personality Inventory for Children (PIC) Revised Format.* Los Angeles: Western Psychological Services.

Wise, S. L., & Plake, B. S. (1990). Computer-based testing in higher education. *Measurement and Evaluation in Counseling and Development, 23,* 3–10.

Wonderlic Personnel Test, Inc. (1992). *Wonderlic Personnel Test user's manual.* Libertyville, IL: Author.

Woodcock, R. W., & Johnson, M. B. (1989, 1990). *Woodcock-Johnson Psycho-Educational Battery-Revised.* Chicago: Riverside.

Worthen, B. R. (1995). Review of the Strong Interest Inventory. In J. C. Conoley & J. J. Kramer (Eds.), *Twelfth mental measurements yearbook* (pp. 999–1002). Lincoln, NB: The University of Nebraska Press.

Worthington, E. L., McCullough, M. E., Shortz, J. L. Mindes, E. J., Sandage, S. J., & Chartrand, J. M. (1995). Can couples assessment and feedback improve relationships? Assessment as a brief relationship enrichment procedure. *Journal of Counseling Psychology, 42,* 466–475.

Yansen, E. D., & Shulman, E. L. (1996). Language assessment; Multicultural assessment. In L. A. Suzuki, P. J. Meller, & J. G. Ponterotto (Eds.), *Handbook of multicultural assessement: Clinical, psychological, and educational applications* (pp. 3–28). San Francisco: Jossey-Bass.

Zytowski, D. G. (1992). Three generations: The continuing evolution of Frederic Kuder's interest inventories. *Journal of Counseling and Development, 71,* 245–248.

INDEX